Praise for *Always Eat After 7 PM*

"Turning your health around should never mean starving yourself, especially at the times when you're hungriest. *Always Eat After 7 PM* provides a refreshing approach to weight loss by prioritizing healthy habits and listening to your body's signals—crucial steps for anyone's well-being."

—Heidi Powell, celebrity trainer and star of ABC's *Extreme Weight Loss*

"Backed on the latest findings in nutrition science and filled with practical advice, *Always Eat After 7 PM* will change your life. Stop stressing about food and start on a realistic path to your optimal health—Joel's wisdom in this book will help you every step of the way."

—Rashad Jennings, *New York Times* bestselling author of *The IF in Life*, former NFL running back, and *Dancing with the Stars* champion

"What I love most about this book is the integration of the mental side of transformation for both achieving and sustaining results. No doubt Joel's nutrition recommendations will help many, but the mental success strategies covered will be the true game-changer for those who adopt the contents of this powerful book."

—Lewis Howes, *New York Times* bestselling author of *The School of Greatness* and podcast host

"In *Always Eat After 7 PM*, Joel Marion tackles one of the biggest diet myths in the fitness industry and provides a flexible tool for those looking for more balance in this overly complicated diet world."

—Drew Manning, *New York Times* bestselling author of *Fit2Fat2Fit*

"Joel Marion knows from experience how important it is to pay attention to what your body *needs* rather than following the latest trendy diet advice. His regimen in this book is a straightforward, scientific plan that can help anyone reach their health and weight-loss goals."

—Todd Durkin, celebrity trainer and bestselling author of *The IMPACT Body Plan*

"Having trained many of the world's top athletes, I've witnessed the power of mental toughness in achieving elite results. Joel Marion exemplifies those principles of mental toughness day in and day out, and if you do the work, he can help you achieve your goals."

—Tim Grover, *New York Times* bestselling author of *Relentless*

"When you are hungry, you should eat! This statement should never be controversial or at odds with any diet or weight-loss plan. *Always Eat After 7 PM* will set you on the path to the best health of your life—without the BS rules or gimmicks."

—John Romaniello, *New York Times* bestselling author of *Engineering the Alpha*

"*Always Eat After 7 PM* is spot on! I couldn't stop reading and finished it in one sitting. There are so many myths out there, and this book will answer all your questions. Joel, thank you so much for educating us and providing a TON of value. This book is a MUST read.

—Josh York, Inc. 500 founder and CEO of GYMGUYZ®

"If you're serious about losing weight, you need to drop the fads and focus on habits that are scientifically proven to help you get healthier. That's where *Always Eat After 7 PM* comes in. The title says it all: Ignore the old myths and do what's best for your body. Joel Marion will help you get there!"

—Steve Weatherford, NFL Super Bowl Champion

"Ninety-nine percent of fitness and nutrition experts are dead WRONG when it comes to burning fat. Just like you don't have to do long, slow, boring cardio to lose weight, the truth is that you don't have to starve yourself at dinner—or deny yourself an indulgent snack—any night you want. Thank you, Joel Marion, for clearing up this disastrous diet myth."

—Craig Ballantyne, *Wall Street Journal* bestselling author of *The Perfect Day Formula*

"*Always Eat After 7 PM* has been the missing link for everyone wanting to lose weight and keep it off. The program is very instinctive, it doesn't deprive you of food when you want it most (at dinner time), and best of all it's all backed by science. Plus I literally tried every recipe in the book and they're all so delicious. This is a game changer!"

—Bedros Keuilian, *Wall Street Journal* bestselling author of *Man Up*, and founder and CEO Fit Body Boot Camp

"How many times have we all heard that we should deprive ourselves in the evening if we want to slim down?! That 'rule' sets so many of us up to fail, in addition to being totally unhealthy to begin with. I'm so glad to see *Always Eat After 7 PM* tackling this harmful misconception head-on."

—Heath Evans, NFL Super Bowl Champion

"Achieving your best health shouldn't be a painful process. I commend Joel on creating a simple yet science-based approach to physical and mental transformation, and especially his inclusion of the power morning routine I've been teaching my high performance clients for years. You'll benefit greatly from this book."

—Jim Kwik, celebrity brain fitness and memory coach and host of the podcast KwikBrain

ALWAYS

EAT AFTER 7 PM

Also by Joel Marion

The Cheat to Lose Diet: Cheat BIG with the Foods You Love, Lose Fat Faster Than Ever Before, and Enjoy Keeping It Off!

ALWAYS EAT AFTER 7 PM

The Revolutionary Rule-Breaking Diet That Lets You **Enjoy Huge Dinners, Desserts, and Indulgent Snacks**—While Burning Fat Overnight

Joel Marion

with Recipes by Diana Keuilian

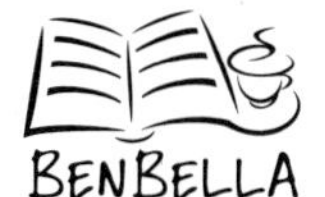

BenBella Books, Inc.
Dallas, TX

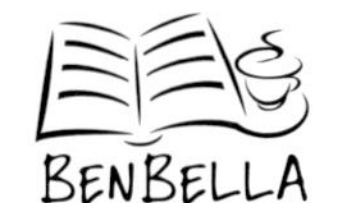

BenBella Books, Inc.
10440 N. Central Expressway, Suite 800
Dallas, TX 75231
www.benbellabooks.com
Send feedback to feedback@benbellabooks.com

Printed in the United States of America
10 9 8 7 6 5 4 3 2 1

Library of Congress Control Number: 2019031912
ISBN 9781948836524 (trade paper)
ISBN 9781948836777 (electronic)

Editing by Claire Schulz
Copyediting by Jennifer Brett Greenstein
Proofreading by Karen Wise and Cape Cod Compositors, Inc.
Indexing by WordCo Indexing Services, Inc.
Text design and composition by Aaron Edmiston
Cover design by Perception LLC
Cover photo © Marazen - Dreamstime
Photographs of Joel Marion courtesy of the author
Printed by Versa Press

Distributed to the trade by Two Rivers Distribution, an Ingram brand
www.tworiversdistribution.com

To my wife, Lisa, and my two daughters, Lily and Gabby. You are everything.

Contents

Introduction

It's nine o'clock at night. Your stomach is rumbling. Food is calling your name. But you're on a diet, and that means eating now is against the rules, right?

Ever felt this way? Ever wondered, if you broke the rules, could you still lose weight? I'm sure you have. Nighttime hunger happens to just about everyone. Even so, for years we've been told that if we want to lose weight, we have to avoid carbs and eat a "sensible" dinner. Then we're forced to starve ourselves until bedtime—which is when our most intense cravings hit.

So . . . should you tough it out and follow the popular rule of avoiding food each night for fear of putting on pounds? Or should you answer the call of the fridge?

Let me answer that for you: you *should* head to the fridge.

Okay, you probably think I'm crazy. We've all heard that we should avoid nighttime eating because if we eat food late in the evening—when we're physically inactive—we'll pack away those calories as fat rather than burning them for energy. But truth be told, there's just not much proof to definitively support this advice. (In fact, recent scientific research shows the exact opposite is true.)

For example, when nutritional scientists scrutinized the diet habits and body weights of more than 7,400 men and women for 10 years, they found that the calories that their research subjects ate after 5 PM had no effect on their weight. In short, they did not put on any weight because they ate in the evening. This study was published in the *International Journal of Obesity and Related Metabolism Disorders*.

This finding and the other research that I'll share in this book provide compelling evidence that you *can*, in fact, eat at night—and you will *not* put on pounds.

It's time for a late-night eating rethink.

And that's where this book comes in.

HOW I DISCOVERED THAT DIETING RULES WERE MADE TO BE BROKEN

I've always been a bit of a maverick. I don't like rules. Sure, there are lots of rules we should follow in life. If you see a sign that says "Do Not Enter" or "Do Not Feed the Alligators," there's usually a pretty good reason for it. However, some warnings based on eating and dieting from decades ago simply don't apply today.

It took me a long time to find this out. As much as I hate to admit it, I wasn't always the fit and healthy guy I am today. Though I started my fitness career more than 15 years ago, during that time I had my own struggles with weight gain and dieting.

It all began after I launched my nutritional supplement company, BioTrust Nutrition, and I started working 12- to 16-hour days and pulling all-nighters building the brand. In just the first 16 months, we got to over $100 million in sales, but I was pushing myself hard. As a result, I experienced some pretty intense, even uncontrollable cravings for unhealthy food—particularly at night. Now, at first I resisted the urge to eat late in the evening because I was misinformed like most people. Well, as the old *Star Trek* saying goes, "Resistance is futile." I eventually caved into my cravings for junk food.

Slowly but surely, over the course of the next few years, my body packed on 10 pounds, then 20, then eventually 50 pounds. As a certified sports nutritionist (CISSN), I knew that any time you're hauling around an extra 50 pounds, you're going to develop some significant health problems.

Around that same time, I met my future bride, Lisa, got married, and started a family. Next thing you know, we had not one, but two little girls, Lily and Gabby. Between work and family obligations, making healthy food choices plunged even farther down my priority list.

My poor food choices took their toll on me mentally too. Every day when I looked at myself in the mirror, I was ashamed. My self-esteem was at an all-time low, and I felt guilty because I was letting my family down day after day after day. These were *terrible* feelings, to say the least.

I eventually realized that I was slowly digging my own grave by not taking time to prioritize my own health. Even though I had helped people around the world get fit with my articles and books, and BioTrust had built a reputation as one of the largest and highest-quality supplement companies in the country, I wasn't walking the talk when it came to my own body. How embarrassing for someone who had such a successful track record helping the world get healthy and fit!

I had hit an all-time low with my health, but it was that low that made me say, "Enough is enough." I needed to get in the driver's seat of my own life again. So I dusted off an old plan from more than 10 years earlier: the same diet plan that had landed me first place in the world's largest body transformation contest when I was 20 years old.

It was a traditional low-fat approach to weight loss, and yes, it worked. But like many diets—especially back then—it wasn't fun, it wasn't easy enough, and it certainly wasn't tasty enough. Eating bland broccoli and chicken day after day made me feel like I was going to choke on my food.

Around the same time, I was hearing one big complaint from my clients who were dieting. They were constantly hungry and not feeling full after their meals, especially at dinnertime and late at night—challenges that were difficult to overcome, challenges I understood because I had personally dealt with them. Deep down, I knew that if my clients couldn't get a grip on their late-night hunger and cravings, they'd have a hard time adhering to any diet.

All of this brought me to the turning point. I knew I had to give my own approach to diet and nutrition a complete overhaul. I had to find a new, innovative method that could stop cravings at night, help people feel full and satisfied at each meal, and let them enjoy lots of their favorite, delicious foods without severely limiting food groups—while still burning fat *fast*.

But was such a plan even possible? Nutritional science offers a wealth of research on eating right, but it can also confuse you with its contradictory findings. I decided to play devil's advocate and question every "rule" I'd ever heard or read about dieting and weight loss. I'm talking about the messages you often hear from the medical establishment and diet industry, such as "Breakfast is the most important meal of the day," "Avoid carbs—especially at night," and "Whatever you do, *never* eat before bedtime."

What if it was okay to eat late at night? What if it was okay to skip breakfast? What if it was okay to snack on carbs at night? I wanted answers.

I'm a science geek, so I dug through peer-reviewed journals and databases. I took a deep dive into the research to learn what really happens in our bodies if we eat late at night. I reached out to my circle of contacts in the natural health field—the doctors, scientists, and innovative experts I've built relationships with over the years, people who stay on top of the latest research studies and cutting-edge information. I even talked to my bodybuilder friends, who tend to be pretty lean. Even *they* were eating late at night, they told me, because it helps develop muscle!

What I was discovering blew my mind. The research was crystal clear: eating your largest meals at night can actually be the hidden key to losing fat quickly and safely and won't necessarily make you gain weight.

I had to experiment on myself first to see if it would work. Well, the results were nothing short of remarkable. I dropped 12 pounds in under two weeks. My abs were significantly flatter. My cravings for unhealthy food vanished. After 16 weeks on my new plan, I had lost a total of 46 pounds. At my next medical checkup, my doctor was shocked at how good my blood work had gotten so quickly.

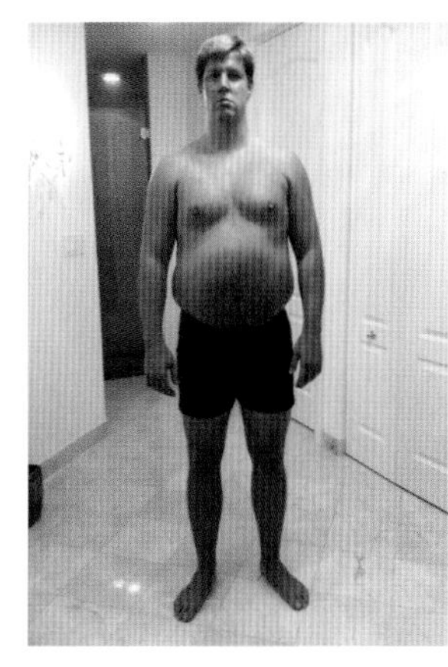

Before

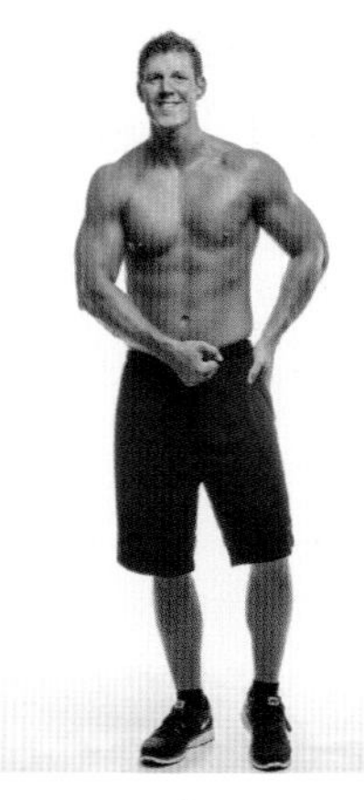

After

And let's not forget the most important part: for the first time in months, I had the energy to keep up with my little girls. I would jump out of bed extra early every morning, excited to get them ready for school. They were finally getting the best version of their daddy. My confidence was back because I felt like a new man!

From there, I went on to use this plan with my clients, and they experienced similar results: amazing fat loss, improved health markers, great energy, and more. And now, I'm sharing this plan with you.

HOW ALWAYS EAT AFTER 7 PM WILL WORK FOR YOU

The wonderful thing about Always Eat After 7 PM is that it lets you eat at night, burn fat at night, and end junk food cravings at night. Along the way, it moves you to a healthier, leaner body and more energy—and it does so quickly.

So stop declaring the kitchen off-limits after 7 PM, and stop feeling guilty about sitting down to a sensible, huge dinner or stressing out if you don't get around to it until 8 or 9 PM. In this program, I'm going to recommend the following: let's break the rules about dieting and late-night eating and start transforming your body with new facts, new strategies, and new science.

Inside this book I've given you everything you need to succeed. First, I'll debunk common myths about eating and weight loss and explain the science behind the program so you can understand how to eat to achieve your weight loss goals. Every strategy is simple to follow, is based on solid science, and produces rapid results. What's more, all the strategies are safe to use even long term as a lifestyle diet that can help you live long and fight off many of today's most deadly diseases. Then, I'll share an easy-to-follow daily meal schedule, as well as six weekly menu plans and 70 delicious recipes from my great friend and top chef Diana Keuilian, aka "The Recipe Hacker."

And so I say all this to motivate you. To challenge you. To inspire you. If I can do this, with my insane work schedule, travel schedule, and family life, anyone can do it. *Anyone*. And that means you. You can change, just like I did.

Joel Marion

PART I
THE FOUNDATION

CHAPTER 1
WHY YOU SHOULD ALWAYS EAT AFTER 7 PM

I'm excited that you picked up this book because the information it contains will change the way you've dieted and tackled weight loss in the past. You will eat large, delicious meals. You will enjoy foods you love. You will not feel deprived. You will enjoy meals and snacks at night. And you will lose weight quickly and safely in the process. No matter what a person's diet history, this is a plan that anyone—and I mean *anyone*—can have success with.

Before we get into the specifics of the diet, it's critical that you understand *why* you're doing *what* you're doing, starting with the science that supports late-night eating for faster weight loss and explains why it is a much more effective solution for fat burning compared to other programs. It's fascinating research that will lay the groundwork for your success. Let's begin with some myth-busting facts and then talk about what distinguishes Always Eat After 7 PM from other diets.

MYTH #1: EATING FOOD AFTER 7 PM MAKES YOU FAT.

It's probably been drilled into your head that eating late at night leads to obesity and excess belly fat. Myths like this one are strangely persistent, even though there's little research to back them up. Randomized scientific trials, however, definitely contradict the notion that late-night eating inevitably leads to weight gain or interferes with weight loss.

For example, in a study published in the journal *Nutrition*, Brazilian researchers randomly assigned obese women to a very low-calorie diet under three separate conditions:

1. Five meals were spread throughout the day.
2. All the meals were consumed between 9 AM and 11 AM.
3. All the meals were consumed between 6 PM and 8 PM (late-night eating).

The study lasted 18 days and was conducted in a hospital. The women ate the same number of calories in each of the conditions. The women in *all three groups* lost weight. After completion, there were no differences in weight loss, body composition, or resting metabolic rate between the groups. This provides evidence that, in a highly controlled setting, when food choices and portion sizes are consistent, eating at night doesn't negatively affect weight loss.

There's also value in eating a large dinner in the evening: Researchers from Israel wanted to test whether eating more at night makes you gain weight. In their six-month study, they randomized people (men and women aged 25 to 55) to one of two groups: the experimental group and a control group. The experimental group was prescribed a standard low-calorie diet (20 percent protein, 30–35 percent fat, 45–50 percent carbohydrates, 1,300–1,500 kcal), including a large dinner with mostly carbs, while the control group received a standard low-calorie diet (20 percent protein, 30–35 percent fat, 45–50 percent carbohydrates, 1,300–1,500 kcal), including carbohydrates throughout the day and a lighter dinner. The experimental group ate a small breakfast, while the control group had a large breakfast. The study was reported in *Nutrition, Metabolism, and Cardiovascular Diseases* in 2013.

The huge-dinner eaters not only lost more fat but also felt more full throughout the entire six-month period and had more favorable changes to their hunger hormones. Compared to the control group, the huge-dinner eaters experienced these specific results:

- They had fewer hunger cravings and were more satisfied with their meals.
- They lost 11 percent more weight.
- They trimmed 10 percent from their waistlines.
- They lost 10.5 percent more body fat.

This study is encouraging because it supports late-night eating as a significant weight loss strategy—one that clearly helps people burn more fat.

MYTH #2: LATE-NIGHT EATING SLOWS DOWN YOUR METABOLISM.

Your metabolism is what enables your cells, tissues, and organs to perform the digestion, respiration, circulation, and other functions that turn food into fuel and keep you alive. Though it seems intuitive that your metabolism might be slowest when you are sleeping, it does not come to a screeching halt, leaving everything you've eaten destined to become unsightly body fat. In fact, research shows that the average person's metabolic rate is no different during sleep than during the day. In short, your metabolism doesn't slow down at night. Nor does your body store fat at the end of the day. Whether it's 8 AM or 8 PM, you use food for energy the same way.

Then there's this amazing physiological reaction called the "thermic effect of food," or TEF for short. No matter when you do it, eating a meal causes the body to burn calories to digest, absorb, and transport the nutrients in that meal. This is the TEF, and it leads to an increased metabolic rate and calorie burn.

Different categories of food have different TEFs. The thermic effect of carbohydrates, for example, is between 5 percent and 15 percent; this means it takes 5 to 15 calories to burn off 100 calories of foods containing carbs. Fat is also between 5 percent and 15 percent. Protein has the highest TEF, around 20 percent (which is why, on this program, you'll eat protein at every meal, including your late-night snack).

Knowing all this, how can anyone argue that a late-night meal or snack slows your metabolism? When you have *any* meal, especially one with protein, your metabolism increases, thanks to the TEF!

I do need to add that there are other factors influencing TEF, according to a review published in the *Journal of the American College of Nutrition* in 2019. The authors pointed out that TEF tends to decrease with age and increase with physical activity, higher-calorie meals, and high-carbohydrate and high-protein meals, as opposed to high-fat meals. In addition, eating plenty of fruits, vegetables, and high-fiber-content meals also seems to have a positive effect on TEF.

MYTH #3: **LATE-NIGHT EATING INTERFERES WITH DIGESTION.**

A common misconception is that food eaten prior to bedtime is not adequately digested. You've probably heard some outdated saying such as "At bedtime, your stomach is closed for business" or "Food eaten at night mostly sits there."

Not true. Recent research clearly demonstrates that the digestive tract is fully functional during sleep; some studies have particularly looked at casein, a protein in milk and cheese, and found that it is quickly digested, absorbed, and put to work to help you build lean muscle when eaten before bed. A study published in the *Journal of Nutrition* in 2017 found that a 40-gram serving of casein protein eaten at night prior to sleep increased overnight muscle protein synthesis in both younger and older men. In essence, late-night feeding helped increase body-contouring muscle overnight!

What's more, researchers have found that nutrients administered during sleep (via nasal infusion) are digested and absorbed just as they would be under normal waking circumstances.

You've also probably heard that optimum digestion requires comfort and relaxation. That's true. What better time to experience those conditions than while you're sleeping?

MYTH #4: **EATING CARBS AFTER 7 PM PACKS ON POUNDS.**

Almost everyone assumes that you should avoid eating large meals with higher-carb foods at dinnertime because they promote weight gain. However, a study in the journal *Nutrition, Metabolism, and Cardiovascular Diseases* in 2013 put this "carb curfew" to rest. Researchers assigned 78 Israeli police officers to one of two diets for six months. Both groups consumed the same number of meals and foods throughout the day. One group followed a "normal" diet with calories and carbohydrates spread out through the day. The other group was assigned to an "experimental" diet in which they consumed a larger percentage of their calories (and carbohydrates) in the evening. Both groups lost weight, body fat, and inches from their waistlines. But here's the kicker: the "experimental" group, which ate most of their carbs in the evening (presumably after 6 PM), experienced significantly greater improvements in all three areas. What was particularly intriguing was that this strategy of eating more carbs later in the day led to improved profiles of hormones related to hunger, satiety, and metabolism such as leptin and ghrelin.

Late-night eating also curbs calorie intake the next day. In a four-week study, dieters added a snack to their daily regimen 90 minutes after dinner every night, and check this out: late-night eaters ate an average of 397 *fewer* calories per day. This study was published in 2004 in the *Journal of the American College of Nutrition*.

What's more, eating carbs at night induces deeper sleep. A research paper published in *Sports Medicine* in 2014 showed that people who eat the majority of their carbs at dinner actually sleep better. Carb-induced, quality sleep decreases cortisol (a fat-storing hormone) and ramps up the production of your sleep hormones, serotonin and melatonin. Restorative sleep increases fat-burning hormones—the main one being growth hormone—overnight.

It's important to note that not all carbs are created equal, and on this program we'll prioritize what I call "Super Carbs." These are natural, wholesome plant foods such as rice, potatoes, yams, and squash that support metabolism and fat burning.

Yes, one of the best dinner carbs is white rice. Are you surprised? Most people have no clue that this Super Carb is a gluten-free starch from nature that is rich in glucose, which triggers deeper sleep, fuels your activities for the next day, and prevents your metabolism from slowing down. So even though we've all been advised to cut back on white rice, or never eat it at all, if we want to avoid fat storage and disease, it's really a nutritionally power-packed dinnertime Super Carb that can help you burn more fat.

The Okinawans of Japan are living proof of this science. They generally get 69 percent of their calories from evening Super Carbs, frequently eating high-carb dinners with rice as late as 10 PM. We often think of rice as "fattening," and yet, older Okinawans have a typical body mass index (BMI) of 18 to 22, compared to a typical BMI of 26 or 27 for adults over the age of 60 in the U.S. In fact, not only are they lean, but they are also more likely to reach 100 years of age than anyone else in the world.

Kitavan Islanders are another perfect example of folks who defy this diet myth. Their diet consists of more than 50 percent Super Carbs, most of which are fruits like berries and starchy sweet potatoes. Yet, despite their unusually high-carb diet, they have great blood sugar control and amazing blood lipid profiles, have a low incidence of metabolic syndrome (a precursor to diabetes), and are completely free of cardiovascular disease (a precursor to stroke, congestive heart failure, dementia, and high blood pressure). They thrive on eating mostly Super Carbs without becoming obese.

Specific higher-carbohydrate foods (including berries and cherries) support your fat-burning metabolism while you sleep, providing your body with a steady stream of fuel throughout the night. The trick is knowing how to *combine* them with other evening and pre-bedtime fat-burning foods to fuel your metabolism as you sleep. As an example, a high-protein and/or high-fat snack combined with berries, such as Greek yogurt with walnuts and blueberries, is ideal to fight cravings and burn fat. You'll learn more about how to do this in chapter four.

By now, you know that there's just not a lot of truth behind some of the most common dieting rules. With Always Eat After 7 PM, you'll get a whole new approach to eating that is completely unlike any other diet.

WHY OTHER DIETS MAY HAVE FAILED YOU

If you're like a lot of people I've met and worked with, you've probably spent tons of time, energy, and money buying special foods, purchasing diet programs, or joining diet clubs—but with zero results. I've heard from people who are shattered because conventional diets have utterly failed to bring them any lasting weight loss. I know one woman who tried to subsist on one meal a day, another woman who ate only lettuce and cottage cheese, and a guy who worked out three hours a day to burn off calories (and ended up with swollen joints in the process). I remember a woman who got so hungry late at night that she regularly raided her fridge for anything that tamed her cravings.

People everywhere subject themselves to lives of starvation dieting and exercising hell, and none of it is working. They crave food, walk around hungry all day, and miss out on one of life's great pleasures—eating good food. And when they fail, as most dieters will, they feel guilty and full of self-hatred. But they haven't failed. Those diets have failed them.

Typical "dieting" is perhaps one of the most frustrating practices that just about *everyone* has attempted at one point or another. It's not fun, it gets old, and it rarely works. There are a few reasons for that.

Traditional diets are boring and lack variety.

I don't know about you, but I'm not into eating dried-out chicken breast and bland veggies day after day, week after week, month after mind-numbing month.

But that's dieting! Fact is, most diets are extremely narrow with regard to food choices and variety, and many even limit entire macronutrients altogether over the course of the entire program (think low-carb and low-fat diets).

Three months with no carbs? No thanks. Such practices not only are entirely unnecessary, but make for a miserable, unsustainable experience.

Traditional diets require that you give up your favorite foods, and that's simply unrealistic.

Virtually all traditional diets can be summarized by one word: *restriction*. They're all about what you *can't* have, and very little about what you can have (and most of the time, the "allowed" choices are unappetizing).

To make matters worse, they forbid you to eat your favorite foods. No pizza or chocolate chip cookies for months while you try to shed those 30 pounds! That's never going to work in real life. When the inevitable *does* happen and you cheat, you end up feeling terrible, guilty, and like a failure.

Traditional diets yield results that aren't substantial enough to warrant the sacrifice.

Who wants to work hard with no reward? Not me! If you're busting your butt day in and day out and then hop on the scale at week's end only to find *nothing's changed*, that's extremely disheartening and discouraging—and believe me, I feel your pain.

You know what hard work with no reward brings? Quitting, that's what. And I don't blame you (or me, because I did it plenty of times myself). It's not that you "just don't have what it takes"; it's that *no one* is going to continue to work hard without some payoff. Always Eat After 7 PM is different. With this program, you won't have to completely give up your favorite foods, *and* you'll see amazing results that will keep you motivated.

EXPERIENCE YOUR FASTEST FAT LOSS *EVER* USING THREE SIMPLE PHASES

Always Eat After 7 PM is a three-phase program that teaches you how to lose big by strategically *eating big* when you are naturally hungriest—in the evening. This may sound too good to be true, but let me assure you it is no gimmick. It's all about making strategic and smart food swaps, and you can still eat your favorite foods.

Here's a brief summary of how the three phases work:

Phase 1: The Acceleration Phase. This phase is designed to give you rapid results in weight loss in the first 14 days. You'll transition from eating a big meal at breakfast to my 3-Minute Fat-Burning Morning Ritual, and lunches and dinners will be based primarily on proteins and non-starchy vegetables. Think of this as a short, dedicated "sprint" to get things going quickly; it's not meant to be sustained, but a sprint will burn more energy per second than a moderate jog. The faster results you'll see in the first two weeks really kick-start the program. Some of my clients have lost as much as a pound a day during this phase.

Phase 2: The Main Phase. This phase allows for larger portions and calorie intake compared to the Acceleration Phase. During this phase, you continue with the 3-Minute Fat-Burning Ritual in the mornings, filling lunches and dinners with lean proteins and lots of fruits and vegetables, and evening meals with Super Carbs. (You also get to cheat once a week!) It is meant to be sustainable for an extended period of time, for weeks or even months, until you reach your goal weight. Your weight loss will slow down a bit during this phase, but don't be surprised if you drop two to five pounds a week.

Phase 3: The Lifestyle Phase. This is a more laid-back version of the Main Phase with more liberties, more food, and even fewer restrictions, to let you transition into a healthy long-term lifestyle that follows the Always Eat After 7 PM principles. If Phase 1 is a sprint and Phase 2 is a moderate jog, Phase 3 is a leisurely walk in the park grounded in the habits formed in the other stages of the program.

NOT JUST ANOTHER DIET

If it looks like I'm handing you another restrictive diet, let me be clear: Always Eat After 7 PM is totally unlike other programs. It defies the most common dietary rules (like "no snacking" and "no carbs") and is specifically designed to work with your body's natural hormonal systems, instead of working against them (you'll learn more about this in chapter two).

Take a look at the chart on the following page to see how Always Eat After 7 PM differs from popular diets you may have tried to follow.

To wind up, Always Eat After 7 PM is a much more enjoyable, realistic way to lose weight and achieve your goals compared to today's most popular diets. You eat the most when you are naturally hungry, you don't go to bed hungry, and you can even indulge your sweet and salty cravings before bedtime.

As you begin this plan and go through its three phases, you'll experience firsthand what a truly effective diet it is in your quest to lose weight and get healthier. The next chapters outline the fundamentals of how to time your meals and snacks to achieve your weight loss goals. This now brings us to something you've probably never been told before: the real truth about breakfast.

	Always Eat After 7 PM	Paleo	Keto	Atkins	Commercial Diets (diet food for purchase)	Mediterranean
Allows carbs	Yes	Yes—but no grains	Yes, but strictly limited	No	Yes	Yes
Allows dairy	Yes	No	Yes	Yes—but limited to cream, cream cheese, and butter	Yes	Yes
Allows fruit	Yes	Yes—but limited	No	No	Yes	Yes
Late-night snacking	Yes	No	No	No	No	No
Controls hunger hormones	Yes	No	No	No	No	No
Encourages off-plan cheat meals	Yes	No	No	No	No	No
Nutritionally balanced	Yes	No	No	No	No; made up of primarily processed diet meals with additives	Yes
Absence of side effects (such as fatigue, moodiness)	Yes	No	No	No	No	Yes
High in fiber	Yes	No	No	No	No	Yes
Sustainable for life	Yes	No	No	No	No	Yes

CHAPTER 2
THE *REAL* TRUTH ABOUT BREAKFAST

Always Eat After 7 PM is all about what foods you're eating and when. The timing of your meals and snacks throughout the day is incredibly important for reaching your weight loss goal and keeping your body in shape. In the following chapters, I'll first walk you through some common myths surrounding meals. This information will completely change the way you look at dieting! Then I'll outline the principles of how to structure your meals and snacks, from morning to evening, focusing on positive behaviors that will help you get into the best shape of your life. Let's begin with breakfast.

Of all the eating and dieting myths we've tackled so far, what we're told about breakfast might be some of the most misleading. We've all heard that breakfast is the most important meal of the day because it boosts your metabolism, prevents midday hunger, and helps us lose more weight. Right?

Well, it turns out that this universal advice is dead wrong. Our strong belief in the power of breakfast is generally based on some pretty biased studies. In fact, many of these studies are funded by the breakfast food industry, which is clearly biased!

Not coincidentally, the Kellogg Company, for example, paid for a well-publicized study concluding that eating cereal for breakfast makes you thinner! The researchers wrote: "This analysis provides evidence that skipping breakfast is not an effective way to manage weight. Eating cereal (ready-to-eat or cooked cereal) or quick breads for breakfast is associated with significantly lower body mass index compared to skipping breakfast or eating meats and/or eggs for breakfast."

You really have to look at who is sponsoring such studies. Who are they fooling? The conclusions tend to favor the food companies!

So before you do—or don't—dig in to your bacon, eggs, and toast, here's a reality check on the five biggest myths surrounding breakfast.

MYTH #1: YOU SHOULD *NEVER* SKIP BREAKFAST BECAUSE IT'S THE MOST IMPORTANT MEAL OF THE DAY.

Most days of the week, I don't eat breakfast. It's not that I don't like eggs, oatmeal, bacon, sausage, and other breakfast foods. It's just that I'm rarely hungry until around lunchtime. So, other than a morning cup of coffee or a fat-burning beverage, I don't eat much before noon.

Heresy, I know. Who in the world would not eat breakfast?

The advice that breakfast is the most important meal of the day is in the same category as many old wives' tales. There's not enough evidence to prove it matters.

Case in point: One of the latest words on this comes from a review article published in the *British Medical Journal* in 2019. In this study, researchers analyzed 13 randomized controlled trials that took place over the past 30 years, mainly from the United States or the United Kingdom.

The volunteers in the trials were of various weights, and some were regular breakfast eaters, while others were not. The studies monitored people for as little as a day or as long as 16 weeks.

Those who ate breakfast ended up eating about 260 calories more a day, the review found. Those who skipped breakfast were about one pound lighter than those who ate breakfast. These findings led the researchers to conclude that eating breakfast isn't necessarily a good strategy for losing weight.

The science about the importance of eating breakfast isn't really there. Breakfast could very well be the least important meal of the day!

MYTH #2: BREAKFAST EATERS LOSE MORE WEIGHT.

In a study published in the *American Journal of Clinical Nutrition*, researchers assigned more than 300 overweight and obese (but otherwise healthy) adults, ages 20 to 65, to either the control group (they continued with their normal eating habits), a group that was told to eat breakfast, or a group that was instructed to skip breakfast. After tracking their weight for 16 weeks, the scientists found that those who ate breakfast didn't lose any more weight than the breakfast skippers.

Eating breakfast just doesn't have a big effect on weight loss.

MYTH #3: BREAKFAST INCREASES YOUR METABOLISM.

Some experts claim that eating breakfast "kick-starts" the metabolism, but this is another misconception. They're generally talking about the thermic effect of food, which we discussed on page 7—the bump in calories burned after you eat any meal, including breakfast. A very protein-rich breakfast will increase TEF because protein has the highest TEF of all three macronutrients, but the typical American breakfast of doughnuts or bagels or sugary cereal will not.

What's more, studies show that there is no metabolic difference in calories burned over 24 hours between people who eat breakfast and those who skip it. So the whole idea that skipping breakfast will somehow *slow down* your metabolism is simply not true.

MYTH #4: EATING BREAKFAST REDUCES DAYTIME AND NIGHTTIME HUNGER.

In fact, the exact opposite happens. Typical breakfast foods such as orange juice, processed cereals, and wheat toast can spike your insulin levels. Elevated insulin churns out fat-storage hormones and makes you so hungry that you could devour every item on a fast-food menu.

Trust me: even if you skip breakfast, you will tame your appetite later in the day. German researchers put this to the test. They examined the breakfast habits of 400 obese and normal-weight people. Over two weeks, the participants were asked to log everything they ate and drank. The researchers analyzed the logs and discovered that those who ate bigger breakfasts did not cut back their food intake at other meals, as is commonly believed. By contrast, those who consumed a small breakfast, or skipped it altogether, ate fewer calories later.

The take-home message: breakfast is not an appetite suppressant!

MYTH #5: SKIPPING BREAKFAST MAKES YOU GAIN WEIGHT.

Right away, this statement is paradoxical. How can *not* eating make you gain more weight? Fact is, research has revealed that cutting out breakfast may curb your overall calorie intake by up to 400 calories a day. This seems logical, because you are effectively removing an entire meal from your diet each day. Skipping breakfast, in reality, helps you lose weight!

So what's the bottom line? The evidence for the importance of breakfast is not very convincing. You shouldn't feel bad if you'd rather skip it, and don't listen to those who lecture you. Breakfast has no magical powers.

What does have some pretty amazing benefits, however, is intermittent fasting.

INTERMITTENT FASTING

Going without breakfast is part of intermittent fasting (IF), also called time-restricted feeding (TRF). IF is a pattern of food consumption that cycles between fasting and eating in specific time periods. There are various ways to do it; one of the most common is the 16/8 protocol, which involves 16 hours of fasting—typically done overnight—with an 8-hour window in which to eat each day.

I started intermittent fasting about 10 years ago, long before it was popular or very well researched. When I practice intermittent fasting, I find that I rarely get hungry during the fast period and skipping breakfast doesn't even faze me.

The science on this phenomenon has since exploded on the scene. IF has been shown to effectively reduce calorie intake, increase weight loss, and improve metabolic health. Published research from Dr. Krista Varady's lab at the University of Illinois has shown that intermittent fasting is beneficial for overweight and obese individuals because it helps burn pure fat while maintaining lean muscle tissue. Additional research published in the scientific journal *Cell Metabolism* has found that alternate-day fasting can improve LDL cholesterol and triglyceride levels in people who are obese. And that's to name just a few of IF's benefits.

THE BENEFITS OF INTERMITTENT FASTING

- Natural increase in growth hormone levels without exercising
- Increased metabolic rate and fat burning
- Lowered risk of diabetes and insulin resistance
- Reduced inflammation
- Prevention of disease, including reduced risk of cancer
- Improved heart health
- Better brain health and protection against dementia and Alzheimer's disease
- Longevity and anti-aging
- Maintenance of skeletal muscle mass (lean muscle)
- Younger, clearer-looking skin

Intermittent fasting really shines when it comes to improving the hormones that directly affect your hunger, blood sugar, and metabolism. One is insulin. IF combats insulin resistance, meaning that it helps your body use insulin more normally, thereby lowering your diabetes risk and boosting your metabolism.

Intermittent fasting also regulates ghrelin. Ghrelin is nicknamed the hunger hormone. When you get hungry, especially when you have those nagging food cravings that just won't go away, ghrelin is to blame. You may think it's a lack of willpower, but in reality it's an abundance of ghrelin.

Generally, ghrelin levels go up when you're not eating or between meals, and they go down after you eat. With intermittent fasting, though, ghrelin levels actually *decrease* rather than continually going up, which banishes cravings and uncontrollable hunger—even though you haven't eaten. And surprisingly, the positive changes in ghrelin that occur during IF elevate dopamine levels in the brain. Dopamine is a feel-good brain chemical that increases mental alertness, triggers quick thinking, boosts mental energy, and enhances the ability to solve problems.

Physically, IF helps drain your muscles and liver of glycogen so that your body is then forced to burn fat for fuel. Mentally, it can break you of bad emotional habits or negative *neuro-associations* you may have with food and provide you with newfound energy and focus.

As with many great tactics, *more is not better*. If you abuse this strategy, your body may start shedding lean muscle—which in turn slows down your metabolism—and the result will be the loss of calorie-burning muscle. Essentially, your body thinks you are starving yourself so it will have to use amino acids from precious muscle tissue to survive.

That's why I recommend that you follow the 16/8 protocol (16 hours of fasting, 8 hours of feeding*) on this plan. It is easy to adhere to for lengthy periods. Plus, research shows that fasting for 14 to 16 hours increases many of the fat-burning and anti-aging benefits of intermittent fasting.

That said, your strategic fasting periods do not have to be exactly 16 hours. They could be 17 or 18 hours or they could be 12 to 14 hours. As long as you're fasting for at *least* 12 hours, you're still within range of the health-improving and fat-burning results created by IF.

You can follow this protocol five to six days per week. I personally like doing it Monday through Friday because it gives me a break and a chance to eat an early-morning breakfast with my wife and two daughters on the weekends.

INTERMITTENT FASTING DAILY MEAL TIMING TEMPLATE—16 HOURS FASTING, 8 HOURS FEEDING

If you eat your last meal of the day at . . .	. . . then you'll eat your first meal the next day at
6 PM	10 AM
7 PM	11 AM
8 PM	Noon
9 PM	1 PM
10 PM	2 PM

When you're fasting, you will:

- keep insulin super low.
- naturally boost fat-burning hormones (leptin, growth hormone, adrenaline, and glucagon).
- regulate your hunger hormone, ghrelin.
- have more daily energy.
- increase productivity and focus.
- give your digestive system and body a break from frequent feeding.
- burn significantly more fat.

* By "8 hours of feeding," I don't mean eating continuously for 8 hours. I'm referring to an 8-hour window in which you eat lunch, dinner, and your late-night snack.

Although intermittent fasting is very safe, it is not for everyone. You should avoid fasting completely if you:

- have a history of eating disorders.
- are sensitive to drops in blood sugar levels.
- are pregnant or nursing.
- are a teenager or child.
- have type 1 diabetes.
- are malnourished, are underweight, or have known nutrient deficiencies.
- are trying to conceive or have issues with fertility.

If any of these apply to you, turn to page 25 for a list of Smart Snacks you can enjoy at breakfast.

Initially, fasting may seem like a huge challenge, but remember to focus on the reward. It makes it possible to get leaner while eating bigger meals at night, enjoying a few glasses of red wine, and even having your cheat meals each week.

Your brain will release the neurotransmitters and hormones that will help you regulate your hormones and burn more stored fat each day. You don't have to be burdened with trying to eat every few hours. With intermittent fasting, dieting becomes *much* easier to adhere to and the benefits are remarkable.

And if fasting scares you or sounds unappealing, rest assured that you are not totally banned from the kitchen before your fast is up! Each day on the plan incorporates a 3-Minute Fat-Burning Morning Ritual.

THE 3-MINUTE FAT-BURNING MORNING RITUAL

As a part of intermittent fasting and in place of breakfast, you'll begin each day with the 3-Minute Fat-Burning Morning Ritual. It primes your metabolism for the highest energy levels and fastest fat loss possible. It also provides your body with everything it needs to power you through your morning *without* being hungry or relying on caffeinated sodas or sugary snacks.

Here's how it works: in the morning, have any of the following easy-to-fix fat-burning drinks.

Lemon Water

One of the simplest 3-Minute Fat-Burning Morning Rituals, lemon water is a glass of water mixed with the juice of half of a lemon. This drink provides all the benefits of regular drinking water, which supports weight loss, digestive health, physical performance, and cognitive function. You want to be sure you're getting enough water, and mixing in some lemon juice can indeed provide a flavorful alternative to plain water, with only a negligible addition of calories and natural sugar.

Although their nutritional characteristics are sometimes overstated, lemons are an excellent source of vitamin C. Like other citrus fruits, lemons are also a good source of phytonutrients, which possess a variety of antioxidant and anti-inflammatory properties. Lemons also contain natural compounds called citrus flavonoids, which are known to help activate fat burning, according to a 2016 report published in *Pharmacology & Therapeutics*.

Just squeeze half of a medium to large lemon into 8 ounces of filtered water and enjoy the benefits during your fast.

HOT OR COLD?

Some may say to drink lemon water (or other "fat-burning" drinks) cold, as cool beverages are purported to burn extra calories, while others suggest warm water as a means to improve digestion. Unfortunately, there's very little—if any—evidence to support either of these suggestions; thus, the temperature of the water is unlikely to make any significant difference.

Mint Citrus Water

Similar to lemon water, mint citrus water is a tasty, refreshing, low-calorie, low-sugar alternative to plain water. Because it is also mostly water, it too provides all the health benefits that you can expect from drinking regular water. For the citrus part of the drink, you can use lemons and/or limes, which are an excellent source of vitamin C and also contain phytonutrients that help the body protect cells.

The mint flavor comes from peppermint leaves, which have long been used in folk medicine and aromatherapy. The leaves contain an oil known for its ability to soothe digestive discomfort and freshen breath through the day. A 2018 review published in the *Journal of Family Practice* notes that there is strong evidence that peppermint helps alleviates the symptoms of irritable bowel syndrome.

There is also evidence that in addition to soothing digestion, peppermint tea may help you eat less. Studies have shown that the smell of peppermint can help curb appetite. In one randomized, crossover study published in the journal *Appetite* and conducted by Bryan Raudenbush at Wheeling Jesuit University, 40 volunteers sniffed peppermint every two hours for five days. For another five days, they did the same with a placebo. When they sniffed the peppermint, they consumed 1,800 fewer calories (over the five days)—about 360 fewer calories each day.

Here's a simple recipe for mint citrus water:

Ingredients

- 2 limes, sliced
- 4–5 fresh peppermint leaves
- 24 ounces water

Directions

- Place the limes and mint in a 32-ounce Mason jar.
- Add the water and cover with the lid.
- Drink immediately or let sit for 30 minutes or longer to let the flavor develop.
- This recipe makes two large servings; refrigerate the second serving for the next morning.

Cinnamon and Apple Cider Vinegar Drink

Both cinnamon and apple cider vinegar (ACV) provide potential health benefits.

For instance, studies consistently show that cinnamon powder (provided in amounts ranging from 1 to 2 teaspoons daily) is markedly effective at acutely improving carbohydrate tolerance and individual glycemic response.

In addition to its impact on blood sugar control and carbohydrate management, cinnamon may also exert additional anti-obesity effects. In a study published in the journal *Scientific Reports*, researchers from Switzerland found that certain compounds in cinnamon may increase fat burning and reduce production of ghrelin.

Cassia cinnamon (*Cinnamomum cassia*) is typically the form used in human trials and has been shown to be both safe and effective for most people. However, it tends to be high in coumarin, a natural plant chemical that acts as a blood thinner. If you are taking a prescription blood thinner, are preparing to undergo a surgical or dental procedure, or are considered to be at a high risk of bleeding, you probably shouldn't consume cassia cinnamon. Instead, look for "true" cinnamon—called Ceylon cinnamon (*Cinnamomum verum* or *Cinnamomum zeylanicum*)—when purchasing; this is likely a better option for you because its coumarin content is negligible.

Apple cider vinegar has been shown in research to help improve insulin sensitivity so that you minimize fat storage and keep your body in a fat-burning environment. In fact, one study showed that ACV can reduce blood sugar by a whopping 34 percent after eating 50 grams of white bread.

ACV has also been shown to aid in heart health and weight loss by detoxifying the liver, increasing metabolism, and suppressing hunger levels. While this concoction may not be the "miracle" that some proponents may lead you to believe, cinnamon, apple cider vinegar, and water do possess numerous health benefits and may be used as part of an overall healthy weight loss program. I recommend that you drink this just like taking a shot because apple cider vinegar has a pungent taste that some can find unpleasant. Also, make sure you rinse thoroughly, use mouthwash, or brush your teeth afterward because apple cider vinegar can be harmful to tooth enamel.

Here's a simple recipe you can use:

Ingredients

- 2 teaspoons Ceylon cinnamon
- 4 ounces hot water
- 1 teaspoon apple cider vinegar

Directions

- Steep the cinnamon in the hot water for 30 minutes.
- Once the water has cooled, add the apple cider vinegar.
- Drink immediately.

Super Greens (MetaboGreens™) Drink

Another pick for your morning ritual is a "green drink" powder, mixed with 8 ounces of water to whip up an instant nutritional beverage. Green powder supplements contain an array of pulverized veggies, healthy bacteria, and beneficial algae. Their energy-boosting, digestion-aiding, and detoxifying qualities are among their reported benefits. The powder I recommend is MetaboGreens, and I cover it in more detail in chapter seven.

Here's a simple recipe you can use:

Ingredients

- 1 scoop MetaboGreens
- 8 ounces water

Directions

- Stir the MetaboGreens powder into the water until well mixed. Alternatively, place the water and powder in a blender, and blend on low speed for 30 seconds.

Black Coffee

Coffee is one of the world's most popular drinks, second only to water and tea. Despite its popularity, coffee seems to be a somewhat contentious beverage, as it is frequently considered "unhealthy."

But research suggests the opposite. There are multiple health benefits associated with drinking coffee; among them is an increase in metabolic rate. Studies over the past several years suggest that drinking coffee may protect against type 2 diabetes, Parkinson's disease, liver cancer, and liver cirrhosis.

Coffee is also a very complex beverage with hundreds and hundreds of different compounds in it. In fact, a cup of coffee contains all of the following essential nutrients:

- pantothenic acid (vitamin B5)
- riboflavin (vitamin B2)
- niacin (vitamin B3)
- thiamine (vitamin B1)
- potassium
- manganese

What's more, coffee is loaded with antioxidants. In fact, studies show that coffee is the single greatest dietary source of antioxidants—outweighing even fruits and vegetables.

Of course, coffee contains the drug caffeine. It too offers a slew of benefits: alertness, greater energy, and better mental performance. Caffeine is also a metabolism booster—a benefit you can get from drinking just one cup of coffee.

Caffeine has also been widely studied from a sports performance standpoint, and it has been shown to significantly improve physical performance and reduce perceived levels of exertion (how difficult or how easy an exercise is) when taken before exercise.

But how much is too much? The Mayo Clinic advises that up to 400 milligrams of caffeine a day appears to be safe for most healthy adults. That's roughly the amount of caffeine in four cups of brewed coffee. Drinking more than that may bring on side effects such as headaches, insomnia, nervousness, stomach upset, and fast heartbeat.

To use coffee as your 3-Minute Fat-Burning Morning Ritual, drink 1 to 2 cups of black coffee, hot or iced. Feel free to add organic stevia or erythritol (Swerve) for a sweetener, but avoid creamers, sugar, and other sweeteners like Splenda, Truvia, monk fruit extracts, and sugar alcohols because they can affect insulin and will potentially break your fast.

Green Tea

Green tea leaves are processed differently than most other teas, which leaves them with a higher concentration of beneficial polyphenols called catechins. These compounds have noteworthy anti-inflammatory and antioxidant properties, and they also seem to have quite a potent effect on metabolism and fat burning. What's more, they may also suppress appetite and decrease the absorption of calories.

Studies consistently show that green tea extract (standardized for the catechin epigallocatechin gallate, or EGCG) increases the body's use of fat for fuel. It does so by helping fat-burning hormones such as norepinephrine do their job. In other words, green tea can help make a good fat loss program even more effective.

Researchers also suggest that in addition to increasing metabolism, calorie expenditure, and fat burning, green tea extract can help control energy balance by suppressing appetite.

To use green tea for your 3-Minute Fat-Burning Morning Ritual, drink 1 to 2 cups, hot or iced. Feel free to add organic stevia for a sweetener.

DON'T FORGET WATER: THE LONG-FORGOTTEN FAT-BURNING NUTRIENT

When the plants or flowers in your yard are not watered, they quickly droop and shrivel up. Similarly, without sufficient water, your body may counter with a sluggish, droopy feeling. In other words, you're dehydrated. It's important to drink water all day long.

Water helps digest your food, expel wastes, regulate your temperature, protect your tissues, cushion your joints, and protect your spinal column, among many other vital functions. It is through water that hormones flow to the proper organs, that nutrients reach all cells, and that toxins are diluted and removed from the body.

Water is also a metabolism booster. Researchers in Germany reported in the *Journal of Clinical Endocrinology & Metabolism* in 2003 that drinking adequate water revs up the rate at which the body burns calories. Involved in the study were seven men and seven women who were healthy and of normal weight. After consuming approximately 17 ounces of water, their metabolic rates increased by 30 percent. These elevations occurred within 10 minutes of water consumption and hit a maximum after 30 to 40 minutes.

The researchers then calculated that annually a person who drinks 1.5 liters a day (about 6 cups) automatically burns an extra 17,400 calories a year—which could result in a weight loss of approximately five pounds in a year.

HOW MUCH?

One of the most common mistakes people make is drinking water only when they're thirsty. But your thirst mechanism isn't usually a good indication that you need water. When you're thirsty, chances are that you could already be mildly dehydrated. Not drinking enough water causes your blood to become heavy with salt and other substances. These pull water out of your salivary glands, causing thirst. So don't wait until you're thirsty to drink water.

A good rule of thumb is to consume 50 percent of your total body weight in ounces each day. So if you weigh 150 pounds, then you should be shooting for a minimum of 75 ounces daily—especially if you exercise. If you sweat a lot, are highly active, or are an older adult, the water you need daily goes up.

One easy way to track your water intake is to fill a 2-liter bottle in the morning and make sure it's empty by the end of the day. Start drinking water as soon as you wake up in the morning—have a glass with your breakfast. Then keep sipping throughout the day.

Some advice: Although tap water is convenient, I no longer recommend it after reading a study from the University of Kent and published in the *Journal of Epidemiology and Community Health*. It pointed out that the fluoride in our water supply may cause hypothyroidism, even at levels that are much lower than the highest level allowed by the U.S. Environmental Protection Agency (EPA). Other research indicates that fluoride *inhibits* the body's ability to use iodine, which is needed to produce thyroid hormones.

Bottled water isn't the best choice either, because of the chemicals that leach into the water from the plastic and the environmental problems caused by plastic water bottles.

I suggest that you invest in a high-quality water filter, limit your intake of bottled water, and avoid drinking water straight from the tap at all costs.

ENERGIZING BREAKFAST "SMART SNACKS" FOR PEOPLE WHO CAN'T (OR WON'T) SKIP BREAKFAST

If the idea of skipping breakfast or consuming one of the morning beverages still seems too difficult, or you can't do it for health reasons, don't worry.

During the first seven days of the Acceleration Phase, you do not have to forgo breakfast. I want to ease you into that part of the program.

For the first week (as well as on any days later in the plan in which you do not fast and do not use the 3-Minute Fat-Burning Morning Ritual), you can eat a breakfast and *still* see some of these results. The same goes if you're unable to use intermittent fasting at any point in the program, though you may see slower results.

The key is to avoid all carbs in the morning. That will keep insulin at bay early in the day for more efficient fat burning. The only two exceptions to this guideline are berries and cherries, because both are very low in carbohydrates and minimally affect insulin secretion.

Here are some examples to choose from:

- 3 hard-boiled eggs (with sea salt and black pepper, to taste)
- ½ cup low-fat cottage cheese or full-fat Greek yogurt (use nonflavored varieties) with a handful of nuts or seeds or ½ cup berries or cherries
- Protein shake using unsweetened almond milk or water as a base with ½ cup frozen berries or cherries
- Celery sticks with 2 tablespoons nut butter
- 2–3 scrambled eggs with a sprinkle of cheese (raw, organic cheese preferred)
- 2–3 pieces of beef jerky (grass-fed beef is preferred) with a handful of nuts
- Breakfast wrap: 2 scrambled eggs with ½ avocado, a sprinkle of cheese, and optional hot sauce rolled into a coconut wrap
- Organic cherries with a handful of nuts
- *Instant Pot Egg White Bites* or *Bacon and Caramelized Onion Egg Muffins* from the Breakfast Smart Snacks on pages 112 and pages 115

If you're serious about your body, you'll get serious about forgoing breakfast—not the most important meal after all—and replace it with my 3-Minute Fat-Burning Morning Ritual (or a Breakfast Smart Snack) and make intermittent fasting part of your nutritional lifestyle. Breaking the breakfast rule is your first step toward fast, painless fat loss.

Each day, after your intermittent fasting window has ended, you'll move on to your two large meals of the day. Read on to learn how lunch and dinner work on the plan.

CHAPTER 3
ENERGIZING LUNCHES AND FAT-BURNING DINNERS WITH PORTION VOLUMIZATION

You've learned how intermittent fasting can put you on the right path to achieving your weight loss goals. Now that you know that the timing of your meals is key on Always Eat After 7 PM, I'll show you how to get more mileage out of your food. You might be surprised to learn that you can likely eat *more* food on the plan than you do now—while still losing fat and quickly slimming down.

How do you do it? The key to planning the perfect lunch and dinner on this program is Portion Volumization™. With this technique, you'll seek out nutrient-dense, delicious foods that fill you up and give you a "free pass" to eat 5 to 10 times the amount of food you'd normally eat, while consuming considerably fewer calories.

To drive this point home, here is a perfect example of two food choices:

1. Whole-wheat spaghetti
2. Spaghetti squash

Whole-wheat spaghetti can be a healthier choice than regular pasta, but one large (1½-cup) serving packs a whopping 264 calories and 57 grams of insulin-spiking carbs. Compare that to the same amount of the Portion Volumization pasta substitute, spaghetti squash, which has only 63 calories and 15 grams of carbs in 1½ cups. It takes more than 5 cups to match the calories in whole-wheat pasta. That means, if you wanted to, you could eat *more than three times as much food* and still consume fewer carbs, while also getting more fiber, minerals, and vitamins.

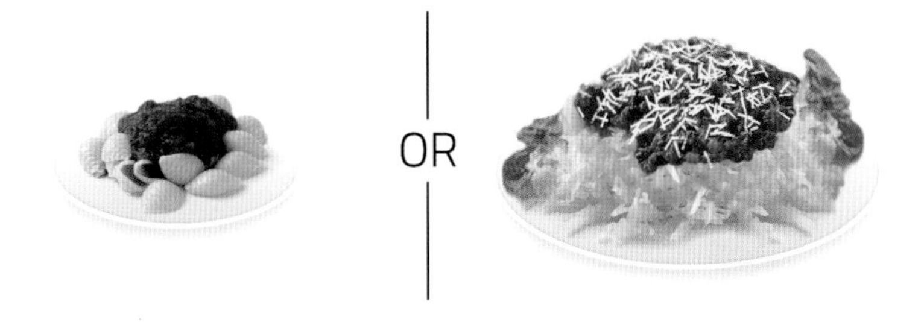

Three times as much food but lighter in carbs **and much healthier**

This is just one simplified version of dozens and dozens of healthy food swaps that can be made to consistently achieve your goals without the sacrifice and hunger that typically accompany every rapid fat loss diet.

Look at the food comparison chart on the next page. On the left, you'll see the normal artery-hardening, fattening foods that many people eat on a daily basis; on the right are meals made up of healthier Portion Volumizing choices. All these meal options have about the same number of calories. As you can clearly see, the difference is profound.

Just ask yourself: *Which meals would you rather eat?*

Love French fries? Swap them out for an even larger portion of boiled redskin potatoes. How about pasta? Put your meatballs and marinara sauce over a huge plate of cooked spaghetti squash or "zoodles," strands of shredded zucchini. Love to spend evenings with two of America's favorite guys, Ben and Jerry? Whip up a frozen banana or pineapple with a little milk for a super-satisfying, super-healthy ice cream. The point is, if you cut calories by simply eating less, you'll feel hungry and deprived. (Who wants to stop at half a burger?) But Portion Volumizing foods help you feel satisfied while you're reducing calories, so you can stick with this plan for the long term.

Best of all, long-term research reveals that diets that emphasize Portion Volumizing foods also promote rapid weight loss. In fact, studies lasting longer than six months show that folks who eat more of these foods experience *three times* greater weight loss than people who simply opt to reduce calories but keep eating the same foods as before.

Sound good? Take a look at all the Portion Volumizing foods you'll eat on Always Eat After 7 PM. These are your food choices for both lunch and dinner.

PROTEINS

To get a lot of bang for your buck with any meal, be generous with protein. Beyond its role in this program, protein is an absolute necessity for life because it provides all the building blocks from

500-CALORIE MEAL COMPARISON

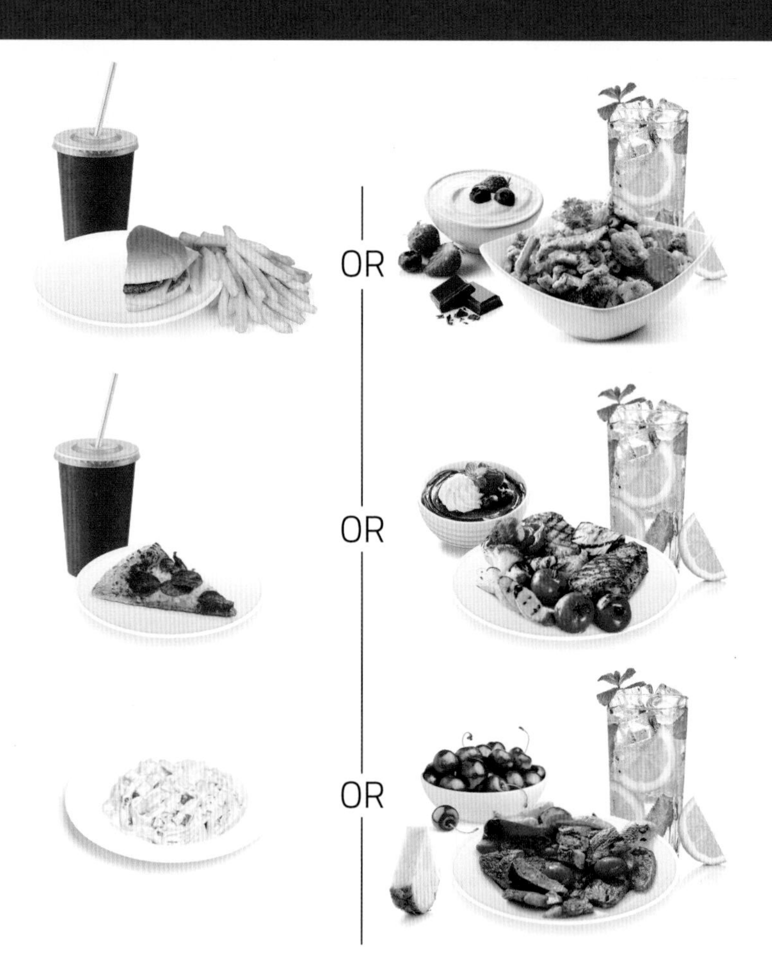

By learning how to choose Portion Volumizing foods at each meal, you can eat much more while consuming fewer calories each day.

which your tissues are made. It helps form hormones and immune cells and rebuilds, repairs, and regenerates your organs on a day-to-day basis. Without sufficient amounts of protein in your diet, your body will not be able to repair and rebuild the tissues that are required for optimal function.

From a fat loss and fitness perspective, protein is probably the most powerful nutrient to include in any diet. Here are six reasons you should eat protein at every meal:

1. Protein has a higher thermic effect of food (TEF) than carbs or fat, which means you'll burn more calories digesting protein compared to other nutrients.

2. Protein helps reduce your hunger hormone, ghrelin, while coaxing the body to release more glucagon. Glucagon is a peptide hormone that "unlocks" your fat cells, allowing stored fat to be used as fuel.
3. Protein preserves lean tissue (muscle) that might otherwise be sacrificed on a weight loss diet. The loss of calorie-burning muscle tends to lead to the dreaded trifecta of decreased metabolic rate, looking "skinny fat" (a phrase used to describe people who look fit and healthy on the surface yet carry mostly fat and very little muscle on their frames), and weight regain. Thus, you want to develop and save as much lean muscle as you can. The more muscle you have, the more efficient your fat-burning systems are.
4. Protein stabilizes blood sugar so that you don't get wild swings and dips in energy—which can lead to cravings. Keeping your blood glucose levels stable throughout the day is a necessity for optimal weight control and prevention of diabetes.
5. Protein boosts your metabolism because it revs up the action of your thyroid gland (one of its jobs is to regulate metabolism).
6. Protein fills you up. It acts like an appetite suppressant so that you don't crave or overeat fattening foods. In fact, protein is the most satiating of the three macronutrients.

And if you've ever heard that protein is harmful to your body, is acidic or inflammatory, or leaches calcium from your bones, there is plenty of evidence, including long-term published studies, showing otherwise.

TOP PROTEIN CHOICES

Beef

You have a huge variety of beef choices on this plan—ground beef, steak, roasts, and more. Despite a bad rap in certain circles, beef is a nutrient-dense all-star. However, not all beef is created equal. I believe that grass-fed beef is a superior option over standard grain-fed options. Depending on the breed of cow, grass-fed beef contains up to five times more omega-3 fatty acids than grain-fed beef. The average ratio of omega-6 to omega-3 fatty acids in grass-fed beef is 1.5:1, which is essentially ideal. On the contrary, in grain-fed beef, this ratio jumps all the way up to nearly 8:1.

Seafood

Another excellent protein choice is wild-caught, cold-water fish such as salmon, sardines, anchovies, mackerel, halibut, and tuna—all loaded with protein and omega-3 fatty acids. In addition to their brain and cardiovascular health benefits, these essential fats have been shown to have beneficial effects on metabolism and body composition.

Chicken

Let's not forget another protein all-star: chicken. Chicken is best known for its high protein content, and at up to 35 grams of protein per 4-ounce (cooked) portion, it is indeed an excellent source.

I like chicken because it contains a weapon in the war on fat—leucine. It's an amino acid that has long been praised by athletes for the way it keeps their muscles toned. Scientists have found that while it maintains muscle, it can also improve the body's ability to shed fat.

In addition to its leucine and protein content, chicken is also a very good source of numerous other vitamins and minerals that are critical to overall health and metabolism. The recipes in this book show you how to turn chicken—which can be a little boring—into amazing dishes.

These are just a few of your protein choices; there are many others. Just be sure to plan balanced meals by including a variety of quality proteins at lunch and dinner.

PORTION VOLUMIZATION: HOW TO GET THE MOST FROM PROTEIN

1. Consume one serving of lean protein at every lunch and dinner (see the list on pages 40–41). Feel free to use a high-quality protein powder like BioTrust Low Carb Protein Powder Blend™ in place of meat, poultry, or seafood, if desired. It makes a great meal replacement when you're on the go and pressed for time.
2. Make sure you choose mostly lean cuts when Portion Volumizing. Although fatty cuts of animal protein are still healthy sources of high-quality protein and friendly fats, selecting lean cuts lets you eat much larger portion sizes without adding unnecessary calories. If you do choose a fattier cut, do not include additional friendly fats with that meal. See page 42 for more on friendly fats.
3. When selecting beef, an easy rule to follow is to choose cuts that have *round*, *chuck*, or *loin* in their names, which means they're lean or extra lean. Round and chuck steaks are often tougher cuts, but you can use a combination of lemon juice, light soy sauce (or coconut aminos), and minced garlic to help tenderize your lean cuts of meat quickly. Do not add oil to your marinades, because this introduces unnecessary fat.
4. Try to choose animal protein sources that are grass-fed, pasture-raised, organic, and hormone- and antibiotic-free. When choosing fish, make sure to select wild-caught.

SUPER CARBS

Carbohydrates tend to get a bad rap. There's a lot of misleading information out there, and many people believe carbs are responsible for obesity and deadly diseases. And, to some degree, they are—but only because of poor carb choices. For example, many of the carbohydrates we eat are full of sugar and heavily processed, causing unhealthy blood glucose fluctuations that can increase fat storage and risk for diabetes.

But not all carbohydrates are bad. Many carbohydrate-containing foods are jam-packed with vitamins, minerals, antioxidants, and fiber.

Carbs come in various types, and you get to enjoy most of them—*even to the point of filling up on certain types*. First, there are starches, including dried beans, lentils, carrots, peas, beets, oats, grains, certain breads, and even some pastas. These are what I call Super Carbs—more on these below.

Second, there are fruits. Yes, fruit has sugar, but it also supplies fiber—a natural blood sugar–balancing nutrient—and a variety of other vitamins. Because you'll be eating meals with plenty of protein and vegetables, your body won't have trouble with the sugar in fruit and will definitely profit from its nutrients.

The third carb category is the non-starchy vegetables. Non-starchy vegetables are those that are low in calories and high in water and fiber, both of which help fill you up. In fact, many of these veggies are 90 percent fiber, which is important for weight loss and digestive health; as noted above, it also helps avoid spikes in blood sugar. Plus, non-starchy vegetables have the highest concentration of vitamins, minerals, and phytochemicals of any foods out there.

Refined sugars and starches, however, are not on the menu. I'm talking about sugar, white bread, white pasta, snack foods, sugary cereals, fruit juices, and sodas, among others. Too much of this stuff raises levels of chronic inflammation and blocks your fat-burning ability.

THE BENEFITS OF EATING *LOTS* OF SUPER CARBS

You're probably thinking, "But I thought going low carb was the way to burn fat and lose weight." Not according to important scientific evidence. So that's another misguided diet "rule" that I encourage you to break on Always Eat After 7 PM. You see, low-carb dieting interferes with leptin, a hormone that is produced in the body's fat cells and monitors incoming energy as well as total body fat stores. When either incoming energy or body fat stores start to decline (as is often the case on low-carb or low-calorie fat loss diets), a series of reactions is set off in the body. As your leptin levels decline, you'll experience a downward spiral of negative side effects (see the box on the next page).

By feeding your body properly with the right Portion Volumization Super Carbs and other carbs, you can reverse virtually every one of the negative side effects listed in the box.

Super Carbs have some amazing benefits when it comes to fat burning and weight control:

1. They provide energy to the brain and body for increased mental function and exercise performance.
2. They increase metabolic rate by preventing metabolic slowdown while dieting.
3. They optimize thyroid hormones for more efficient fat burning.
4. They maintain leptin levels and improve leptin sensitivity, thus preventing weight loss plateaus.

NEGATIVE SIDE EFFECTS OF LOW-CARB DIETS AND DECREASED LEPTIN LEVELS

- Slower metabolic rate (metabolic slowdown)
- Uncontrolled cravings and hunger
- Fatigue and lethargy
- Insomnia and restless sleep
- Sharp decline in libido levels
- Anxiousness, irritability, and depression

There's more. Glucose-based starches, like rice and potatoes, are great sources of anaerobic fuel for exercisers; they can help increase ATP (energy) production, enhance recovery, build muscle, increase metabolic rate, and optimize hormones.

If you select Super Carbs and combine them with lots of protein and moderate to low fats, they can dramatically improve your body's fat-burning efficiency and overall metabolic health.

YOU MUST EAT SUPER CARBS AT NIGHT!

Eating carbs at night does not spell disaster for your waistline. In fact, they're actually good for controlling your weight. I'm super serious about this: it is absolutely vital to eat carbs in the evening. Let's dig a little deeper into the "why."

Your body follows a circadian rhythm—an internal metabolic clock—in which hormone levels fluctuate throughout the day. Cortisol is one of these hormones. Under normal circumstances, it is naturally elevated in the morning to get you alert and ready to go. Over the course of the day, it naturally falls. As cortisol drops, the sleep hormones, melatonin and serotonin, rise. They, along with growth hormones, support nightly healing and repair, helping us look and feel younger.

Your circadian rhythm can get turned upside down if you are stressed out or eliminate carbs at night. When your rhythm is disrupted, cortisol goes *up* in the evening and floods your system, making you anxious, unable to sleep, and prone to gaining belly fat (when your cortisol levels are elevated for too long, the amount of fat you keep in your belly can increase).

The solution is to eat slow-digesting, unrefined Super Carbs in the evening. They cause insulin levels to rise gradually instead of dramatically and blood sugar levels to remain steady. Insulin is an antagonist to cortisol, and consequently cortisol levels do not skyrocket.

Having carbs in the evening is also a great weight loss strategy. When you're active, your body burns mainly carbohydrates and muscle glycogen for energy. By eating carbs at night, you allow your body to use them to restore glycogen for energy the next day and provide your body with the glucose it needs to regulate your blood sugar levels during sleep.

Also, including slow-digesting carbs at night helps keep you feeling fuller for longer and banishes those dreaded "after-dinner munchies" that ultimately pack on pounds.

Further, avoiding carbohydrates and restricting calories later in the day can have an adverse effect on your thyroid hormones, which play a major role in metabolism. When the thyroid fails to secrete enough of the hormones that control metabolism, this can trigger symptoms like fatigue, depression, weight gain, thinning hair, and dry skin.

There are two forms of thyroid hormone in the body: an inactive form, called T4, and an active form, called T3. T4 is transported through the blood, and once it reaches each cell, it is converted to the active T3 form. It can do its job only if the conversion process works as it should.

A key part of that process is the availability of carbs. You see, carbs supply glucose, the number-one building block of thyroid hormones. Glucose (from Super Carbs) and thyroid hormones rely on each other synergistically, so without the right carbs, your body cannot convert T4 into the active hormone T3. But when you eat Super Carbs, you increase your thyroid hormones and support the conversion, so that you can quickly (and permanently) regulate your metabolism and quickly melt stubborn fat.

So, despite all the bad press over the years, certain carbohydrates play an important role in balancing your hormones and regulating your metabolic rate, while avoiding the dreaded weight loss plateaus that accompany conventional diets. Furthermore, when you eat these carbohydrates, you'll feel much better than you would if you were following a traditional diet.

In Phases 2 and 3 of Always Eat After 7 PM, eating Portion Volumizing Super Carbs for

BEST CARB PRACTICES FOR PORTION VOLUMIZATION

- Always combine Super Carbs and fruits with high-quality protein and moderate to low friendly fats to help keep blood sugar levels stable.
- Try to consume your largest Super Carb serving of the day after you exercise or for dinner to increase insulin sensitivity and optimize hormones.
- Avoid and limit any type of processed carbohydrate (unless it's a cheat meal or cheat day).
- Familiarize yourself with calculating net carbs when reading food labels. Net carbs refers to carbs that are absorbed by the body. To calculate net carbs in a food, simply subtract the fiber from the total carbs to get the net carbs.

lunch and dinner every day with a high-quality protein source will help you further boost your metabolism. Just make sure you follow best carb practices.

Bottom line: cutting carbs is not a short- or long-term strategy to meet your weight loss goals. Follow these guidelines and your favorite carbs will be a powerful tool in helping you achieve your goals.

PORTION VOLUMIZATION: HOW TO BULK UP YOUR MEALS WITH SUPER CARBS, FRUIT, AND NON-STARCHY VEGETABLES

1. In Phases 2 and 3, consume at least one serving of Super Carbs at dinner, such as squash, potatoes, carrots, rice, quinoa, beans or legumes, oats, or sprouted or sourdough breads. Feel free to increase portion sizes of all squashes. See the list on page 41 for my recommended Super Carbs.
2. Consume one serving of low-sugar fruits or berries *or* 2 to 4 squares of 70 percent cocoa dark chocolate for dessert each night while on the Acceleration Phase, and other fruits and Super Carbs on the Main and Lifestyle Phases. (If it's tough to keep all this straight, don't worry—we'll go in depth into each phase in part two.)
3. One serving from the approved (non-starchy) vegetables list on page 42 can be added to any lunch or dinner. This will allow you to meet your total calorie and macronutrient needs for each day. Make sure to take into account additional calories from any butter or oil added to vegetables. Salads can be counted as a serving of vegetables, but make sure to use very small amounts of oils and dressings.
4. Exercisers can feel free to increase carb servings by 25 percent if they are eaten in the post-workout meal (carbs can be fruits or starches).

WHITE POTATOES—FEAR NOT!

As for the much-maligned white potatoes, if you're worried that eating them will make you fatter, you'll be pleasantly surprised to hear this true story. After the USDA proposed eliminating the potato from federal feeding and nutrition programs, Chris Voigt, the executive director of the Washington State Potato Commission, staged a protest by eating nothing but 20 potatoes per day for two whole months. Even though he wasn't trying to lose weight, he did. Not only that, but Chris, who was in his forties at the time, had dramatic improvements in other areas of his health as well:

Starting weight: 197 pounds	Ending weight: 176 pounds
Starting blood glucose: 104 mg/dL	Ending blood glucose: 94 mg/dL
Starting cholesterol: 214 mg/dL	Ending cholesterol: 147 mg/dL
Starting triglycerides: 135 mg/dL	Ending triglycerides: 75 mg/dL

What's more, his ending blood pressure was 112 over 70—an ideal level.

These numbers indicate that Chris dramatically *reduced* his risk for heart disease and diabetes eating nothing but potatoes. His health improvements from the potato diet were in fact far *greater* than what we normally see from prescription drugs and many intensive lifestyle programs.

Potatoes supply your body with 100 percent all-natural glucose. Every cell in your body, even your brain, utilizes glucose. In fact, in terms of human evolution, glucose has a long history as a fuel. Our bodies have been using glucose as a primary fuel source since the caveman days. And get this: on average, only 1 out of every 120 calories from glucose gets stored as fat.

So 95 percent of the time your body burns up glucose immediately after you consume it. Glucose from potatoes has also been shown to suppress the hunger hormone ghrelin to help us crush late-night cravings without fat storage.

While I would *never* recommend an all-potato diet for anyone, Chris Voigt's stunt proves once and for all that in spite of all the bad press, starchy vegetables like potatoes do not make you fat, as long as you cook them in a healthy way and don't pile butter, sour cream, cheese, or creamy sauces on top of them—or deep-fry them, of course.

So roast them. Bake them. Fry them in small amounts of healthy oil. Add them to soups, stews, and scrambles, or just have them as a side dish.

FRIENDLY FATS

For years and years, we've been told by doctors, public health authorities, and the diet food industry that we should avoid high-fat foods. Unfortunately, this low-fat craze has dominated the world of nutrition for too long. Many of us have come to believe that we should shun fats altogether, but research shows otherwise.

A review published in the *American Journal of Clinical Nutrition* in 2010 gathered data from 21 studies and included nearly 348,000 adults. It found no difference in the risks of heart disease and stroke among people who consumed the lowest and highest intakes of "friendly" saturated fat. Countless other studies support this finding, now proving that saturated fats from the right food sources have *nothing* to do with heart disease and sickness.

There are certain types of fats, such as all vegetable oils and trans fats, which should be avoided altogether. Friendly fats, however, play a vital role in weight loss and overall health improvement. And they offer some amazing health benefits.

1. Friendly fats optimize neurotransmitters (brain chemicals), brain health, and memory.
2. They help maintain healthy skin and nerves.
3. Fats provide the building blocks for hormones. (The primary sex hormones, estrogen and testosterone, are largely made up of dietary fat, so when you cut out friendly fat sources, you put yourself at risk for muscle loss, accelerated aging, and fat storage.)
4. Friendly fats help lower inflammation.
5. Fats transport fat-soluble vitamins such as A, D, E, and K through the body, thereby helping to keep these vitamins at healthy levels in the body.
6. They improve cholesterol profiles, reducing your risk of heart disease.
7. Friendly fats balance blood sugar levels and help prevent hunger between meals.
8. They protect the body from cell-damaging oxidative stress to fight aging.

THREE TYPES OF FRIENDLY FATS

There are three types of fats you should be incorporating into your nutrition plan consistently: saturated, monounsaturated, and polyunsaturated. To be sure you're getting the healthiest options, look for fats from these sources:

- Saturated fats should come from healthy animal fats (such as grass-fed beef, grass-fed butter, ghee, and tallow) and coconut oil (which is plant based).

- Monounsaturated fats should come from mixed nuts, nut butters, avocado, olives, and olive oil.
- Polyunsaturated fats should come from fish and fish oils (wild-caught salmon, for example, or quality fish oil and/or krill oil supplements), flaxseed oil, and hemp.

There is a fourth type of fat: trans fats. These are oils that have been turned into solids via a process called hydrogenation (they often appear in food ingredient lists as "partially hydrogenated" oils). Trans fats are the worst kinds of fats for us and they should be avoided.

PORTION VOLUMIZATION: HOW TO DO IT WITH FRIENDLY FATS

1. Be very mindful of portion sizes when consuming friendly fats and oils since they yield over twice the calories (9 calories per gram) of proteins and carbs (4 calories per gram).
2. Consume one serving of friendly fats with lunch and dinner. Here are some examples of how to properly add friendly fats to your Portion Volumizing meals:
    - Drizzle olive or avocado oil on a salad.
    - Serve melted grass-fed butter or ghee on your vegetables.
    - Pan-fry or sear proteins, veggies, and carbs in ghee, grass-fed butter, tallow, duck fat, or avocado, coconut, or olive oil.
    - Sprinkle nuts on a salad or add them to a dinner recipe.
    - Slice half an avocado and add it to a salad.
    - Use coconut oil in a protein smoothie or milkshake that is eaten as a lunch meal replacement.
3. Always try to buy raw or roasted nuts and nut butters, along with cold-pressed oils.
4. Make sure you don't add additional friendly fats to meals that contain fatty cuts of meat. These cuts will function as your serving of friendly fats for that particular meal.

ADDITIONAL FOODS AND NUTRIENTS TO AVOID WHEN USING PORTION VOLUMIZATION

It's pretty obvious these days what foods need to be avoided for the most part. But a lot of misinformation (read: "lies") is still out there, along with labeling loopholes that allow food companies to tout certain foods as "healthy," when in reality they're far from it.

Of course, there are the obvious offenders as well. Here's a list of foods to either avoid altogether or limit your consumption of (that is, eat them only in cheat meals and on cheat days).

- **Low-fat and sugar-free diet foods or nutrition bars:** These are highly processed and often high in unhealthy preservatives, carbs, sugar, or sugar alcohols.
- **Conventional (non-organic) milk:** If you tolerate dairy, you can use small amounts of regular milk, but make sure you take into account its milk sugars and fat content. When choosing dairy products in general, I recommend organic (see page 46 for more).
- **Some condiments or sauces:** These food products contain hidden sugars and other harmful preservatives.
- **Excessive beer, wine, or sugary cocktails:** Due to beer's carb content, excessive beer consumption is obviously not recommended. Vodka, gin, rum, and red wine can all be consumed in moderation after the first week, but I recommend that you do so on weekends only or as part of your cheat meal.
- **Artificial sweeteners:** Limit your intake of sucralose, aspartame, saccharine, and other forms of fake sugar. They trick your body into thinking it needs sweets, and you can wind up craving sugary foods.

PUTTING IT ALL TOGETHER: HOW TO CREATE PORTION VOLUMIZING LUNCHES AND DINNERS

Based on these food categories, it's simple to structure your meals. Part two of the book will get into plan guidelines in more detail. Selections and portion sizes will vary depending on what phase you're in. (In the Acceleration Phase, for example, you don't eat any Super Carbs.)

In general, meals are made up of certain components no matter what phase you're in. To give you a preview, lunch is:

- One serving of protein
- One serving of Super Carbs (starchy carbs) or one serving of fruit (not both)—in the Main Phase and the Lifestyle Phase
- One serving of non-starchy vegetables
- One serving of friendly fat

A lunch like this breaks down into 300 to 500 calories, 40 percent carbohydrates, 40 percent protein, and 20 percent fat.

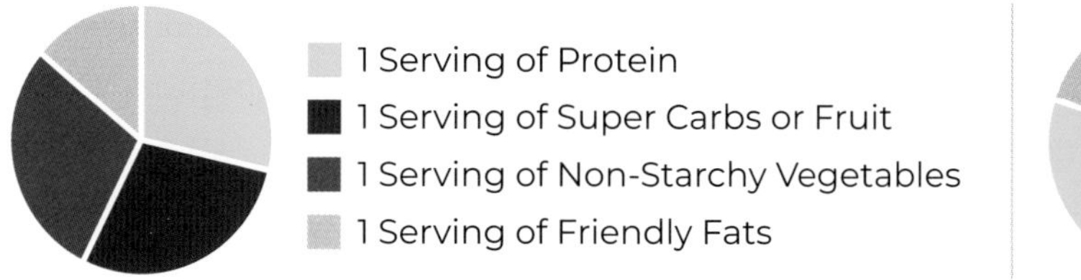

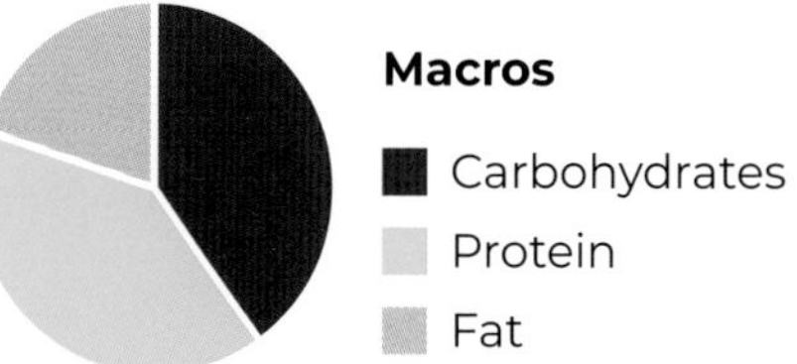

Translating these category names into real food, your energizing lunch might be one serving of grilled chicken, one serving of chickpeas, and one generous serving of leafy greens and salad vegetables, drizzled with olive oil.

Or it might be a roast beef sandwich on Ezekiel bread, with avocado slices, lettuce, and tomato.

Then, in the evening, dinner is:

- One serving of protein
- One serving of Super Carbs (starchy carbs) or one serving of fruit in the Main Phase and the Lifestyle Phase
- One or two servings of non-starchy vegetables
- One serving of friendly fat
- Dessert: one serving of low-sugar fruit or berries, *or* 2 to 4 squares of 70 percent cocoa dark chocolate.

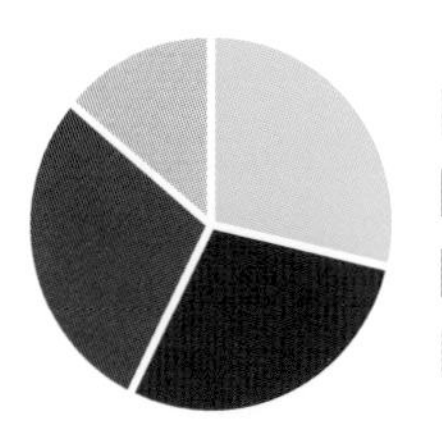

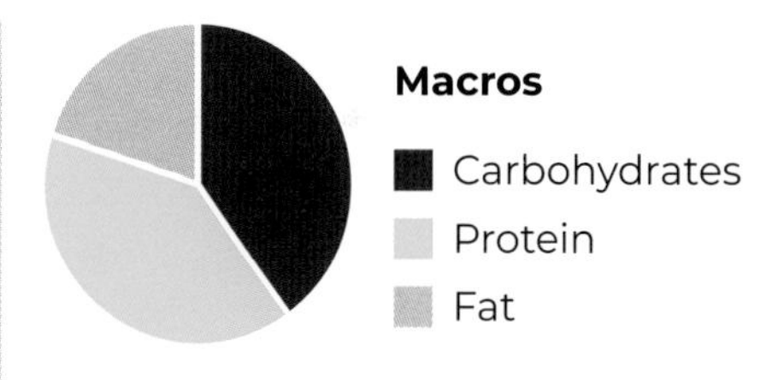

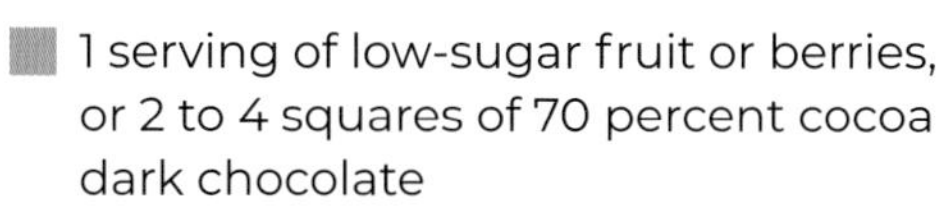

A dinner like this breaks down into about 300 to 500 calories, 40 percent carbohydrates, 40 percent protein, and 20 percent fat. Your healthy dessert should be around 200 calories.

Translating these categories into real food, your huge dinner might be one serving of roasted pork tenderloin, one medium baked sweet potato, steamed green beans, a dinner salad with olive oil dressing, and four squares of dark chocolate for dessert.

For other options, take a look at the many delicious recipes to enjoy for lunch and dinner in part three.

After you feel satisfied, comfortably full, and energized from your power-packed lunch and dinner, your metabolism will be primed for even faster fat burning. In the next chapter, we'll get to one of the best parts of this plan: the fat-burning bedtime snacks.

PORTION VOLUMIZATION FOOD LISTS

Protein		
Choose lots of lean cuts and low-fat dairy, including:	**Choose limited fattier protein choices, including:** (Note: If eating protein from this list, do not include additional friendly fats with that meal.)	**Avoid most processed proteins, including:**
Red meat		
Sirloin tip, top sirloin, top round, eye of round steak, bottom of round steak, filet mignon, beef brisket, venison (all or most cuts are lean), bison (all or most cuts are lean), veal (all or most cuts are lean)	Ribeye steak, rib roast, prime rib, New York strip, T-bone steak, Delmonico steak, flank or skirt steak, lamb, beef or bison jerky	Processed meats such as cold cuts that contain sugar and preservatives, any fried and/or breaded meat and poultry
Poultry		
Chicken breast, turkey breast, Cornish hens	Chicken thighs/legs, turkey thighs/legs, duck, all chicken and turkey sausages (without breadings, added sugar, or fillers)	Processed meats such as cold cuts that contain sugar and preservatives, any fried and/or breaded meat and poultry
Pork		
Pork tenderloin, top loin chop, top loin roast	Pork chops, bacon (without added sugar), ham (without added sugar), ribs, ground pork, picnic pork, all pork sausages (Italian sausages, chorizo, etc., without breadings, added sugar, or fillers)	Processed meats such as cold cuts that contain sugar and preservatives, any fried and/or breaded meat and poultry
Dairy		
Egg whites, low-fat unflavored cottage cheese, low-fat unflavored Greek yogurt	Whole eggs, full-fat cottage cheese, full-fat unflavored Greek yogurt	Flavored, sweetened, or fruit-added cottage cheese or Greek yogurt

Fish and seafood		
Bass, bluefish, catfish, cod, flounder, grouper, haddock, halibut, mahi mahi, monkfish, mullet, orange roughy, perch, pike, pollock, snapper, swordfish, trout, tuna	Anchovies, butterfish, carp, Chilean sea bass, herring, mackerel, pompano, sablefish, salmon, sardines (in olive oil is best), shad, smelt, whitefish, eel, squid, oysters	Farm-raised fish, fried and/or breaded fish
Shellfish		
Clams, conch, crab, lobster, mussels, scallops, shrimp		

Super Carbs	
Choose lots of slow-digesting unrefined starches, such as:	**Avoid processed carbs, such as:**
Sweet potatoes, yams, potato varieties Gluten-free slow-cooking oats and oatmeal (Irish oatmeal, steel-cut oatmeal) Beets, peas, carrots Starchy squashes (acorn, butternut, calabaza) Legumes (kidney beans, black beans, black-eyed peas, lima beans, red beans, chickpeas, pinto beans, butter beans, navy beans, lentils) Wild rice, brown rice, black rice, white rice (note: rice should be steamed or boiled, not fried) Quinoa Healthier refined carbohydrates including healthy pastas (black bean pasta, chickpea pasta, brown rice pasta, whole-wheat pasta [for those who tolerate gluten]); acceptable breads (Ezekiel brand breads, millet, rice, sprouted grain sourdough); acceptable wraps (Ezekiel or gluten-free: rice flour, sprouted grain, cassava flour) Corn (use only locally farmed, and limit intake)	Refined sugar, high-fructose corn syrup, all white pastas, all white bread (except sprouted grain sourdough), packaged breakfast cereal, packaged granola and granola bars, all deep-fried foods (French fries, etc.), potato chips Excessive alcohol (beer, wine, liquor)

Fruits	
Choose lots of fresh fruits, including:	**Avoid fruit products, such as:**
Apples, apricots, bananas, blackberries, blueberries, cantaloupe, cherries, clementines, cranberries, grapes, grapefruit, kiwifruit, mango, nectarines, oranges, papaya, pears, pineapple, plums, raspberries, strawberries, tangerines, watermelon	Fruit juices, dried fruit, bottled fruit smoothies, fruit-flavored yogurts, frozen fruits with sugar added, canned fruits with sugar added and prepackaged fruit cups

Vegetables	
Choose lots of non-starchy vegetables, including:	**Choose limited unhealthier veggies, such as:**
Artichokes, arugula, asparagus, broccoli, Brussels sprouts, cabbage (all varieties), cauliflower, celery, collard greens, cucumber, eggplant, green beans, kale, kimchi (marinated cabbage), leeks, lettuces and greens (all varieties—think romaine, packaged spring mix, etc.), mushrooms, onions, parsnips, peppers, pickles, radishes, sauerkraut (raw, unfermented), sea vegetables (seaweed, kelp, sea lettuce, etc.), spinach, squashes (non-starchy varieties such as spaghetti, yellow, summer, Hubbard, kabocha, pumpkin, zucchini), Swiss chard, tomatoes, turnips	Deep-fried vegetables, any processed vegetables, veggie chips, frozen vegetables with sauces, commercial vegetable juices

Fats	
Choose limited quantities of friendly fats from sources like:	**Avoid processed fats and trans fats, including:**
Avocado, coconut meat or flakes, olives, raw cheese, grass-fed butter, ghee, tallow, lard, duck fat	Canola oil; corn oil; cottonseed oil; peanut butter that contains sugar, added oils, and other additives; safflower oil; soybean oil; sunflower oil
Oils	
Olive oil, coconut oil, avocado oil, cold-pressed grapeseed oil, cold-pressed macadamia nut oil, cold-pressed hemp oil	
Nuts	
Almonds, Brazil nuts (limit to 3 or 4 per day), cashews, macadamia nuts, pecans, pistachios, walnuts	
Seeds	
Chia seeds, flaxseeds, hemp seeds, pumpkin seeds, sunflower seeds	
Nut Butters and Seed Butters*	
Almond butter (natural and unsweetened), cashew butter (natural and unsweetened), coconut butter, peanut butter (natural and unsweetened), sunflower seed butter (natural and unsweetened), walnut butter (natural and unsweetened)	
*Raw, freshly ground nut and seed butters are preferable, because they contain no additives or trans fats.	

CHAPTER 4
THE POWER OF LATE-NIGHT SNACKS

Now we come to the part of the plan I know you've been waiting for: your pre-bedtime, fat-burning snacks. Almost every other diet plan would tell you that after dinner, the kitchen is closed until the next day. Well, not this plan. The no-snacks rule is one you should *definitely* break if you want to bust cravings and keep burning fat overnight.

Before we continue, let me clarify something: this means neither that you should binge eat at night nor that you have a license to eat whatever you want. What it does mean is that when the right foods are chosen in the right amounts, eating at night will not inherently lead to fat gain for most people. In fact, choosing certain foods can positively affect body composition and fat loss.

Before delving into some of the best food choices and recipes for the ultimate pre-bedtime meal, I'd like to share some helpful tips that may be useful in guiding your late-night eating habits.

FOUR KEYS TO EATING BEFORE BEDTIME FOR FASTER FAT LOSS

1. Focus on protein, particularly sources that are slow-digesting.

Protein should be the centerpiece of your pre-bedtime meal. As I mentioned in the last chapter, protein plays a tremendous role in improving body composition, promoting overall health, and supporting a healthy metabolism. What's more, high-protein meals boost satiety, which means that protein-dense foods are much more likely to make you feel full and satisfied—a real plus when those late-night hunger pangs hit.

Scientists have established that consuming at least 20 grams of protein stimulates muscle protein synthesis for two to five hours after eating a meal. However, recent research also shows that protein synthesis drops to unexpectedly low levels during sleep, even if you eat ample protein during and after evening exercise. This has led researchers to speculate that this process may fall off during sleep if you don't eat protein prior to bedtime.

You can counter this problem by eating 20 grams of slow-digesting protein prior to sleep. That's the amount found in three eggs, ¾ cup of cottage cheese, a cup of Greek yogurt, *or* a scoop of protein powder. This amount has been shown to significantly increase muscle building at night and improve overnight recovery from exercise.

One of the best nighttime proteins is casein, a slow-digesting protein that is a constituent of milk, cottage cheese, and many protein powders. It delivers amino acids into your system more slowly and for longer periods of time.

Supplementing with casein prior to bedtime has been shown to stimulate overnight muscle growth in older men, who are prone to muscle loss, according to a study from the *Journal of Nutrition*. Many other studies of casein taken prior to bedtime have shown similar results, especially in people who work out with weights.

2. Choose Portion Volumizing foods.

It's tough going to bed on an empty stomach. And it's not rocket science that when you feel full and satisfied, you no longer want to eat. With that in mind, it's important to select Portion Volumizing foods as part of your late-night meal. Nearly all non-starchy vegetables and many fruits count as Portion Volumizing foods. In the next section, I'll provide several examples of the best Portion Volumizing foods for bedtime.

3. Include late-night Super Carbs.

We've talked about why you need Super Carbs at dinner—to reduce fat-storing cortisol, support thyroid hormone production, and improve sleep—but what about your late-night meal? Should you include Super Carbs then?

The answer is yes—especially when the Super Carbs are combined with protein and friendly fats, in order to slow digestion, regulate blood sugar, and promote satiety.

As I mentioned earlier, Super Carbs promote the release of serotonin, a sleep-inducing neurotransmitter, and along those lines, research also suggests that consuming Super Carbs improves sleep quality, helps you fall asleep faster, and stabilizes morning blood sugar levels.

4. Add a few friendly fats.

Friendly fats—like those found in avocados, nuts, certain oils, and fatty fish—are also good additions to your pre-bedtime meal. On one hand, fats can help slow the rate of gastric emptying, and when combined with carbohydrates, fat may help reduce the glycemic response of the meal (that is, how quickly carbohydrates appear in the bloodstream).

In general, healthy fats can also help increase feelings of fullness and satisfaction because they regulate appetite through a number of mechanisms, including the release of appetite hormones. What's more, combining fat with fiber has been shown to further increase the satiating potential of fat. The satiating power of fats is often one explanation offered to describe why some weight loss trials have shown that low-carbohydrate (and higher-fat) diets tend to lead to greater weight loss than low-fat diets.

THE TOP 12 PRE-BEDTIME FAT-BURNING FOODS

In general, many of the choices in the Portion Volumization Food Lists (pages 40–42) are suitable for any time, including before bed. That said, there are certain foods that are especially beneficial as bedtime snacks because they keep burning fat even as you sleep. These 12 are my go-to pre-bedtime choices. (And you'll also find recipes for delicious bedtime snacks on pages 187–198.)

1 and 2. Greek Yogurt and Cottage Cheese

Complete milk proteins from dairy are composed of 20 percent whey protein, which is rapidly digested, and 80 percent casein, which is digested much more slowly. For this reason alone, protein-dense dairy foods like Greek yogurt and cottage cheese are excellent choices for a pre-bedtime meal. What's more, both of these foods are considered Portion Volumizing foods and help fill you up.

Greek yogurt contains more than double the protein of regular yogurt and only about one-third the amount of sugar. What's more, authentic strained Greek yogurt is rich in multiple sources of probiotics, which are hugely beneficial for your gut flora (also known as your gut microbiome, or the inner bacterial ecosystem that helps control your weight, combat infections, and more). Research indicates that the gut flora of obese folks differs significantly from that of thin people. Along these lines, recent research published in the *British Journal of Nutrition* suggests that certain probiotics from the *Lactobacillus* genus of bacteria, which are prominent in Greek yogurt, may help you lose weight and keep it off.

When choosing a Greek yogurt, opt for plain unsweetened versions. Flavored varieties can have over three times as much sugar. Instead, add some berries to your plain yogurt; they will provide a nutrient-dense source of fiber, vitamins, and antioxidant phytochemicals.

Cottage cheese offers many of the same benefits as Greek yogurt. Cottage cheese packs a whopping 28 grams of protein per single cup, and it is also a good source of calcium, riboflavin, vitamin B12, selenium, and phosphorus. Cottage cheese is rich in casein protein.

One cup of cottage cheese also packs a healthy punch of branched-chain amino acids (BCAAs), including over 2.5 grams of leucine, which is essential for fat burning and is considered to be the "anabolic trigger" for muscle recovery and growth following exercise. BCAAs are crucial to exercise performance and maintenance of blood sugar levels.

While dairy seems to have gained a negative reputation in certain circles, a number of studies have demonstrated that dairy consumption helps promote body-firming muscle and burn fat.

If eating dairy foods causes mild intestinal discomfort, gradually increase your consumption of these foods or try supplementing with digestive enzymes. Although most supplemental enzymes tend to supply only the lactase enzyme—which is necessary for the proper breakdown of lactose, the sugar found in milk—it's a better idea to consider a full-spectrum product that also includes proteolytic enzymes to help with the digestion of the proteins, which may be the culprits in digestive discomfort.

Also, consider using a milk-based protein supplement that includes casein and/or milk protein concentrate.

SHOULD I GO ORGANIC?

If you can, I recommend that you choose organic sources of Greek yogurt, cottage cheese, and other forms of dairy. Organic dairy has a significantly different fatty acid profile when compared to conventional dairy. Specifically, studies comparing organic to conventional have reported that organic dairy contains:

- 25 percent fewer omega-6 fatty acids, which promote inflammation.
- 62 percent more omega-3 fatty acids, which fight inflammation.
- a 2.5 times lower omega-6 to omega-3 fatty acid ratio, which is much closer to optimal.
- 32 percent more EPA and 19 percent more DHA, which are two omega-3 fatty acids crucial for nervous system function, cardiovascular health, pain management, hormonal regulation, body composition, feelings of well-being, and more.
- 18 percent more conjugated linoleic acid (CLA), which has been shown to reduce body fat, increase lean body mass, and improve body composition.

3. Eggs

Eggs are one of the highest-quality whole food proteins you can get. Egg protein is slow-digesting—which makes it perfect for a late-night snack. Eggs also contain melatonin, a hormone that plays an important role in our circadian rhythm and is needed to help us not only fall asleep but stay asleep.

Choose eggs from pasture-raised hens, if possible. They are lower in cholesterol and higher in omega-3 fats and various vitamins.

4. Lean Animal Proteins

Proteins such as beef, poultry, and fish are beneficial late-night snacks, especially if you're trying to gain or preserve muscle while losing weight. Protein at night helps your muscles recover from workouts (the recovery period is when new muscle tissue is formed) and helps keep your metabolism running efficiently. You will not be tempted to raid the fridge, either, when you make protein a part of your late-night snack. Numerous studies show that snacks of protein and veggies promote feelings of fullness.

5. Cruciferous Vegetables

Eating more cruciferous vegetables is a healthy habit at any time during the day. The reason they also make a great late-night snack is that these veggies contain lots of fiber, which helps you feel full and satisfied overnight. Choose from the following:

- Arugula
- Bok choy
- Broccoli
- Brussels sprouts
- Cabbage
- Cauliflower
- Collard greens
- Kale
- Radishes
- Rutabaga
- Swiss chard
- Turnips
- Watercress

These veggies contain a powerful plant compound called sulforaphane, which can prevent DNA damage and cancer spread, help fight pathogens, and boost liver detox enzymes (and that's just a short list!). What's more, sulforaphane ramps up the activity of a key fat-burning enzyme called hormone-sensitive lipase (HSL). HSL plays an important role in the breakdown of fats for fuel. Sulforaphane has also been shown in research to both inhibit the body's ability to create new fat cells (adipogenesis) as well as suppress the body's ability to store fat (lipogenesis). Burn more fat and store less—sounds like a winner!

Cruciferous vegetables have other natural chemicals that detoxify bad estrogens (absorbed from the environment) and reduce the risk of breast cancer. Women who consume a lot of cruciferous vegetables as part of their meals have as much as a 40 percent lower risk of breast cancer than those who eat few, if any, of these health-protective veggies.

6. Dark Leafy Greens

Kale, mustard greens, and spinach are rich in calcium, which helps your body use tryptophan to build sleep-inducing melatonin. According to the USDA National Nutrient Database, 2 cups of chopped kale contains about 200 milligrams of calcium, which is the same amount found in a 4-ounce container of plain low-fat yogurt.

Dark leafy greens are also loaded with vitamins, minerals, phytonutrients, and antioxidants, such as the carotenoids lutein, zeaxanthin, neoxanthin, and violaxanthin. The phytonutrients and antioxidants in these foods work hard to scavenge free radicals and fight chronic inflammation.

Along these lines, the research is becoming abundantly clear that inflammation plays an important role in obesity, and vice versa. Thus, including anti-inflammatory foods like spinach in your nutrition arsenal is important for optimizing overall health and body weight.

7. Blueberries and Other Berries

Blueberries, raspberries, blackberries, strawberries, and cranberries are packed with antioxidants and add some fun color to your meals. Antioxidant-rich berries can help reduce your overall stress, which can help you get better rest. Berries are also a great source of fiber and vitamin C. They're rich in phytonutrients that protect cells, preventing damage and reducing the risk of cancer, namely colon, esophageal, oral, and skin cancers.

Blueberries are reported to be particularly good for fat burning. Researchers from Texas Woman's University demonstrated that the polyphenols in blueberries might play a significant role in reducing body fat. Specifically, the researchers found that these compounds block the formation of fat cells.

Plus, researchers from New Zealand found that eating blueberries may also accelerate muscle recovery when combined with exercise. Specifically, folks who consumed a blueberry smoothie before and after exercise experienced reduced muscle soreness and accelerated recovery of strength, which translates to more frequent exercise and improved performance. That also adds up to helping prevent the loss of calorie-burning muscle when dieting. Simply put, muscle loss contributes to decreased metabolism, looking "skinny fat," and rapid rebound weight gain when resuming a "normal" eating routine after a diet—all things you don't want.

Anthocyanins, the colorful antioxidant pigments that give blueberries and other berries their rich color, have been shown to have a unique effect on fat cells, and this has led researchers to state that they may play an intricate role in improving metabolic health. As a matter of fact, researchers investigating the effects of anthocyanins on fat cells (adipocytes) concluded, "Anthocyanins have a significant potency of anti-obesity and ameliorate adipocyte function" and they also have "important implications for preventing metabolic syndrome." Their study was published in the *Journal of Agricultural and Food Chemistry* in 2008.

8. Cherries

Like berries, cherries are rich in antioxidants and phytochemicals. An important late-night benefit of cherries is that they may help promote sleep because they contain melatonin. A review of the health benefits of cherries published in *Nutrients* in 2018 reported that melatonin is found in both sweet and tart cherries; its concentration is slightly higher in sweet cherries.

The influence of cherries on sleep was documented in a study conducted by a group of Spanish researchers. Middle-aged and elderly volunteers consumed about 1 cup of cherries (a variety of different types of cherries were consumed across the group) twice daily at lunch and dinner for three days. The researchers found that cherry consumption increased sleep time significantly and reduced the number of awakenings. This study was published in the *Journals of Gerontology* in 2010.

9. Kiwifruit

Kiwifruit is another serotonin-boosting fruit that has been shown to have beneficial effects on sleep. In a study published in the *Asia Pacific Journal of Clinical Nutrition*, researchers from Taiwan found that middle-aged adults who consumed two kiwifruits one hour before bedtime every night for four weeks experienced significantly improved sleep—both total sleep time as well as sleep efficiency. The researchers concluded, "Kiwifruit consumption may improve sleep onset, duration, and efficiency in adults with self-reported sleep disturbances."

Kiwifruit is low in calories and high in water content, making it a great Portion Volumizing food and a solid option for your pre-bedtime meal. It is also a good source of fiber, particularly because it provides what's referred to as prebiotic fiber. Prebiotics are "food" for probiotics, helping them grow and thus stimulating more healthy bacteria in the gut. Both prebiotic- and probiotic-containing foods are supported with years of sound science, showing that they can help manage obesity, diabetes, and other illnesses.

With this in mind, taking steps to improve the balance of healthy gut bacteria—which includes providing important support nutrients like the prebiotic fiber found in kiwifruit—has serious implications for reducing body fat and optimizing weight management.

10. Grapefruit

Grapefruit is a cortisol fighter due to its high content of vitamin C, which lessens the effect of this hormone in the body. As I explained earlier, cortisol is one of the body's primary stress hormones. When elevated at night, it can interfere with sleep, making grapefruit a helpful late-night snack.

Grapefruits are a good source of fiber, which helps slow gastric emptying and increase feelings of fullness, making them a great choice to keep those late-night hunger pangs at bay. Grapefruits also have a very high water content (around 91 percent), and consequently they are considered a Portion Volumizing, hunger-controlling food.

In a study published in the *Journal of Medicinal Food*, researchers from the Scripps Clinic in California found that overweight folks consuming fresh grapefruit three times daily before meals lost *five times* more weight than the placebo group (which ate no grapefruit) over the course of 12 weeks. Not only that, but the researchers also found that the addition of grapefruit significantly improved insulin sensitivity, which is intimately tied to carbohydrate metabolism and weight management.

Grapefruit has one more trick up its sleeve: naringin, which is a potent antioxidant that helps protect cells from free radicals. Free radicals lead to oxidative stress, which is associated with aging, reduced carbohydrate tolerance, and obesity.

In the body, naringin is broken down into naringenin, a compound that has been shown to activate an important enzyme called AMPK, which drives carbs into muscles to be used for energy (instead of being stored as fat).

If that's not enough, naringenin has also been shown to reduce a process called adipogenesis—a fancy name for the creation of new fat cells—as well as increase fat burning.

11. Avocados

Although avocados are delicious any time of the day, they contain high levels of potassium and magnesium, natural muscle relaxers that calm your body and get it ready for sleep.

In general, avocados are nutrient-dense fruits, containing upwards of 20 essential nutrients that are crucial to optimizing your health and stoking your fat-burning furnace, including fiber, vitamin K, folate, vitamin B6, vitamin C, vitamin E, pantothenic acid, potassium, riboflavin, and niacin. Avocados are loaded with monounsaturated fatty acids (MUFAs), including oleic acid, which seems to have a potent impact on appetite regulation.

Researchers from the University of California, Irvine, found that oleic acid stimulates the production of a compound called oleoylethanolamide (OEA) by the cells of the small intestine. OEA helps suppress appetite by activating specific sites in the brain that help curb hunger. Previously, this group of researchers found that increasing OEA levels reduces appetite, increases weight loss, and improves various metabolic parameters. Their report appeared in the journal *Cellular and Molecular Life Sciences* in 2005.

In a study published in *Nutrition Journal* in 2013, researchers examined the dietary habits of over 17,000 men and women, and they found that folks who regularly consumed avocados were more likely to have a lower body weight, body mass index (BMI), and waist circumference.

12. Mixed Nuts

Nuts are a source of two important sleep-inducing nutrients: melatonin and magnesium. Plus, nuts are filling—perfect for fighting nighttime food cravings. As you already know, protein, fiber, and healthy fats like those found in nuts signal powerful satiety hormones. Researchers also believe that the sensory characteristics of nuts, specifically the fact that they're crunchy, also have satiety value. That is, the mechanical aspect of chewing crunchy nuts generates a satiety signal.

These little powerhouses are rich in MUFAs, which are known for their heart-healthy benefits. Just like avocados, nuts are rich in a specific MUFA called oleic acid. As a result, one of the many potential benefits of consuming nuts is an improvement in appetite regulation.

Although predominantly a fat-dense food, nuts also contain a healthy dose of fiber and some protein, and they are also a rich source of essential nutrients (such as minerals and fat-soluble vitamins) and phytonutrients.

Overall, a collection of evidence suggests that people who regularly consume nuts have a lower BMI than those who do not. Regular nut consumption has been shown to boost metabolism by as much as 11 percent and increase fat burning by up to 50 percent.

Because of their diverse nutrient profiles, consider trying a variety of nuts for your late-night snack, including:

- Almonds
- Brazil nuts
- Cashews
- Pecans
- Pistachios
- Walnuts

STRUCTURING YOUR LATE-NIGHT FAT-BURNING SNACKS

Using the foods listed above, there are several food combinations that will ignite fat burning while you sleep, providing your body with a steady stream of fuel during the night. Here are some combinations that will help structure your late-night snack:

- Protein + berries + fat: Greek yogurt, blueberries, and mixed nuts; or cottage cheese, kiwifruit, and mixed nuts
  OR
- Protein + non-starchy vegetable + fat: hard-boiled egg, cruciferous vegetable, and slice of avocado; or tuna, spinach, and slice of avocado
  OR
- One of my late-night snack recipes on pages 187–198.

So now that you have a good idea what the best foods are to enjoy before turning in for the night, let's move on to some other strategies that ensure success on the Always Eat After 7 PM plan.

CHAPTER 5
CHEAT YOUR WAY THIN

Not only do you get to eat after 7 PM on this plan, but you also have a license to cheat if you want to. I'm talking about treating yourself to pizza and ice cream or your other favorite indulgent foods (for me, it's my mom's famous chocolate chip cookies or my grandma's mac 'n' cheese). That's right—after you complete the 14-day Acceleration Phase, each week you are encouraged to enjoy your favorite foods.

How's that for breaking the rules? And best of all, you will still burn fat, achieve a flatter belly, and drop pounds, even if you periodically cheat, or "overfeed," as it's technically called.

I know you're wondering, "How in the world can I cheat and still get to my ideal weight?" Well, it all has to do with a weight control hormone called leptin.

LEPTIN: THE HORMONE THAT LETS YOU CHEAT

The major player in fat burning and fat storing is the hormone leptin. Its name is derived from the Greek word *leptos*, meaning "thin," and it's without a doubt the most important hormone you've probably never heard of.

While other hormones play a role in regulating fat metabolism, leptin is the master hormone, regulating all other collateral hormones involved in fat metabolism (such as insulin, thyroid hormone, adiponectin, cortisol, estrogen, progesterone, and testosterone).

Sometimes called "the fullness hormone," leptin is one of the two primary hunger hormones, the other being ghrelin. Released primarily in the stomach, ghrelin increases your appetite and plays a role in regulating your body weight. Normally, ghrelin rises dramatically before you eat; this signals hunger. It then goes down for about three hours after your meal.

Produced in your fat cells, leptin is the bigger player of the two. In fact, some researchers believe that leptin regulates ghrelin. Leptin sends signals to your brain to tip you off that you can stop eating, that you're full. At the same time, leptin sends signals to your brain to "turn on" your metabolism and thus start converting food to energy.

As leptin levels rise, you experience a diminished appetite; as leptin levels decrease, the result is a feeling of hunger. Likewise, rising leptin levels will increase your rate of metabolism, while falling levels will slow your metabolism.

In short, leptin regulates both your appetite and your metabolism. When leptin levels are in a normal range, your brain gets the message that your food intake is adequate. Your metabolism stays in gear, and your body is primed to burn fat.

Leptin levels are regulated by two factors. The first is the amount of body fat you carry. All else being equal, people with more body fat have higher leptin levels than those with less body fat. The second mediator of leptin levels is your calorie intake. Unfortunately, when you diet to lose fat and cut calories, your body responds accordingly by lowering your leptin levels (levels plummet by 50 percent or more after only one week on a calorie-restricted diet). Because leptin is the number-one fat-burning powerhouse, metabolism then slows down. This slowdown thwarts weight loss. (*Hello,* belly fat.)

Then your thyroid hormones, which are extremely important to metabolism, respond by taking a nosedive, and the fat-storing stress hormone cortisol skyrockets measurably.

And if that wasn't bad enough, ghrelin and two other appetite-stimulating hormones, neuropeptide Y and anandamide, all hop on board to make your life even more miserable. If all that sounds too technical, just remember that when leptin drops, you get seriously hungry.

There are other hormonal problems related to leptin: insulin resistance and leptin resistance. If you're in the habit of eating a lot of sugar and sugary junk foods, you might develop insulin resistance, meaning your cells can no longer accept glucose for energy. Insulin then just hangs around in the blood, wreaking all kinds of havoc on cells and tissues. High insulin levels block leptin signals to the brain, and leptin resistance ensues. If you develop leptin resistance, your body's ability to "hear" that it is full and should stop eating gets blocked and your metabolism slows down. There are a number of ways through which we become leptin resistant—poor diet, depression, stress, dehydration, and a sedentary lifestyle. A lack of sleep is another factor in leptin resistance. Leptin resistance is believed to be the leading driver of fat gain in humans.

HOW TO BOOST LEPTIN PRODUCTION AND BURN MORE FAT

Wouldn't it be wonderful if you could banish hungry feelings, balance your hormones, and create a metabolism geared for fat burning while dieting? It would seemingly solve all your problems. In order to do this, you'd have to somehow maintain your leptin levels.

So, how about "supplementing" with leptin?

Not so fast. Leptin is a protein-based hormone. If you took it orally, it would simply be digested. So that rules out a leptin supplement.

What about leptin injections? Well, they do exist, and they work mainly by reversing the metabolic adaptations to dieting and "starvation" even while a person continues to restrict calories.

But there's a big problem here too. Daily leptin injections are super pricey, costing thousands of bucks a week. Not to mention, the treatment requires giving yourself an injection daily. So we can pretty much rule out supplemental leptin as a solution.

The good news—no, the great news—is that you can manipulate your leptin production naturally. In fact, we'll swap the injections and mounds of cash for a more budget-friendly (and tastier) option: more calories and more carbs.

A LICENSE FOR (STRATEGIC) CHEATING

There is a direct, linear relationship between leptin levels and the amount of food you eat. As I mentioned, leptin levels decrease by about 50 percent after only one week of dieting. Fat loss slows down, and you feel bad psychologically. But because the relationship is linear, the opposite is also true: an increase in calorie intake results in an increase in leptin levels. And fortunately, it doesn't take *nearly* as long for leptin to bump back up with a substantial increase in caloric intake—only about 12 to 24 hours. That's right. It takes only one day of overfeeding or "cheating" to bring levels back up to baseline.

So the solution to our leptin dilemma is this: every seventh day, enjoy one "cheat day" or "cheat meal" that is rich in both carbohydrates and fats. This alternation of foods increases your sensitivity to leptin, and your fat burning will be more sustained. Cheat meals also provide a much-needed mental break from dieting. Essentially, the sanctioned cheat days on Always Eat After 7 PM are everything "typical" dieting isn't. And the fact that the program uses pizza and other cheat foods to strip away fat faster certainly hasn't brought in any complaints!

Don't worry, either. You won't stall your progress. Each week, you start fresh with baseline levels of leptin and a hormonal environment primed for burning fat. And forget about psychological feelings like guilt, failure, anxiety, or discouragement. Best of all, you need not feel guilty when you cheat. Instead, you can feel good about choosing to cheat—because you know that when you do, you're accelerating your progress.

CHEAT DAY GUIDELINES

1. Employ a cheat day or cheat meal only after you've completed the 14 days of the Acceleration Phase.
2. Exercisers are allowed one cheat day per week and non-exercisers are allowed one cheat meal per week with a dessert. You can cheat any day of the week as long as you have completed six clean-eating days in a row.
3. Avoid alcohol during the Acceleration Phase. During the other two phases, you may add it, but do it in moderation (1 to 2 drinks) with your cheat meal.

Sidestep excess beer, and try to stick with red wine or clear liquors (vodka, tequila, rum, or gin).

4. Don't binge or stuff yourself while eating your cheat meal or when having a cheat day.
5. Drink extra water before, during, and after your cheat meals. Staying well hydrated helps digestion, prevents overeating, and stimulates glycogen replenishment from the extra carb intake.
6. Perform some type of low-intensity cardio or 15-minute high-intensity interval training (HIIT) workout an hour or two before your cheat meals to help minimize fat storage and enhance absorption of nutrients.

There are other natural ways to boost leptin, and these involve specific food choices to combat leptin resistance.

FOODS THAT FIGHT LEPTIN RESISTANCE

Recent scientific literature published in *Molecular Nutrition & Food Research* tells us that there are potentially valuable nutrients and food components in what we eat that can reverse leptin resistance. These nutrients just happen to be very prevalent in Always Eat After 7 PM. This means that the program itself, day in and day out, is fueling your body with food that makes your cells more sensitive to leptin and thus more prone to burning fat. These nutrients and food components include:

Resveratrol. Found in red grapes, wine, blueberries, and cranberries, resveratrol is an antioxidant that helps restore leptin in the body and assists in breaking down fat.

Taurine. This is an essential amino acid found in all dairy products, meat, poultry, and fish. In studies, taurine has been shown to battle leptin resistance.

Vitamin A. Foods such as sweet potatoes, carrots, squash, fish, and dairy products are excellent sources of vitamin A. Sufficient amounts of this vitamin ensure high leptin concentrations in the body.

Vitamin D. Available from sunlight and found in mushrooms and fortified dairy products, vitamin D is an extremely

In the recipe section of this book, you'll find a selection of delicious Cheat Day Treats (pages 205–210)—which are healthier versions of typical breakfast and snack foods. Choose these when you're looking for smarter choices, even when indulging!

important nutrient and is vital for the prevention of many diseases, from heart disease to cancer. A lack of vitamin D interferes with leptin, leading to an out-of-control appetite and cravings, and as a consequence, weight gain.

Pectin. One animal study (such as the one reported in 2015 in *Molecular Nutrition & Food Research*) has shown that pectin—a fiber in apples—may be effective in fighting leptin resistance. Adult rats were given pectin supplements for one month; the pectin decreased body fat and improved insulin and leptin resistance, overall contributing to better metabolic health. Whether the same holds true for humans, we'll see—stay tuned.

All of these leptin-stimulating foods and nutrients are allowed, and encouraged, on this plan. Because they can have a dramatically positive effect on leptin levels, incorporating more of these foods in your diet gives you a better chance of burning fat, including stubborn belly fat.

REVERSE CARBOHYDRATE TAPERING: KEEP YOUR LEPTIN LEVELS UP EVEN AFTER CHEAT DAY

A downside to cheating is that the bump in leptin doesn't last long. Leptin levels again decline once you return to the plan. That being the case, what can be done to combat falling leptin levels throughout the week?

Make sure you do not eliminate Super Carbs as you resume the plan after your cheat day. Of any nutrient, carbohydrates have the greatest net effect on leptin levels. After a cheat day, when leptin starts to decline, eat a few additional Super Carbs—like 10 to 20 grams—each day until your next cheat day. (Twenty grams of Super Carbs is equal to a few bites of rice or oatmeal or half of a medium baked potato.)

This introduction of a small amount of Super Carbs into your diet is called "reverse carbohydrate tapering." It keeps leptin levels from falling too fast.

The extra leptin is more beneficial if you also take steps to continually improve your body's sensitivity to this hormone. As mentioned previously, leptin resistance is extremely common if you've been overweight or obese for a long time or have habitually eaten lots of processed foods. Leptin resistance makes your body unresponsive to leptin, even at high levels. This is like having a car with a full tank of gas and a broken starter; it won't run as it should.

Fortunately, you can immediately begin repairing this situation as soon as today by eating the leptin-stimulating foods I listed on page 55.

Now before we launch into the plan, let's talk about key thought patterns and characteristics held by people who are in phenomenal shape—and how to adopt these patterns to create your own amazing transformation.

CHAPTER 6
SUCCESS BEGINS IN THE MIND (DON'T SKIP THIS CHAPTER!)

Are you ready to experience the life-changing, fat-burning, health-boosting results of Always Eat After 7 PM? I'm sure you are, and I'm excited for you! But before you're able to truly do that, we must cover some prerequisites to ensure your long-term success.

Up to now, we've focused on the science that explains why the diet works, because when things make sense logically, you're much more likely to get excited and actually start (because you believe it will work). You're also likely to stick with the program much longer than if you were blindly going through the motions without fully understanding how everything you are doing is contributing to your ultimate success.

Even more important to your success than addressing the why of the program, however, is taking time to prepare your mind for the journey that you're about to embark on. So, before we get into the how of the program, I want to share some principles to help get you in the mind-set to succeed. Simply put, as with everything worth pursuing and accomplishing, there will be plenty of challenges and obstacles and setbacks along the way. And if you're not mentally prepared and relentlessly tough from the neck up, you'll have a hard time achieving *anything* great in life, including long-term weight loss on this program.

The advice in this chapter is drawn from both my fitness and entrepreneurial background. It outlines the principles that helped me achieve my personal transformation and also the many lessons learned while building one of the largest nutritional supplement companies in the United States. Additionally, through my podcast *Born to Impact* (which you can find on iTunes), I've had the pleasure to sit down with many of the world's elite coaches, athletes, and business leaders, learning the secrets *they've* used to build a life worth remembering; I'll share some of their stories here as well.

I believe these to be the 10 most essential mind-set strategies relating to your success on this program, and even more, your life as a whole. Let's get started.

1. Believe you can, and lose the excuses.

Here's the deal: if you aren't *one thousand* percent sure that you are going to achieve your goals, somehow, some way, then you might as well quit right now. It may sound harsh, but it's the truth. As my good friend Ed Mylett teaches, before starting, you absolutely *must* make the commitment that there is no plan B. Ed is a super-successful entrepreneur who's become an author, speaker, philanthropist, and coach. He describes a mind-set that's critically important: you have to say that no matter what, you aren't going to stop moving toward the life you want to live, and that your will to win will *never* be for sale.

If you don't do this, you're all but guaranteed to sell out on your will to win at some point—probably sooner rather than later. An obstacle comes, results don't occur as quickly or as easily as you had anticipated, or you have a physical or emotional setback—a "life interruption," as recovery coach Tim Storey calls it—and next thing you know, you're coming up with reason after reason why abandoning your goals is justified.

You know what those reasons are called? Excuses.

There is no person who inspired me to drop any and all excuses more than my friend Nick Santonastasso, who's a competitive bodybuilder and an international motivational speaker.

At birth, Nick was brought into this world with an extremely rare genetic condition that caused three out of four of his limbs to never develop. He has no legs and only one arm, and attached to that arm is an underdeveloped hand with one finger. And yes, you read that last paragraph right: he is a competitive bodybuilder.

You see, Nick had *every* reason to feel sorry for himself, to play the "bad genetics" card (which in his case would have been completely justified), to live a life of mediocrity, to never pursue anything great in life. But today, he thrives. He's an athlete. He speaks all over the world, inspiring crowds of thousands. If you want to be inspired to drop every excuse for the rest of your life and achieve greatness no matter what you're up against, check out episode 5 of the *Born to Impact* podcast, "No Legs, One Arm, ZERO Limits." Your life will never be the same.

Bottom line: you may be starting with more obstacles in front of you than someone else is, but you probably aren't up against anything close to the magnitude of Nick's obstacles. If he's making it happen, so can you. But you have to believe it. Deep down in your core, you have to know you will achieve your goals and dreams, and there is no plan B. It may be a little bit harder than you thought, it may take a little bit longer than you'd like, but if you keep going, you know (and you should know) that you will get there.

2. Excommunicate negative people from your life.

Once you've laid the foundation—you completely believe in yourself and have made up your mind that quitting is not an option—your next step is to get rid of people who don't support that belief.

But what if they are close friends or family members? Listen, I'm not saying to completely drop people who have been a significant part of much of your life, but I am saying to severely limit your contact with them when it comes to anything and everything related to your dreams, goals, and ambitions.

Simply put, people who don't support you will *drain* you, and you have to protect your dreams, ambitions, and goals. My longtime friend Bedros Keuilian, who founded the ultra-successful fitness franchise Fit Body Boot Camp, calls these people crabs: people with a negative, scarcity mind-set who will constantly try to drag you back down to their level. The true issue at hand is that they don't believe in themselves.

Maybe you have a friend who isn't overly negative about *you*, per se, but instead is exceptionally negative about *everything*. Sour grapes every time you talk to them. Nothing good ever happens to them. Complaint after complaint after complaint. Is that person helping you in any way? No. And the reality is that you aren't going to bring that person up; they are only going to bring you down.

My point is this: you have to protect your future self and guard your dreams from negative people who will steal your zeal, deflate your ambition, and take the wind out of the sails of your drive to succeed. Your dreams are too important. Don't open them up to anyone who is less than 100 percent on board with not only your pursuit of them but also your achievement of them.

3. Live in the present.

To quote the pastor, futurist, and designer Erwin McManus from his book *The Way of the Warrior*, "We will never know peace if we lose the present because we are trapped in the past and paralyzed by the future. This is in no small part why we live in a culture crippled by depression and anxiety. Depression is rooted in your past; anxiety is rooted in your future . . . The path to freedom from your past and freedom to your future is the connectedness that comes from living in the moment, fully present."

How incredibly true and relevant is this? So many people fail to achieve their goals and their dreams because they are riddled with self-doubt related to their past: who they *were*. And because of this past, they experience intense anxiety about the future, because they believe that who they were is who they will continue to be.

The past is the past; it's over, and there's nothing you can do to change it. The only thing you *do* have control over is the future, and the only moment that is relevant for creating the narrative that you desire for your future is the present moment.

Bottom line: stop living in the past and allowing your past experiences, past mistakes, and past failures to play a role in how you view your future. Beyond that, there's no point in worrying and experiencing anxiety about your future (anxiety that is anchored in your past) when the only moment you truly control is the now. Embrace the present, live in the moment, and make the choice to progress further toward the person you want to become, today.

For more on this topic and a ton more, listen to my whole conversation with Erwin McManus in episode 21 of *Born to Impact*, "Worry, Fear, & the True Path to Inner Peace."

4. Redefine who you are.

As my friend James Clear, entrepreneur author of the *New York Times* best-selling book *Atomic Habits*, states, "True behavior change is identity change."

Here's the thing: unless you do the deep work to change who you are, achieving a goal will be nothing more than a momentary change, instead of the lasting change that you desire. For example, if you focus on losing 20 pounds, you might, but how long will you actually keep those 20 pounds "lost"? Statistics show that less than 6 percent of people continue to keep the weight off.

Why does this happen? It happens because the change is outcome based, not identity based—and once you achieve the outcome of losing 20 pounds, you have no real motivation to continue making healthy choices. The goal is the motivator. You hit the goal. You are no longer motivated.

But what if the goal is not to lose 20 pounds but rather to become a healthy person? What if you ask yourself before making exercise and nutrition choices, "What would a healthy person do?" And then what if you take it a step further and say, "I am a healthy person. What would a healthy person like me choose?" Then you make that choice.

Before long, you'll have more than enough evidence—every positive choice you've made—to show that you are in fact a healthy person.

You see, when you focus on becoming the person you want to become, and *do the work* to change your identity so that you are that type of person, you will be much more successful with creating change that lasts. I can't tell you how much this helped me. Fact is, I was notorious for setting a goal, crushing it, and then falling back into old habits. Why? Because the goal was the motivator, and I didn't do the deep work.

Since then, I've taken huge steps to change my overall identity as it relates to my goals. If you want to dive deeper into this topic and successful goal achievement, check out episode 13 of *Born to Impact* with James Clear, "Why Goals Suck."

5. Start!

Nothing happens without action, period. You can buy the book, read the book, buy the supplements, and do your grocery shopping, but if you don't actually start putting one foot in front of the other on the actual execution of the game plan, you will never, ever achieve success.

As a business coach and life coach, I am amazed at the number of people who will spend top dollar on education and coaching but never actually do anything with it. Do you want to think about success, or do you actually want to experience it? The latter only comes with action.

And here's another phrase that you need to eliminate: "I'll start when . . ."

"I'll start when my kids start school again."

"I'll start when I get back from my vacation at the end of next month."

"I'll start when life calms down a bit."

"I'll start when I can afford to buy organic."

"I'll start when everything is perfect and the stars align and God audibly speaks to me, telling me to begin."

"I'll start when . . ." Stop! Change that immediately to "I'll start *today*." Then figure the rest out. Here's another great quote from my friend Ed Mylett: "Turn your 'one day' into 'day one.'" And start today. There will never be a perfect time, so stop waiting for it.

6. Develop a simple morning routine.

My friends Tim Ferriss (the author of *The 4-Hour Body*), Lewis Howes (the author of *The School of Greatness*), and Jim Kwik (a celebrity brain coach) are all huge proponents of morning routines. Why? Because often, as our morning goes, so the rest of our day follows. As Jim says, "Getting up and adhering to a success-driven morning routine creates positive momentum and vision for the rest of your day to also be successful."

Here are some of my favorite aspects of Jim's morning routine:

A. **Make the bed.** Making the bed is a success habit, and how you do anything is how you do everything. Even more, when you return to your bed in the evening, you're guaranteed to end your day with success.
B. **Take a premium probiotic to feed your gut, like BioTrust Pro-X10™.** Your gut is your second brain, and there is an incredible number of nerve cells in your gut, so make sure they are fed.
C. **Meditate and practice deep breathing for 10 to 15 minutes.** Breathing techniques oxygenate your body and meditation clears your mind as you enter the day. Jim recommends the Wim Hof method for breathing at www.wimhofmethod.com and the Headspace app for guided meditation.
D. **Move.** Two minutes of morning exercise is all that is needed to get your heart rate up and to significantly increase your level of alertness. Try jumping jacks, push-ups, and/or bodyweight squats for simplicity and efficacy.
E. **Journal with pen and paper.** The act of writing stimulates your brain to a much higher degree than typing, and nothing beats gratitude journaling to start off your day with positivity.
F. **Fuel your brain.** My favorite way to do this is with any of the drinks in my 3-Minute Fat-Burning Morning Ritual (explained in detail on pages 19–23), particularly BioTrust MetaboGreens 45X. Its antioxidants, energy, fiber, digestive enzymes, and super greens will make a huge difference in the way

you feel. For an even more pronounced boost in brain health and function, try BioTrust Brain Bright™, washed down with one of the beverages from the 3-Minute Fat-Burning Morning Ritual. (I'll cover the how and why of using supplements in chapter ten.)

7. Allow yourself bad moments, not bad days.

Ever had a bad morning that caused you to be miserable for the rest of the day? Or maybe a temporary diet mistake that caused you to write off the rest of the day and continue to make bad diet decision after bad diet decision? We all have. But author Levi Lusko tells readers in his book *I Declare War*, "No matter how much of the day has been spent, it's not too late to change course—not tomorrow, but right now."

Simply put, a bad morning doesn't have to turn into a bad day. A bad diet decision at lunch doesn't have to turn into a completely catastrophic evening of bingeing. No, that's self-sabotage at its best, and the fact is, you can change the course of the day at *any* moment—as Levi says, "not tomorrow, but right now."

Listen, we all have bad moments, but the key is not allowing a bad moment to negatively affect the entire day. Rein it in, get back in control, and begin moving forward again.

If you don't? That bad morning could turn into a string of bad days. That momentary 500-calorie diet slip-up could turn into tens of thousands of calories you weren't supposed to eat. And guess what? Now you've gained weight instead of moving toward your goals.

One doughnut isn't going to be the difference between losing weight one week and not, but a doughnut-turned-binge will be. Regain control. We all make mistakes. Don't let a single mistake turn into anything more than that. For more on this and so much more, tune in to episode 11 of *Born to Impact* with Levi Lusko, "Declaring War on Your Thoughts."

8. Recognize failure as a teacher, not a final destination.

As my longtime friend Lewis Howes notes, "Failure is feedback." Lewis is a former pro football player who's now an entrepreneur, athlete, author, and podcaster—yet he's had his share of setbacks and obstacles to overcome. Here's reality: no one gets it right the first time. We fail, and either we quit or we look at the feedback (why the failure occurred), course-correct, and try again. The latter is how any "successful" person actually achieves success.

If you make a mistake, if you screw up, if you don't achieve the desired outcome, analyze why it happened and how you can avoid the cause next time. For example, maybe you get swamped at work and wind up working late. When you finally leave, you're starving, and you head to the fast-food place on the other side of the parking lot and order some fries. Yes, you "failed" on adhering to your diet plan, but let's look at *why* this happened and figure out how it could have been prevented.

Cause: no healthy food or snack options were available at work, causing you to be overly hungry when finally leaving the office, and ultimately you made a poor food choice while you were hungry.

Solution: always have some healthy food or snack options in your purse, backpack, or desk.

You see, if you learn from the failure, you won't find yourself at the fast-food joint in the parking lot chowing down on fries ever again because you're overhungry. Instead, you'll satisfy your hunger with a smart snack choice and then enjoy your next scheduled healthy meal at home.

When things don't go as planned, don't get discouraged—get analytical. Figure out the cause, and plan to avoid it in the future. Failure is feedback; listen to it.

9. Own your results.

Your place in life is a direct reflection and culmination of your decisions, period. Maybe you faced some difficulties that certain other people did not, but you chose how to react to those difficulties—either to allow them to define your future or to adamantly find a way to overcome them. Another great quote from my friend Erwin McManus: "Even if it's not your fault, it's still your responsibility."

You see, when you blame someone or something else, you abdicate responsibility for your own life. But more important, not only do you abdicate responsibility, but you also abdicate your power. After all, if someone or something else is responsible for your situation, they are the only one who can fix it, and you become dependent on them to change it for you. Essentially, you become powerless.

As the ex–Navy SEAL Jocko Willink writes in his book *Extreme Ownership*, "Leaders must own everything in their world. There is no one else to blame."

Are you powerful or powerless? Are you the leader of your life? If you *aren't* powerless, and if you *are* indeed the leader of your life, then you must take responsibility for every failure or shortcoming, taking control to turn each of them around. Whatever the reason why you didn't achieve the desired outcome, take steps to fix it. Own it, fix it. It really is that simple; it has to be that simple.

10. Briefly celebrate success, then move on.

There's nothing worse you can do after hitting a goal than to ease off the gas. Keep moving.

My friend Tim Grover is known around the world for his work training three of the greatest basketball players of all time, Michael Jordan, Kobe Bryant, and Dwayne Wade. Tim teaches even these elite athletes that after they hit a milestone—it could be something as major as winning a world championship—they should say, "Done. Next."

Tim truly is the master of mental toughness, and his best-selling book *Relentless* really epitomizes everything this chapter is all about: being mentally prepared for every battle to ensure that in the end, you are successful. If you want to take your mental toughness to an entire new level, be sure to check out *Born to Impact* episode 9, "Becoming Mentally Unstoppable," where I talk with Tim Grover for more than two hours.

To close, am I saying that you can never celebrate or recognize an accomplishment? No, but make it brief, and then get right back to business.

THIS CHAPTER WILL EITHER MAKE OR BREAK ALL THE OTHERS

Honestly, you just read the most important chapter of the book. It's the prerequisite to achieving anything and everything with all the other information included from here on out. I recommend returning to this chapter from time to time and taking notes on what is resonating with you (perhaps as part of the morning journaling Jim Kwik recommends). When you've really internalized these mind-set principles, then it's time to get started.

PART II
BURN FAT IN THREE EASY PHASES

CHAPTER 7
THE ACCELERATION PHASE

Always Eat After 7 PM is a three-part plan that begins with a 14-day Acceleration Phase. As I mentioned before, you can think of this part of the program as a short sprint to get you started. I call this phase "Acceleration" because its focus is to activate your fastest weight loss in a healthy way with lots of nutrient-packed foods. Here's what this phase does for you:

- cuts back on calories and carbohydrates to quickly get your body to start burning fat for energy (this is sometimes called becoming "fat adapted")
- ramps up protein intake for more efficient fat burning and lean muscle preservation
- emphasizes high-fiber vegetables to keep you satisfied, fight cravings, and increase your digestive health
- fuels your motivation and desire to continue because of the rapid results you'll see on your scale

Get ready to drop up to one pound per day. That's what I've seen with some clients. Although everyone is different, expect to be impressed with your own results over the next 14 days.

During this phase, you get to eat a variety of protein choices and many different kinds of veggies. You'll be limiting your calories and carb intake a bit so that your body shifts quickly into fat-burning mode; this is the only phase in which you won't eat Super Carbs. You do get to enjoy berries, cherries, and dark chocolate, though, along with friendly fats, all of which supply energy and help you feel satisfied.

THE POWER OF RAPID FAT LOSS

For years, many weight loss experts have sermonized on the dangers of rapid weight loss diets. But a plan that delivers fast results *can* be healthy if designed correctly. What's more, though it sounds counterintuitive, research over the past few years suggests that the faster you lose weight, the longer you keep it off.

For example, in 2010 a study published in the *International Journal of Behavioral Medicine* showed that "slow and steady" weight loss doesn't necessarily win the race. For the study, researchers at the University of Florida analyzed data from 262 dieters who were enrolled in an obesity treatment trial. It included obese middle-aged women, with an average age of 59 and an average body mass index (BMI) of 36.8 (30 and above is considered obese).

The researchers divided the women into three groups based on diets that were designed to produce fast, moderate, or slow weight loss. Sixty-nine were in the "fast" group, 104 were in the "moderate" group, and 89 were in the "slow" group. At six months, the fast group had lost an average of about 30 pounds; the moderate group, 20; and the slow group, 11. After 18 months, the fast group had maintained their losses better than the other groups.

Rapid weight loss is also good for trimming belly fat, according to a 2003 Finnish study published in the *International Journal of Obesity*. Researchers found that a fast weight loss diet, followed for six weeks, shed visceral abdominal fat by 25 percent and abdominal subcutaneous fat by 16 percent. Visceral fat is the type that collects around our organs and raises the risk of hypertension, heart disease, and diabetes. Subcutaneous fat is just under the skin and is responsible for "spare tires" and "muffin tops."

Researchers say that one reason rapid weight loss diets lead to such positive results is the motivation factor. There's a definite psychological benefit—as well as a physical one—to losing weight in the early stages. You feel encouraged because you can see improvements in your appearance, in how your clothes fit, or in how light you feel.

So, with the way I've set things up, you'll experience two weeks of rapid progress. Not only will you see rapid results on the scale, but you'll observe a noticeable difference in how you look in the mirror.

The Acceleration Phase is also an important weight control tool. If your weight creeps up in the future for whatever reason, simply follow the Acceleration Phase for another 14 days to get the scale moving downward again. This is a great strategy for staying on track and maintaining a great body.

COUNTING MACROS FOR WEIGHT LOSS

In all three phases of Always Eat After 7 PM, you'll keep a close eye on your macronutrients (aka macros). Macronutrients are the three types of nutrients that provide you with most of your energy: carbohydrates, protein, and fat. (Micronutrients, on the other hand, are the types of nutrients that your body uses in smaller amounts—think vitamins and minerals.)

The idea behind macro dieting is pretty simple: instead of simply staying under a set calorie threshold, you focus on getting a certain ratio of macronutrients—protein, carbohydrates, and fat—to make sure you're getting enough for fat burning and overall well-being.

Always Eat After 7 PM sets specific macro targets for you in each phase of the plan. The meal plans offer specific suggestions that have the right balance of all three macros. But let's look at the math behind this so that you understand the process and can make up your own meals if you wish. The actual number of macros you need is calculated in three steps:

1. Establish your approximate calorie needs for a particular meal. Needs will vary for men and women and by phase of the diet. For now, let's use the example of a 500-calorie lunch.
2. Tally macro percentages to determine how many grams of protein, fat, and carbs to eat at each meal. This involves a little bit of math.

   Say the macro breakdown for lunch in your phase of the diet is 40 percent carbs, 40 percent protein, and 20 percent fat. This means that if your lunch is 500 calories, then about 200 calories would come from carbs, another 200 would come from protein, and the remaining 100 would come from fat.

   The math looks like this:

   Carbs: 40 percent of 500 calories = 500 × .4 = 200 calories from carbs
   Protein: 40 percent of 500 calories = 500 × .4 = 200 calories from protein
   Fat: 20 percent of 500 = 500 × .2 = 100 calories from fat
3. Figure out how many grams of each macro to aim for. This means you need to know how many calories are in a particular gram of that macro. Using the same numbers from the lunch example:

   Carbs: 200 calories ÷ 4 calories/gram = 50 grams of carbs
   Protein: 200 calories ÷ 4 calories/gram = 50 grams of protein
   Fat: 100 calories ÷ 9 calories/gram = 11 grams of fat

When you know roughly how many grams of each macro to aim for, you can plan your meals accordingly to reach those numbers and ensure that you're getting enough carbs, protein, and fat at each meal. Sure, you may not hit these exactly, but you'll be close.

And for those of you who hate math, remember that macros are already figured into the meal plans. You can also use apps such as My Macros+, MyFitnessPal, Carb Manager, or Cron-o-Meter to easily track your macros.

IMPORTANT DAILY MEAL PLAN GUIDELINES FOR THE ACCELERATION PHASE

1. Weeks 1 and 2 are specifically designed to be lower in calorie and carb intake

to get your body adapted to burning fat as a fuel source. You do not eat Super Carbs during the Acceleration Phase. This phase also kick-starts rapid weight loss, preparing your body for week 3 and beyond, in which you will introduce Portion Volumizing Super Carbs.

2. Week 1 is designed to phase you out of eating breakfast so you can employ intermittent fasting in week 2 and beyond with my recommended 3-Minute Fat-Burning Morning Ritual drinks for breakfast. Avoid all creamers and artificial sweeteners while fasting.
3. If you're a breakfast eater or you have to eat after you wake up, please select from the Breakfast Smart Snacks on pages 112–115.
4. The target calorie goals for the Acceleration Phase are 1,100 calories a day for women and 1,400 to 1,600 calories a day for men. Calorie counts are automatically figured into the meal plans.
5. If you don't exercise, reduce your lunch portion sizes by 25 percent—a 100- to 150-calorie restriction.
6. You may add 1 cup of non-starchy cruciferous veggies or a small side salad with veggies, olive oil, and apple cider vinegar to your lunches and dinners. Use just a small amount of olive oil.
7. No cheat meals or cheat days are allowed for weeks 1 and 2, but you'll be happy to know that cheat days are allowed for exercisers and a weekly cheat meal is allowed for non-exercisers in week 3 and beyond.
8. Do not drink alcoholic beverages during the Acceleration Phase.
9. Stay hydrated with filtered or spring water, and drink 50 percent of your total body weight in ounces of water each day (for example, if you weigh 200 pounds, drink 100 ounces of water each day).
10. Review the information on supplements in chapter ten. If you opt to supplement, take the following recommended dietary supplements:
    - Morning supplements: During week 1, one of your breakfast snacks can be a protein shake with 2–3 scoops of BioTrust Low Carb Protein Powder Blend or 2 scoops of Harvest™ Complete Vegan Plant Protein Powder Blend and 1 scoop of MetaboGreens. After week 1, in place of one of the 3-Minute Fat-Burning Morning Ritual choices, you may substitute 8 ounces of water mixed with 1 scoop of MetaboGreens as part of the intermittent fasting protocol.
    - Between 8 AM and noon: Add 1 scoop of Ageless Multi-Collagen Protein Powder™ or 1 scoop of Keto Elevate™ to a cup of coffee or a protein shake.
    - Lunch supplements: 1 Pro-X10 capsule and 3 OmegaKrill 5X™ softgel capsules

- Dinner supplement: 1 Pro-X10 capsule
- Pre-bedtime snacks: Consider a protein shake made with 2–3 scoops of BioTrust Low Carb Protein Powder Blend or 2 scoops of Harvest Complete Vegan Plant Protein Powder Blend. Feel free to add 1 scoop of Ageless Multi-Collagen Protein Powder or 1 scoop of Keto Elevate.

THE ACCELERATION PHASE OVERVIEW AND MEAL TEMPLATE

During the Acceleration Phase, you may use the following meal template and plan accordingly, selecting from the food lists on pages 40–42 or the recipes on pages 112–204—look for the .

MEASURING SERVING SIZES

While I have given approximate measurements and total calorie counts for each meal in each phase, these should be considered guidelines more than a strict rule—everyone will have slightly different calorie needs based on their height and how active they are. To figure out how much to eat, you can use your hand for reference. People of larger stature can eat larger portions, and they often have a proportionally larger hand size. You can visually compare portion sizes to your hand, fist, palm, or fingertip.

A serving of protein, for example, is about equal to the size and thickness of the palm of your hand. This could be a cut of meat, fish, or poultry, or even something as simple as eggs or cottage cheese.

A portion of carbs equates to the size of your clenched fist. This could be a serving of rice or other grain, a side of lentils or beans, a single potato or sweet potato, carrots, corn, pasta, or even fruits or green vegetables.

Last are fats. Servings of fats or oils can be matched to the size of the end of your thumb.

DAILY MENUS ARE GUIDES

On the next pages, you'll find sample menus for each meal of the Acceleration Phase. **Remember, these are just guidelines.** You have dozens of options to choose from! I suggest using the recipes within the meal plans, but I also understand that a lot of people don't really like to cook, so I've also provided simple options that most people would be able to whip up without a recipe.

Meals	Serving Sizes for Women	Serving Sizes for Men	Macro % Target
Breakfast Smart Snack—week 1 only* 3-Minute Fat-Burning Morning Ritual Drink	See the Breakfast Smart Snack choices on page 25. See the drink choices on pages 19–23.		n/a
Portion Volumizing Lunch: Protein + Vegetable + Fat	3 ounces protein (¾ palm-sized serving); 1 cup non-starchy vegetables (1 clenched fist); 1 tablespoon friendly fat, oil, or nut butter (end of thumb) Aim for around 300 calories	5 ounces protein (¾ palm-sized serving); 1½ cups non-starchy vegetables (1½ clenched fists); 2 tablespoons friendly fat, oil, or nut butter (end of thumb × 2) Aim for around 400 calories	15% carbs 50% protein 35% fat
Huge Portion Volumizing Dinner: Protein + Vegetable + Fat	4–5 ounces protein (1¼ palm-sized servings); 1 cup non-starchy vegetables (1 clenched fist); 1 tablespoon friendly fat, oil, or nut butter (end of thumb) Aim for around 400 calories	6–7 ounces protein (1¼ palm-sized servings); 1½ cups non-starchy vegetables (1½ clenched fists); 2 tablespoons friendly fat, oil, or nut butter (end of thumb × 2) Aim for around 600 calories	15% carbs 50% protein 35% fat
Healthy Dessert: Berries or cherries OR 70% cocoa dark chocolate OR Fat-Burning Dessert from the recipes on pages 174–186	1 cup berries or cherries (1 clenched fist) OR 2–4 squares of 70% cocoa dark chocolate OR 1 serving of any of the Fat-Burning Dessert recipes Up to 200 calories	1½ cups berries or cherries (1½ clenched fists) OR 2–4 squares of 70% cocoa dark chocolate OR 1 serving of any of the Fat-Burning Dessert recipes Up to 200 calories	n/a
Pre-bedtime Fat-Burning Snack: Protein/Berries/Fat OR Protein/Vegetable/Fat	1 small protein serving (2 ounces) or 1 hard-boiled egg or ½ cup cottage cheese or yogurt + ½ cup berries or cherries + fat (slice of avocado or ¼ cup nuts or seeds or 1 tablespoon friendly fat) OR 1 small protein serving (2 ounces) or 1 hard-boiled egg or ½ cup cottage cheese or yogurt + ½ cup non-starchy vegetables + fat (slice of avocado or ¼ cup nuts or seeds or 1 tablespoon friendly fat) OR Pre-bedtime Acceleration Phase approved snack 200–300 calories		15% carbs 50% protein 35% fat

*In week 1, you are allowed a breakfast snack, as noted. Try to wean yourself off it through the week, however, and switch yourself over to one of the 3-Minute Fat-Burning Morning Ritual drinks, which are required beginning in week 2.

SAMPLE MEAL PLANS

ACCELERATION PHASE: Days 1–14			
Week 1			
	Day 1	**Day 2**	**Day 3**
Breakfast Smart Snack ***OR*** ***3-Minute Fat-Burning Morning Ritual Drink*** (See page 25 for other suggestions.)	3 hard-boiled eggs OR *Instant Pot Egg White Bites* (2) OR Lemon water or any of my other 3-Minute Fat-Burning Drinks	Protein shake blended with ½ cup frozen berries or cherries OR Leftover *Instant Pot Egg White Bites* (2) OR Lemon water or any of my other 3-Minute Fat-Burning Drinks	2–3 pieces of beef jerky (grass-fed beef preferred) with a handful of raw nuts OR *Creamy Café Mocha Protein Smoothie* OR Lemon water or any of my other 3-Minute Fat-Burning Drinks
Portion Volumizing Energizing Lunch	Tuna atop a bed of mixed greens with chopped raw broccoli and cauliflower, drizzled with 1 tablespoon olive oil and apple cider vinegar OR Tuna atop a bed of mixed greens with *Ground Turkey "Spaghetti" Sauce* over steamed cabbage	Grilled or baked chicken breast with sliced avocado and 1 sliced tomato OR Leftover tuna atop a bed of mixed greens with leftover *Ground Turkey "Spaghetti" Sauce* over steamed cabbage	Steamed or boiled shrimp atop a bed of greens with 1 diced tomato, drizzled with 1 tablespoon olive oil and apple cider vinegar OR *Turkey and Bacon Goulash*
Huge Dinner with Dessert	Steak and steamed asparagus with grass-fed butter or ghee; cherries OR *Braised Cuban Flank Steak*; strawberries	Roast turkey breast and steamed mixed vegetables with grass-fed butter or ghee; cherries OR Leftover *Braised Cuban Flank Steak*; cherries	Pan-fried pork chop and roasted Brussels sprouts topped with chopped garlic with grass-fed butter or ghee; blueberries OR *Honey Garlic Pork Loin* and steamed broccoli; blueberries
Pre-bedtime Fat-Burning Snack	Cottage cheese (low fat) sprinkled with *Chili-Spiced Nuts* (or mixed nuts), and a few pieces of raw broccoli or cauliflower	Leftover roasted turkey or chicken and mixed vegetables OR *Homemade Beef Jerky* and pieces of raw vegetables such as broccoli	Greek yogurt (full fat) with blueberries OR Cottage cheese (low fat) with *Chili-Spiced Nuts*

ACCELERATION PHASE: Days 1–14			
Week 1			
Day 4	**Day 5**	**Day 6**	**Day 7**
Celery sticks with raw nut butter OR *Chocolate Nut Butter Smoothie* OR Lemon water or any of my other 3-Minute Fat-Burning Drinks	Cottage cheese or Greek yogurt with a handful of raw nuts or seeds or ½ cup of berries or cherries OR *Bacon and Caramelized Onion Egg Muffins* (2) OR Lemon water or any of my other 3-Minute Fat-Burning Drinks	Breakfast wrap: 2 scrambled eggs with ½ avocado, sprinkle of cheese, and optional hot sauce rolled into a coconut wrap OR Leftover *Bacon and Caramelized Onion Egg Muffins* (2) OR Lemon water or any of my other 3-Minute Fat-Burning Drinks	2–3 scrambled eggs with a sprinkle of cheese (raw, organic preferred) OR Leftover *Bacon and Caramelized Onion Egg Muffins* (2) OR Lemon water or any of my other 3-Minute Fat-Burning Drinks
Turkey burger topped with grilled onions and mushrooms and drizzled with 1 tablespoon olive oil OR Leftover *Turkey and Bacon Goulash*	2 chopped hard-boiled eggs and 2 slices crumbled cooked bacon atop a bed of raw spinach with chopped onions, grape tomatoes, and chopped cucumbers, drizzled with 1 tablespoon olive oil and apple cider vinegar OR *Chicken "Spaghetti" Skillet* (men can eat 2 servings)	Hamburger patty topped with steamed spinach and sun-dried tomatoes (with olive oil) OR Leftover *Chicken "Spaghetti" Skillet* (men can eat 2 servings)	Canned salmon atop a bed of mixed greens with grape tomatoes and 2 tablespoons chopped onion, drizzled with 1 tablespoon olive oil and apple cider vinegar OR *Ground Turkey "Spaghetti" Sauce* over cooked cabbage with a side of ½ cup avocado slices
Baked white fish with grass-fed butter or ghee, steamed broccoli, cauliflower, and yellow squash; 2–4 squares of 70% cocoa dark chocolate OR *Spiced Tilapia* (men can eat 2 servings) and steamed broccoli topped with minced garlic; *Frozen Dessert Bark*	Grilled salmon and steamed asparagus with grass-fed butter or ghee; cherries OR *One-Pan Garlic Roasted Salmon and Broccoli*; cherries	Chicken tenders stir-fried in olive oil with broccoli florets, chopped onion, bean sprouts, sliced red pepper, and sliced mushrooms; 2–4 squares of 70% cocoa dark chocolate OR Leftover *Spiced Tilapia* (men can eat 2 servings) and steamed broccoli topped with minced garlic; 2–4 squares of 70% cocoa dark chocolate	Steak and steamed green beans with grass-fed butter or ghee; cherries OR *BBQ Carnitas Lettuce Tacos*; cherries
Protein shake with ½ cup frozen blueberries and chia seeds OR *Blackberry Chia Seed Pudding*	2 hard-boiled eggs and celery sticks with raw nut butter OR *Frozen Dessert Bark*	Cottage cheese (low fat) sprinkled with *Chili-Spiced Nuts* (or mixed nuts), and a few pieces of raw broccoli or cauliflower	Greek yogurt (full fat) with sliced strawberries sprinkled with mixed nuts or *Chili-Spiced Nuts*

ACCELERATION PHASE: Days 1–14

Week 2

	Day 8	Day 9	Day 10
3-Minute Fat-Burning Morning Ritual Drink (Intermittent Fasting)	Lemon water or any of my other 3-Minute Fat-Burning Drinks	Lemon water or any of my other 3-Minute Fat-Burning Drinks	Lemon water or any of my other 3-Minute Fat-Burning Drinks
Portion Volumizing Energizing Lunch	BLT salad: 3–4 slices of crumbled cooked bacon and diced tomato atop a bed of iceberg lettuce, drizzled with 1 tablespoon olive oil and apple cider vinegar and splashed with optional hot sauce OR Tuna atop mixed greens with *Ground Turkey "Spaghetti" Sauce* over steamed cabbage	Cottage cheese atop a bed of mixed greens and diced tomato, sprinkled with walnut pieces OR Cottage cheese atop mixed greens with leftover *Ground Turkey "Spaghetti" Sauce* over steamed cabbage	Tuna mixed with diced avocado and wrapped in endive sheaths or romaine lettuce leaves OR *Chicken "Spaghetti" Skillet* (men can eat 2 servings)
Huge Dinner with Dessert	Hamburger patty topped with avocado slices and wrapped in large lettuce leaves, served with a side salad, drizzled with 1 tablespoon olive oil and apple cider vinegar; 1 cup sliced strawberries OR Leftover *BBQ Carnitas Lettuce Tacos*; strawberries	Grilled shrimp with lemon butter sauce and steamed asparagus; cherries OR *Slow Cooker Honey Garlic Chicken* and steamed asparagus; cherries	Pork roast and roasted Brussels sprouts, broccoli, and cauliflower, drizzled with olive oil; blueberries OR Leftover *Slow Cooker Honey Garlic Chicken* and steamed asparagus; blueberries
Pre-bedtime Fat-Burning Snack	Greek yogurt (full fat) mixed with sliced strawberries OR *Teriyaki Meatballs* and a few pieces of raw broccoli or cauliflower	Leftover grilled shrimp and cut-up raw broccoli and cauliflower OR *Teriyaki Meatballs* and a few pieces of raw broccoli or cauliflower	Protein shake with ½ cup blueberries OR *Cinnamon Almond Protein Smoothie* and a few pieces of raw broccoli or cauliflower

ACCELERATION PHASE: Days 1–14			
Week 2			
Day 11	**Day 12**	**Day 13**	**Day 14**
Lemon water or any of my other 3-Minute Fat-Burning Drinks	Lemon water or any of my other 3-Minute Fat-Burning Drinks	Lemon water or any of my other 3-Minute Fat-Burning Drinks	Lemon water or any of my other 3-Minute Fat-Burning Drinks
Grilled chicken breast served with a salad of mixed greens, grape tomatoes, and chopped cucumbers, drizzled with 1 tablespoon olive oil and apple cider vinegar OR Leftover *Chicken "Spaghetti" Skillet* (men can eat 2 servings)	Boiled or grilled shrimp served atop kale, slices of red bell pepper, and chopped cucumber, drizzled with 1 tablespoon olive oil and apple cider vinegar OR *Turkey and Bacon Goulash*	2 hard-boiled eggs, avocado slices, several slices of red onion, and a few tablespoons of chopped cucumber atop shredded cabbage, drizzled with balsamic vinegar OR Leftover *Turkey and Bacon Goulash*	Canned salmon mixed with spiralized zucchini and avocado slices, drizzled with 1 tablespoon olive oil and apple cider vinegar OR *Turkey Burgers* (without the *Butternut Buns*) wrapped in lettuce leaves with *Yogurt Sauce*
Baked salmon, coated with chopped nuts and served with baked mashed cauliflower and steamed spinach; cherries OR *One-Pan Garlic Roasted Salmon and Broccoli*; cherries	Roast turkey breast, served with avocado and roasted red bell peppers; 2–4 squares of 70% cocoa dark chocolate OR Leftover *One-Pan Garlic Roasted Salmon and Broccoli*; 2–4 squares of 70% cocoa dark chocolate	Baked Cornish hens with cooked mashed parsnips and a side salad of mixed greens, chopped tomatoes, diced celery, and any leftover roasted red pepper, drizzled with 1 tablespoon olive oil and apple cider vinegar; 2–4 squares of 70% cocoa dark chocolate OR *Caramel Chicken* and mashed cauliflower and side salad tossed with 1 tablespoon olive oil and apple cider vinegar; 2–4 squares of 70% cocoa dark chocolate	Grilled lamb chops and steamed green beans, topped with chopped fresh mint and grass-fed butter or ghee, and baked mashed cauliflower; cherries OR Leftover *Caramel Chicken* and mashed cauliflower and side salad tossed with 1 tablespoon olive oil and apple cider vinegar; cherries
2 hard-boiled eggs and celery sticks with raw nut butter OR *Frozen Dessert Bark*	Cottage cheese (low fat), blueberries, and mixed nuts OR *Cinnamon Almond Protein Smoothie* and a few pieces of raw broccoli or cauliflower	2 hard-boiled eggs, almonds, and cut-up raw cauliflower OR *Chocolate Buttons* with 2 hard-boiled eggs	Greek yogurt (full fat) with sliced strawberries OR *Blackberry Chia Seed Pudding*

CHAPTER 8
THE MAIN PHASE

You have been dropping pounds like crazy for 14 days now. You're looking and feeling lighter, and I hope you're inspired by your progress so far. Once you hit week 3, you've reached the Main Phase of Always Eat After 7 PM. This phase lasts from week 3 until whenever you achieve your weight loss goal.

During each week of the Main Phase, you combat falling leptin levels through the addition of Super Carbs at lunch and dinner—and then conclude each week with a leptin-boosting cheat day for exercisers and a cheat meal for non-exercisers (preferably on the seventh day of the week during the Main Phase). Losing weight is about to become even more pleasant.

By periodically cheating on your diet, you circumvent the negative side effects of calorie restriction. Each week, you start fresh with baseline levels of leptin and a hormonal environment primed for burning fat, not muscle.

There's still an emphasis on protein, non-starchy vegetables, friendly fats, and healthy desserts. You can even have a little alcohol (unless you're driving, pregnant, or washing exterior windows on a skyscraper).

One of the goals of the Main Phase is to help you forge good, solid eating habits so that when you get to the Lifestyle Phase, keeping your weight off will be a breeze.

The Main Phase continues until you reach your target weight. How long you stay on it obviously depends on how much you'd like to lose. For some people, another 14 days will get you there; for others, several more weeks or even months will be needed. Honestly, expect your rate of weight loss to slow down a bit, but it will be steady—so don't blow it off or vow to restart your diet until next January. You'll get to your goal without feeling hungry or waylaid by cravings.

IMPORTANT DAILY MEAL PLAN GUIDELINES FOR THE MAIN PHASE

1. In week 3 and beyond, add Portion Volumizing Super Carbs to your regimen.

2. Intermittent fasting should be used at least six days a week from here on out. It's completely fine to have a social breakfast with friends or coworkers here and there, but try to use intermittent fasting on as many days as you can.
3. If you have to eat breakfast after you wake up due to health or medication reasons, please select from the Breakfast Smart Snacks on page 25. Important: Breakfast eaters should cut their lunch portion sizes in half to balance out daily calories.
4. The target calorie goals for week 3 and beyond are 1,300 to 1,500 calories a day for women and 1,700 to 1,900 calories a day for men. Calorie counts are automatically figured into the meal plans.
5. If you do not exercise, reduce your lunch portion sizes by 25 percent—a 100- to 150-calorie restriction.
6. You may add 1 cup of non-starchy cruciferous veggies or a small side salad with veggies, olive oil, and apple cider vinegar to your lunches and dinner. Use just a small amount of olive oil.
7. Exercisers are allowed one cheat day per week and non-exercisers are allowed one cheat meal with dessert per week in place of dinner and a healthy dessert. Revisit chapter five if you need a refresher on how to strategically cheat for success. Remember, don't binge or stuff yourself.
8. Stay hydrated with filtered or spring water, and drink 50 percent of your total body weight in ounces of water each day (for example, if you weigh 200 pounds, drink 100 ounces of water each day).
9. Moderate amounts of alcohol can be consumed a few days per week during the Main Phase. Make sure you don't binge drink, and try to consume only clear liquors and red wines—preferably on the day(s) of your cheat meal(s).
10. Review the information on supplements in chapter ten. If you opt to supplement, take the following recommended dietary supplements:
    - Morning supplements: During week 1 of the Main Phase, one of your breakfast snacks can be a protein shake with 2–3 scoops of BioTrust Low Carb Protein Powder Blend or 2 scoops of Harvest Complete Vegan Plant Protein Powder Blend and 1 scoop of MetaboGreens. After week 1 of the Main Phase, in place of one of the 3-Minute Fat-Burning Morning Ritual choices, you may substitute 8 ounces of water mixed with 1 scoop of MetaboGreens as part of the intermittent fasting protocol.
    - Between 8 AM and noon: Add 1 scoop of Ageless Multi-Collagen Protein Powder or 1 scoop of Keto Elevate to a cup of coffee or a protein shake.
    - Lunch supplements: 1 Pro-X10 capsule and 3 OmegaKrill 5X softgel capsules

- Dinner supplement: 1 Pro-X10 capsule
- Pre-bedtime snacks: Consider a protein shake made with 2–3 scoops of BioTrust Low Carb Protein Powder Blend or 2 scoops of Harvest Complete Vegan Plant Protein Powder Blend. Feel free to add 1 scoop of Ageless Multi-Collagen Protein Powder or 1 scoop of Keto Elevate.

11. Use the Main Phase until you've reached your goal body weight. Once you've hit that weight, move on to the Lifestyle Phase as your permanent diet. Any time you fall off track and gain unwanted weight, you can always go back and repeat Phases 1 and 2 to accelerate your results.

EATING OUT ON THE PLAN

Food is, and always has been, the centerpiece of our social lives. You'll find it at every social occasion. And the number of restaurants in every town and city seems to prove that eating is truly America's pastime—not baseball!

Many people, though, don't know how to dine out in a healthy way that honors their bodies. They often fail to identify the healthiest items on the menu. And often, they'll finish off whatever arrives on the plate (especially if it's a bargain!) rather than eating only until satisfied. If a dish is marketed as "king-size," "two for one," "whopper," or the like, all the better. And so it goes.

Fortunately, with the Always Eat After 7 PM plan, it's easy to stick to the parameters because the diet offers so many choices. When eating out, simply keep the following basics in mind:

Identify approved foods on the menu. Most restaurants offer foods you can eat on this plan. Look for proteins such as fish, poultry, and meat, and make sure they're not fried or awash in sauces or gravy. For extra fiber and nutrients, order a salad when it's offered. At salad bars, choose toppings such as peas, chickpeas, sunflower seeds, and colorful vegetables. Choose Super Carbs such as rice, baked potatoes, and sweet potatoes when ordering.

Stick to the prescribed portions. You do *not* have to eat everything on your plate. Use your hand to eyeball correct portions. If you have leftovers on your plate, bring the rest home for a quick, reheatable meal the next day.

Keep a check on your drinking. There's always the temptation to enjoy too much wine or too many cocktails while dining out. But be careful. Although alcohol is allowed in Phases 2 and 3, it stimulates your appetite and adds empty calories. Curtail your drinking or avoid alcohol altogether while you're trying to shed pounds.

Go ethnic. Search out ethnic restaurants, which often have a healthy variety of foods. Asian restaurants use lots of vegetables, seaweed, raw fish, sushi, and rice. Middle Eastern restaurants usually have grilled meats, green leafy vegetables, and vegetarian alternatives like hummus and tabbouleh. Mexican restaurants can be great sources of bean protein. If the restaurant is Italian, watch out for pastas that are cooked in buckets of white sauce or butter. A tomato-based marinara sauce served over wheat pasta or spaghetti squash will shave off the calories. Go for salads at Italian eateries.

Go light at fast-food restaurants and delis. At fast-food restaurants, order smaller burgers, grilled chicken, or fruit. Other approved choices are sandwich wraps, salads, and fruit cups. At delis and sandwich shops, ask for leaner meats, less meat, and extra lettuce and tomato, on whole-wheat, oatmeal, or rye bread. Just be careful to avoid anything not on the approved food lists.

Have a buffet strategy. The temptation at a buffet is to pile your plate so high that you can't see over it. It's better to design your plate selectively with lean proteins, vegetables, Super Carbs, and a fruit for dessert, and not roam the buffet for second helpings.

Travel healthy. While staying at a hotel, find out if there is a farmers' market, whole foods grocery, or health food store nearby. All are terrific sources of fresh, wholesome, healthy meals and snacks, in case you don't want to order off a tempting menu.

Skip the appetizers and desserts. Your meal should cover your protein, vegetable, Super Carb, and fat needs, so there's no need to add more via appetizers and desserts. One exception: you can make a meal of a healthy appetizer and side salad with a light dressing.

If you keep the above basic guidelines in mind, you'll never have to turn down an invitation to dine out at a restaurant. Be social, have fun, and enjoy spending time with those you love—all while being healthy. It can be done—especially on this plan—much more easily than you might think.

THE MAIN PHASE OVERVIEW AND MEAL TEMPLATE

In the Main Phase, use the following template and plan your meals accordingly, selecting from the food lists on pages 40–42 or the recipes on pages 112–204.

I've provided two weeks' worth of sample menus for the Main Phase on pages 82–85. Remember, this phase lasts until you reach your target weight, so it might take you longer than two weeks. If repeating the same menus over and over seems unexciting, this is a great opportunity to learn to mix and match your own menus—a skill that will serve you well in the Lifestyle Phase.

Meals	Serving Sizes for Women	Serving Sizes for Men	Macro % Target
3-Minute Fat-Burning Morning Ritual Drink*	See the drink choices on pages 19–23.		n/a
Portion Volumizing Lunch: Carbohydrate + Protein + Fat	4 ounces protein (1 palm-sized serving); 1 cup Super Carbs (1 clenched fist); 1 cup non-starchy vegetables (1 clenched fist); 1 tablespoon friendly fat, oil, or nut butter (end of thumb); ¼ cup nuts and seeds 200–300 calories	6 ounces protein (1 palm-sized serving); 1½ cups Super Carbs (1½ clenched fists); 1½ cups non-starchy vegetables (1½ clenched fists); 2 tablespoons friendly fat, oil, or nut butter (end of thumb × 2); ¼ cup nuts and seeds 400–500 calories	40% carbs 40% protein 20% fat
Huge Portion Volumizing Dinner: Carbohydrate + Protein + Fat + Dessert (see next page)	6 ounces protein (1½ palm-sized servings); 1 cup Super Carbs (1 clenched fist); 1 cup non-starchy vegetables (1 clenched fist); 1 tablespoon friendly fat, oil, or nut butter (end of thumb); ½ cup nuts and seeds (1 cupped hand) 400–500 calories	9 ounces protein (1½ palm-sized servings); 1½ cups Super Carbs (1½ clenched fists); 1½ cups non-starchy vegetables (1½ clenched fists); 2 tablespoons friendly fat, oil, or nut butter (end of thumb × 2); ½–¾ cup nuts and seeds (1 cupped hand) 600 to 700 calories	40% carbs 40% protein 20% fat

*In this phase, you should be using an intermittent fasting protocol along with my 3-Minute Fat-Burning Morning Ritual. For those who can't fast due to health reasons, choose a Breakfast Smart Snack from the options on page 25 (macro target: 10% carbs, 50% protein, 40% fat). Remember, breakfast eaters should cut their lunch portion sizes in half to balance out daily calories.

<table>
<tr><th>Meals</th><th>Serving Sizes for Women</th><th>Serving Sizes for Men</th><th>Macro % Target</th></tr>
<tr><td>Dessert:
Berries, cherries, or piece of fruit
OR
70% cocoa dark chocolate
OR
Fat-Burning Dessert from the recipes on pages 174–186</td><td>1 cup berries, cherries, or other whole fruit (1 clenched fist)
OR
2–4 squares of 70% cocoa dark chocolate
OR
1 serving of any of the Fat-Burning Dessert recipes
Up to 200 calories</td><td>1½ cups berries, cherries, or other whole fruit (1½ clenched fists)
OR
2–4 squares of 70% cocoa dark chocolate
OR
1 serving of any of the Fat-Burning Dessert recipes
Up to 200 calories</td><td>n/a</td></tr>
<tr><td>Pre-bedtime Fat-Burning Snack:
Protein/Berries/Fat
OR
Protein/Vegetable/Fat</td><td colspan="2">1 small protein serving (2 ounces) or 1 hard-boiled egg or ½ cup cottage cheese or yogurt + ½ cup berries or cherries + fat (slice of avocado or ¼ cup nuts or seeds or 1 tablespoon friendly fat)
OR
1 small protein serving (2 ounces) or 1 hard-boiled egg or ½ cup cottage cheese or yogurt + ½ cup non-starchy vegetables + fat (slice of avocado or ¼ cup nuts or seeds or 1 tablespoon friendly fat)
OR
Pre-bedtime approved snack
200–300 calories</td><td>15% carbs
50% protein
35% fat</td></tr>
</table>

SAMPLE MEAL PLANS

THE MAIN PHASE: Days 15–28 (or until you reach your goal)			
Week 3			
	Day 15	**Day 16**	**Day 17**
3-Minute Fat-Burning Morning Ritual Drink (Intermittent Fasting)	Lemon water or any of my other 3-Minute Fat-Burning Drinks	Lemon water or any of my other 3-Minute Fat-Burning Drinks	Lemon water or any of my other 3-Minute Fat-Burning Drinks
Portion Volumizing Energizing Lunch	Sliced turkey on two slices of Ezekiel bread with mustard, lettuce, and avocado slices; sliced tomato OR *Stuffed Bell Peppers* (women can eat 2 stuffed peppers; men can eat 3 stuffed peppers)	Diced baked chicken thighs mixed with diced celery, 1 tablespoon chopped onion, and 1 tablespoon olive oil, served atop mixed greens; baked potato OR Leftover *Stuffed Bell Peppers* (women can eat 2 stuffed peppers; men can eat 3 stuffed peppers)	Canned salmon atop a bed of mixed greens with 1 diced tomato and 2 tablespoons chopped onion, drizzled with 1 tablespoon olive oil and apple cider vinegar; baked sweet potato sprinkled with cinnamon OR *Salmon and Lentils en Papillote*
Huge Dinner with Dessert	Baked chicken thighs, mashed cauliflower, and peas with grass-fed butter or ghee; cubed fresh pineapple or other fresh fruit choice OR *Moroccan Spiced Chicken and Squash* (men can eat 2 servings); 2–4 squares of 70% cocoa dark chocolate	Grilled or boiled shrimp, rice, and steamed green beans with 1 teaspoon grass-fed butter or ghee; 2–4 squares of 70% cocoa dark chocolate OR *Shrimp Curry with Coconut Rice* (men can eat 2 servings); *Frozen Dessert Bark*	Steak, rice, and steamed green beans with grass-fed butter or ghee; apple or other fresh fruit OR *Slow Cooker Braised Pot Roast* (women can eat ½ serving); *Fruit Mini Tarts*
Pre-bedtime Fat-Burning Snack	Greek yogurt (full fat) and blueberries OR *Cinnamon Almond Protein Smoothie* and a few pieces of raw broccoli or cauliflower	Cottage cheese (low fat) with *All-Spiced-Up Roasted Chickpeas* OR *Matcha Protein Smoothie*	Cottage cheese (low fat) and celery sticks with raw nut butter OR *Creamy Apple Celery Salad*

THE MAIN PHASE: Days 15–28 (or until you reach your goal)			
Week 3			
Day 18	**Day 19**	**Day 20**	**Day 21***
Lemon water or any of my other 3-Minute Fat-Burning Drinks	Lemon water or any of my other 3-Minute Fat-Burning Drinks	Lemon water or any of my other 3-Minute Fat-Burning Drinks	Lemon water or any of my other 3-Minute Fat-Burning Drinks OR Breakfast Smart Snack wrap: 2 scrambled eggs with ½ avocado, a sprinkle of cheese, and optional hot sauce, rolled into a coconut wrap OR Cheat Day Breakfast: *Dark Chocolate Granola* with coconut milk
Turkey burger on two slices of Ezekiel bread with mustard, with a side salad, drizzled with olive oil and apple cider vinegar OR *Turkey Burgers with Butternut Buns*, with a side salad, drizzled with 1 tablespoon olive oil and apple cider vinegar	Hamburger patty, baked potato, and stewed tomatoes OR *Classic Chicken Stew* (men can eat 2 servings)	Roasted turkey, acorn or butternut squash, and a side salad, drizzled with olive oil and apple cider vinegar OR *Curried Pumpkin Soup with Chicken and Quinoa* (men can eat 2 servings)	BLT salad: 3–4 slices of crumbled cooked bacon and diced tomato atop a bed of iceberg lettuce, drizzled with 1 tablespoon olive oil and apple cider vinegar and splashed with optional hot sauce; baked potato OR Leftover *Curried Pumpkin Soup with Chicken and Quinoa* (men can eat 2 servings)
Baked ham with a baked sweet potato and steamed broccoli with grass-fed butter or ghee; 2–4 squares of 70% cocoa dark chocolate OR *Moscato-Dijon Ham Roast* (men can eat 2 servings) with a baked sweet potato and steamed broccoli; *Chocolate Chunk Cookies*	Grilled salmon, baked sweet potato, and roasted Brussels sprouts; 2–4 squares of 70% cocoa dark chocolate OR *Greek Salmon Quinoa Bowl*; *Mexican Brownies*	Cooked ground beef mixed with no-sugar-added marinara sauce and served over black bean pasta, with steamed broccoli with grass-fed butter and ghee; 2–4 squares of 70% cocoa dark chocolate OR *Ground Beef Lasagna with Tomato Basil Sauce*; *Chocolate Very Cherry Ice Cream*	***Cheat Dinner: Your choice!***
Cottage cheese (low fat) and cherries, sprinkled with mixed nuts OR *Matcha Protein Smoothie*	Cottage cheese (low fat), raw baby carrots, and avocado slices OR *Homemade Beef Jerky* and raw vegetables such as cut-up raw broccoli and cauliflower	*Spiced Oatmeal Protein Smoothie* or other smoothie	2 hard-boiled eggs with raw carrots and mixed nuts OR Cheat Day Smart Snack: *Chocolate Nut Butter Protein Bar*

*Day 21 is the day on which you can cheat. If you're an exerciser, you may make this a cheat day, meaning all your meals can be "cheats" if you wish. However, make sure you don't binge or stuff yourself, and be sure to limit alcohol intake. If you do not exercise, cheat at only one meal each week. The meals provided in this plan are one example.

Week 4			
	Day 22	**Day 23**	**Day 24**
3-Minute Fat-Burning Morning Ritual Drink (Intermittent Fasting)	Lemon water or any of my other 3-Minute Fat-Burning Drinks	Lemon water or any of my other 3-Minute Fat-Burning Drinks	Lemon water or any of my other 3-Minute Fat-Burning Drinks
Portion Volumizing Energizing Lunch	Baked, skinless chicken thighs, mashed sweet potatoes, and a side salad, drizzled with 1 tablespoon olive oil and apple cider vinegar OR *BBQ Chicken en Papillote* (men can eat 1½ servings)	Baked salmon, mashed sweet potatoes, roasted Brussels sprouts, and sliced avocado OR Leftover *Braised Cuban Flank Steak* with black beans	Tuna atop a bed of mixed greens with 1 cup chopped broccoli and cauliflower, drizzled with 1 tablespoon olive oil and apple cider vinegar; quinoa OR Leftover *Chili-Loaded Baked Potato* (women can eat ½ serving)
Huge Dinner with Dessert	Ground beef stir-fried with veggies and olive oil and served over rice; 1 cup sliced strawberries or other fresh fruit OR *Braised Cuban Flank Steak* with black beans; strawberries or other fresh fruit, or *Salted Dark Chocolate–Dipped PB Cookies*	Grilled shrimp with lemon butter sauce, mashed butternut squash, and steamed asparagus; cherries or other fruit OR *Chili-Loaded Baked Potato*; cherries or other fruit, or *Coconut Panna Cotta*	Pork roast, mashed butternut squash, and roasted veggies such as Brussels sprouts, broccoli, and cauliflower, drizzled with 1 tablespoon olive oil after serving; blueberries or other fruit OR *Pomegranate-Glazed Pork Chops*, mashed butternut squash, and roasted veggies such as Brussels sprouts, broccoli, and cauliflower; blueberries or other fruit, or *No Bake Salted Caramel Bars*
Pre-bedtime Fat-Burning Snack	Greek yogurt (full fat) mixed with sliced strawberries OR *Chocolate Nut Butter Protein Bar*	Leftover grilled shrimp and cut-up raw broccoli and cauliflower OR *Matcha Protein Smoothie*	Protein shake with blueberries OR *Cookie Butter Protein Smoothie* with a few pieces of raw broccoli or cauliflower

Week 4			
Day 25	**Day 26**	**Day 27**	**Day 28***
Lemon water or any of my other 3-Minute Fat-Burning Drinks	Lemon water or any of my other 3-Minute Fat-Burning Drinks	Lemon water or any of my other 3-Minute Fat-Burning Drinks	Lemon water or any of my other 3-Minute Fat-Burning Drinks OR Breakfast Smart Snack wrap: 2 scrambled eggs with ½ avocado, a sprinkle of cheese, and optional hot sauce, rolled into a coconut wrap (see page 25 for other suggestions) OR Cheat Day Breakfast: *Sweet Potato Pancakes*
Grilled chicken served with a salad of mixed greens, grape tomatoes, and chopped cucumbers, drizzled with 1 tablespoon olive oil and apple cider vinegar; quinoa or rice OR Leftover *Pomegranate-Glazed Pork Chops*, mashed butternut squash, and roasted veggies such as Brussels sprouts, broccoli, and cauliflower, drizzled with 1 tablespoon olive oil after serving	Hamburger patty between 2 slices of Ezekiel bread with mustard; kale side salad, drizzled with 1 tablespoon olive oil and apple cider vinegar OR Leftover *Spiced Tilapia* (men can eat 2 servings)	2 hard-boiled eggs, ½ sliced avocado, several slices of red onion, a few tablespoons of chopped cucumber, and quinoa atop shredded cabbage, drizzled with balsamic vinegar OR *Chicken Hash with Kale and Butternut Squash* (men can eat 2 servings)	Sliced turkey on two slices of Ezekiel bread with mustard and sliced avocado; sliced tomato on the side OR *Fiesta Chicken Skillet*
Baked or grilled white fish coated with chopped nuts and served with baked sweet potatoes and sautéed kale; cherries or other fresh fruit OR *Spiced Tilapia* (men can eat 2 servings); cherries or other fresh fruit, or *Chickpea Pecan Blondies*	Roast turkey breast, mashed potatoes with grass-fed butter or ghee, and steamed green beans; 2–4 squares of 70% cocoa dark chocolate OR *Roasted Turkey Roulade* (men can eat 1½–2 servings); 2–4 squares of 70% cocoa dark chocolate or *Chocolate Super-Seed Bark*	Baked Cornish hens with mashed potatoes and a side salad of mixed greens, chopped tomatoes, diced celery, and sliced red pepper, drizzled with 1 tablespoon olive oil and apple cider vinegar; 2–4 squares of 70% cocoa dark chocolate OR *Maple Chicken and Veggies* (men can eat 1½ servings); 2–4 squares of 70% cocoa dark chocolate or *Chocolate Chunk Cookies*	***Cheat Dinner: Your Choice!***
2 hard-boiled eggs and celery sticks with raw nut butter OR 2 hard-boiled eggs and *All-Spiced-Up Roasted Chickpeas*	Protein shake with blueberries OR *Peach Mango Protein Smoothie*	Greek yogurt (full fat) with sliced kiwifruit or other fruit OR *Lemon Blueberry Protein Bar*	Cottage cheese (low fat) with pineapple chunks, sprinkled with mixed nuts OR *Chocolate Buttons* with 2 hard-boiled eggs

*Day 28 is the day on which you can cheat. If you're an exerciser, you may make this a cheat day, meaning all your meals can be "cheats" if you wish. However, make sure you don't binge or stuff yourself, and be sure to limit alcohol intake. If you do not exercise, cheat at only one meal each week. The meals listed in this plan are one example.

CHAPTER 9
THE LIFESTYLE PHASE

Congratulations—you made it!

You began dropping pounds fast on the Acceleration Phase and continued your success on the Main Phase. Now you're at your ideal weight. You've reached your goal. Your body is burning fat and handling calories correctly. The occasional slice of cheesecake or side order of French fries won't send your blood sugar and appetite into a tailspin now that you've retuned your metabolism—as long as these are once-in-a-while indulgences.

This is a huge achievement on your part, and I know you look and feel great.

So, after weeks of healthy eating (even at night!), the extra weight is finally off—now what?

Maintain your weight loss with the Lifestyle Phase! Very few diets have a maintenance component, but Always Eat After 7 PM does. Everyone knows how to lose weight (at least in theory), but what we're never told or filled in on is how to *maintain* weight loss. As you and I well know, that is the most important piece of the weight loss puzzle. Now it comes down to permanently taking control of your health so you'll never again become overweight.

Recall the last time you lost weight. Maybe within a few weeks or months, you gained it back—with interest. You reverted to old habits and old ways of eating. We've all had this experience. It is unlikely to happen, however, on this plan. How do I know? Well, research tells us so. A large European study compared different types of diets and discovered the best way to prevent weight regain: eat lots of lean protein for its fat-burning and satiating potential and stick to Super Carbs because they are slowly digested and slowly converted to blood sugar.

The study, published in the *New England Journal of Medicine*, tested various diets on nearly 800 adults who had dropped pounds on an eight-week diet. For maintenance, the dieters ate lean protein and unrefined carbohydrates (whole, rather than refined, grains and non-starchy vegetables and fruits—in other words, Super Carbs). These choices enabled them to maintain weight loss without going hungry. Those eating a high-carbohydrate/low-protein diet, including a lot of refined, processed carbs, regained the most weight.

Because you worked with your body, training it to rely on fat for fuel and priming your hormones for fat loss, you protected your metabolism, instead of throwing it out of balance like so many commercial diets do. Now you won't have to live in a state of deprivation to keep your weight off.

The Lifestyle Phase is designed to help you stay thin and fit, while avoiding a recurrence of problems with your metabolism or rebound weight gain. While still technically a part of the Always Eat After 7 PM plan, the Lifestyle Phase is more a set of flexible guidelines to live by than a "diet" per se. It is a continuation of all the strategies you've grown used to so far.

During this third and final phase, the basics of the Always Eat After 7 PM plan stay the same. You continue to eat widely from the same approved foods you have been enjoying throughout the diet: proteins, vegetables, fruits, Super Carbs, friendly fats, and desserts.

Also, you've learned how to allow yourself treats through strategic cheating. Continue this strategy to maintain your weight loss. Allowing yourself some leeway each week helps you maintain without temptation. As long as you eat healthfully during the week, for example, you can splurge with cheat days.

The way you've learned how to eat is exactly what to continue to manage your weight permanently.

I also suggest that you periodically watch the scale. Although you may have heard that it's a dirty word, a scale works well for weight control. Most successful maintainers weigh themselves regularly, never allowing a gain of more than five pounds. If this happens to you, there's an easy trick to reversing it: go back on the Acceleration Phase for as long as it takes to get you back to your ideal weight.

One more piece of advice: remember your reason for losing weight in the first place. Is it still important to you? I hope so. You must want to keep your newly acquired body.

IMPORTANT DAILY MEAL PLAN GUIDELINES FOR THE LIFESTYLE PHASE

1. Use the exact same calories and portion guidelines as in the Main Phase. The only difference is that lunch portions in the Lifestyle Phase are 50 percent larger.
2. Intermittent fasting should still be used at least six days per week. It's completely okay to have a social breakfast here and there, but try to use intermittent fasting on as many days as you can.
3. If you have to eat breakfast after you wake up due to health or medication reasons, please select from the Breakfast Smart Snacks on page 25 or the recipes on pages 112–115. Important: Breakfast eaters should cut their lunch portion sizes in half to balance out daily calories.

4. The target calorie goals for the Main Phase are approximately 1,300 to 1,500 calories a day for women and 1,700 to 1,900 calories a day for men. Calories are automatically figured into the sample meal plans.
5. If you do not exercise, reduce your lunch portion sizes by 25 percent—a 100- to 150-calorie restriction.
6. You may add 1 cup of non-starchy cruciferous veggies or a small side salad with veggies, olive oil, and apple cider vinegar to your lunches and dinners. Use just a small amount of olive oil.
7. Exercisers are allowed one cheat day per week and non-exercisers are allowed one cheat meal with dessert per week in place of dinner and a healthy dessert. Don't binge or stuff yourself.
8. Stay hydrated with filtered or spring water, and drink 50 percent of your total body weight in ounces of water each day (for example, if you weigh 200 pounds, drink 100 ounces of water each day).
9. Moderate amounts of alcohol can be consumed a few days per week during the Lifestyle Phase. Make sure you don't binge drink, and try to consume only clear liquors and red wines—preferably on the day(s) of your cheat meal(s).
10. Review the information on supplements in chapter ten. If you opt to supplement, take the supplements I recommend on page 105.

THE LIFESTYLE PHASE OVERVIEW AND MEAL TEMPLATE

In the Lifestyle Phase, use the following guidelines and plan your meals accordingly, selecting from the food lists on pages 40–42 or the recipes on pages 112–204. Your lunch portions should be 50 percent larger than allowed in the first two phases. Because fruit servings double on the Lifestyle Phase, consider splitting up your fruits between meals—such as 1 serving for lunch and the other for dessert after dinner.

I've provided two weeks' worth of meal plans for the Lifestyle Phase on pages 88–93. Since this is a lifestyle that goes well beyond two weeks, learning to plan meals is especially important. Planning your meals also helps ensure that you stay with the program. So use the following template to plan what you will eat each day during this phase.

Meals	Serving Sizes for Women	Serving Sizes for Men	Macro % Target
3-Minute Fat-Burning Morning Ritual Drink*	See the drink choices on pages 19–23		n/a
Portion Volumizing Lunch: Carbohydrate + Protein + Fat	6 ounces protein (1½ palm-sized servings); 1½ cups Super Carbs (1½ clenched fists); 1 cup non-starchy vegetables (1 clenched fist); 1 tablespoon friendly fat, oil, or nut butter (end of thumb); ¼ cup nuts and seeds 200–300 calories	9 ounces protein (1½ palm-sized servings); 1¾ cups Super Carbs (1¾ clenched fists); 1½ cups non-starchy vegetable (1½ clenched fists); 2 tablespoons friendly fat, oil, or nut butter (end of thumb × 2); ¼ cup nuts and seeds 400–500 calories	40% carbs 40% protein 20% fat
Huge Portion Volumizing Dinner: Carbohydrate + Protein + Fat	6 ounces protein (1½ palm-sized servings); 1 cup Super Carbs (1 clenched fist); 1 cup non-starchy vegetables (1 clenched fist); 1 tablespoon friendly fat, oil, or nut butter (end of thumb); ¼ cup nuts and seeds (1 cupped hand) 400–500 calories	9 ounces protein (1½ palm-sized servings); 1½ cups Super Carbs (1½ clenched fists); 1½ cups non-starchy vegetables (1½ clenched fists); 2 tablespoons friendly fat, oil, or nut butter (end of thumb × 2); ¼ cup nuts and seeds (1 cupped hand) 600–700 calories	40% carbs 40% protein 20% fat
Healthy Dessert: Berries, cherries, or piece of fruit OR 70% cocoa dark chocolate OR Fat-Burning Dessert from the recipes on pages 174–186	1½ cups berries, cherries, OR other whole fruit (1½ clenched fists) OR 2 – 4 squares of 70% cocoa dark chocolate OR 1 serving of any of the Fat-Burning Dessert recipes Up to 200 calories	1¾ cups berries, cherries, OR other whole fruit (1¾ clenched fists) OR 2–4 squares of 70% cocoa dark chocolate OR 1 serving of any of the Fat-Burning Dessert recipes Up to 300 calories	n/a
Pre-bedtime Fat-Burning Snack: Protein/Berries/Fat OR Protein/Vegetable/Fat	1 small protein serving (2 ounces) or 1 hard-boiled egg or ½ cup cottage cheese or yogurt + ½ cup berries or cherries + fat (slice of avocado or ¼ cup nuts or seeds or 1 tablespoon friendly fat) OR 1 small protein serving (2 ounces) or 1 hard-boiled egg or ½ cup cottage cheese or yogurt + ½ cup non-starchy vegetables + fat (slice of avocado or ¼ cup nuts or seeds or 1 tablespoon friendly fat) OR Pre-bedtime approved snack 200–300 calories		15% carbs 50% protein 35% fat

*Upon arising, you should follow an intermittent fasting protocol along with my 3-Minute Fat-Burning Morning Ritual. Remember, if you have to eat breakfast after you wake up due to health or medication reasons, please select from the Breakfast Smart Snacks on page 25. Again, breakfast eaters should cut their lunch portion sizes in half to balance out daily calories (macro target: 10% carbs, 50% protein, 40% fat).

14 SAMPLE MENUS FOR THE LIFESTYLE PHASE

	Day 29	Day 30	Day 31
3-Minute Fat-Burning Morning Ritual Drink (Intermittent Fasting)	Lemon water or any of my other 3-Minute Fat-Burning Drinks	Lemon water or any of my other 3-Minute Fat-Burning Drinks	Lemon water or any of my other 3-Minute Fat-Burning Drinks
Portion Volumizing Energizing Lunch	Sliced roast beef on 2 slices of Ezekiel bread with mustard or horseradish, lettuce, and avocado slices; sliced tomato OR *Thai Coconut Shrimp Soup* with a roast beef sandwich	Diced baked leftover chicken breasts mixed with diced celery, 1 tablespoon chopped onion, and olive oil and served atop mixed greens; quinoa OR Leftover *Cheesy Ground Beef Skillet* (women can eat ½ serving)	2 sandwiches: sliced baked ham on 4 slices of Ezekiel bread with mustard, sliced tomato, and lettuce; avocado OR *Orange Shrimp and "Noodles" en Papillote* (men can eat 2 servings)
Huge Dinner with Dessert	Baked chicken breasts, mashed sweet potato, and asparagus with 1 teaspoon grass-fed butter or ghee; 2–4 squares of 70% cocoa dark chocolate OR *Cheesy Ground Beef Skillet* (women can eat ½ serving); *Mexican Brownies*	Grilled or boiled shrimp, rice, and steamed green beans with 1 teaspoon grass-fed butter or ghee; 2–4 squares of 70% cocoa dark chocolate OR *Shrimp Curry with Coconut Rice*; *Frozen Dessert Bark*	Steak, mashed potatoes, and steamed green beans with 1 teaspoon grass-fed butter or ghee; apple or other fresh fruit OR *Braised Cuban Flank Steak* with black beans; *Fruit Mini Tarts*
Pre-bedtime Fat-Burning Snack	Greek yogurt (full fat) with blueberries OR *Chocolate Nut Butter Smoothie*	Greek yogurt (full fat) and ½ grapefruit OR *Nut Butter Banana Protein Smoothie*	Celery sticks and apple slices with raw nut butter OR *Creamy Apple Celery Salad*

Day 32	Day 33	Day 34	Day 35*
Lemon water or any of my other 3-Minute Fat-Burning Drinks	Lemon water or any of my other 3-Minute Fat-Burning Drinks	Lemon water or any of my other 3-Minute Fat-Burning Drinks	Lemon water or any of my other 3-Minute Fat-Burning Drinks OR Breakfast Smart Snack wrap: 2 scrambled eggs with ½ avocado, a sprinkle of cheese, and optional hot sauce, rolled into a coconut wrap OR Cheat Day Breakfast: *Gingerbread-Spiced Waffles*
Hamburger patties, rice, and a side salad, drizzled with 1 tablespoon olive oil and apple cider vinegar OR Leftover *Orange Shrimp and "Noodles" en Papillote* (men can eat 2 servings)	Turkey burgers, rice or quinoa, and a side salad, drizzled with 1 tablespoon olive oil and apple cider vinegar OR *One-Pan "Spaghetti" and Meatballs* and a side salad, drizzled with olive oil and apple cider vinegar	Tuna atop a bed of mixed greens with 1 cup chopped broccoli and cauliflower, drizzled with 1 tablespoon olive oil and apple cider vinegar; quinoa OR Leftover *One-Pan "Spaghetti" and Meatballs* and a side salad, drizzled with olive oil and apple cider vinegar	Chef salad with diced ham, hard-boiled egg, avocado slices, black beans, and diced tomato atop a bed of mixed greens, drizzled with 1 tablespoon olive oil and apple cider vinegar; baked potato OR *Steamed White Fish en Papillote* (men can eat 2 servings)
Baked ham, mashed sweet potatoes, and steamed asparagus with 1 teaspoon grass-fed butter or ghee; 2–4 squares of 70% cocoa dark chocolate OR *Moscato-Dijon Ham Roast* (men can eat 2 servings), mashed sweet potatoes, and steamed asparagus; *Chocolate Very Cherry Ice Cream*	Grilled or baked salmon, mashed butternut squash, and roasted Brussels sprouts with 1 teaspoon grass-fed butter or ghee; 2–4 squares of 70% cocoa dark chocolate OR *Greek Salmon Quinoa Bowl*; *Chocolate Chunk Cookies*	Cooked ground beef mixed with low-carb marinara sauce and served over black bean pasta, with steamed zucchini with 1 teaspoon grass-fed butter and ghee; 2–4 squares of 70% cocoa dark chocolate OR *Ground Beef Lasagna with Tomato Basil Sauce* (men can eat 1½ servings) and *Chocolate Very Cherry Ice Cream*	***Cheat Dinner: Your Choice!***
Cottage cheese (low fat) and sliced banana, sprinkled with mixed nuts OR *Strawberry Banana Protein Smoothie*	Leftover salmon and veggies from dinner OR *Homemade Beef Jerky* and raw vegetables such as cut-up raw broccoli and cauliflower	*Creamy Café Mocha Protein Smoothie* or other smoothie with a few pieces of raw cauliflower or broccoli	Greek yogurt (full fat) with blueberries and *Orange Spiced Granola*

*Day 35 is the day on which you can cheat. If you're an exerciser, you may make this a cheat day, meaning all your meals can be "cheats" if you wish. However, make sure you don't binge or stuff yourself, and be sure to limit alcohol intake. If you do not exercise, cheat at only one meal each week. The meals listed in this plan are one example.

14 SAMPLE MENUS FOR THE LIFESTYLE PHASE

	Day 36	Day 37	Day 38
3-Minute Fat-Burning Morning Ritual Drink (Intermittent Fasting)	Lemon water or any of my other 3-Minute Fat-Burning Drinks	Lemon water or any of my other 3-Minute Fat-Burning Drinks	Lemon water or any of my other 3-Minute Fat-Burning Drinks
Portion Volumizing Energizing Lunch	Chicken thighs, mashed sweet potatoes, and a side salad, drizzled, with 1 tablespoon olive oil and apple cider vinegar OR *Classic Chicken Stew*	Baked salmon, acorn squash, steamed broccoli, and sliced avocado OR *Orange Shrimp and "Noodles" en Papillote* (men can eat 2 servings)	Canned salmon, mixed with diced avocado and wrapped in corn tortillas and served with a sliced tomato OR Leftover *Orange Shrimp and "Noodles" en Papillote* (men can eat 2 servings)
Huge Dinner with Dessert	Grilled red snapper or other white fish, peas and carrots, and mashed cauliflower with grass-fed butter or ghee; 1 cup sliced strawberries or other fresh fruit OR *Spiced Tilapia* (men can eat 2 servings) with baked potato; *Salted Dark Chocolate–Dipped PB Cookies*	Roast beef, mashed potatoes, and steamed green beans; cherries or other fruit OR *Pot Roast Tacos with Chimichurri*; *Coconut Panna Cotta*	Grilled lamb chops, rice, and roasted veggies such as Brussels sprouts, broccoli, and cauliflower; blueberries or other fruit OR *Honey Garlic Pork Loin*, rice, and roasted veggies such as Brussels sprouts, broccoli, and cauliflower; leftover *Coconut Panna Cotta*
Pre-bedtime Fat-Burning Snack	Greek yogurt (full fat) mixed with sliced strawberries OR *Pumpkin Pie Egg Muffins*	Leftover roast beef and vegetables from dinner OR Leftover *Homemade Beef Jerky* and raw vegetables such as cut-up raw broccoli and cauliflower	Protein shake with ½ cup blueberries OR *Piña Colada Protein Smoothie*

Day 39	**Day 40**	**Day 41**	**Day 42***
Lemon water or any of my other 3-Minute Fat-Burning Drinks	Lemon water or any of my other 3-Minute Fat-Burning Drinks	Lemon water or any of my other 3-Minute Fat-Burning Drinks	Lemon water or any of my other 3-Minute Fat-Burning Drinks OR Breakfast Smart Snack wrap: 2 scrambled eggs with ½ avocado, a sprinkle of cheese, and optional hot sauce, rolled into a coconut wrap OR Cheat Day Breakfast: *Coconut Cashew Protein Pancakes*
Roasted turkey, served with a salad of mixed greens, grape tomatoes, and chopped cucumbers, drizzled with 1 tablespoon olive oil and apple cider vinegar; quinoa or rice OR Leftover *Honey Garlic Pork Loin*, rice, and roasted veggies such as Brussels sprouts, broccoli, and cauliflower	Turkey burgers topped with salsa, served with kidney beans and a spinach side salad, drizzled with 1 tablespoon olive oil and apple cider vinegar OR Leftover *One-Pan Garlic Roasted Salmon and Broccoli* (women can eat ½ serving); baked sweet potato	3–4 hard-boiled eggs, 3–4 slices of cooked crumbled bacon, avocado slices, several slices of red onion, a few tablespoons of chopped cucumber, and quinoa atop mixed greens, drizzled with balsamic vinegar OR *Ground Turkey "Spaghetti" Sauce* (men can eat 1½ servings) over black bean pasta	Salad with diced leftover chicken or salmon atop romaine lettuce, Kalamata olives, and slices of red onion, drizzled with 1 tablespoon olive oil and apple cider vinegar; rice or quinoa OR Leftover *Pomegranate-Glazed Pork Chops* (women can eat ½ serving); rice or quinoa
Baked or grilled salmon, rice or couscous, and sautéed kale; cherries or other fresh fruit OR *One-Pan Garlic Roasted Salmon and Broccoli* and baked sweet potato; *Chickpea Pecan Blondies*	Baked ham, mashed sweet potatoes with grass-fed butter or ghee, and steamed green beans; 2–4 squares of 70% cocoa dark chocolate OR *Prosciutto-Wrapped Pork Roast with Roasted Pepper Stuffing*; *Chocolate Super-Seed Bark*	Grilled pork chops, mashed butternut squash, and steamed cauliflower with grass-fed butter or ghee; 2–4 squares of 70% cocoa dark chocolate OR *Pomegranate-Glazed Pork Chops*, mashed butternut squash, and steamed cauliflower; *Chocolate Chunk Cookies*	***Cheat Dinner: Your Choice!***
2 hard-boiled eggs and celery sticks with raw nut butter OR *Lemon Poppy Seed Crepes* and berries	Protein shake with ½ cup strawberries OR *Peach Mango Protein Smoothie*	Cottage cheese (low fat) with sliced strawberries or other fruit, sprinkled with mixed nuts OR *Frozen Dessert Bark*	Greek yogurt (full fat) with pineapple chunks OR *Chocolate Buttons* with 2 hard-boiled eggs

*Day 42 is the day on which you can cheat. If you're an exerciser, you may make this a cheat day, meaning all your meals can be "cheats" if you wish. However, make sure you don't binge or stuff yourself, and be sure to limit alcohol intake. If you do not exercise, cheat at only one meal each week. The meals provided in this plan are one example.

CHAPTER 10
SUPPLEMENT FOR SUCCESS

While adding key dietary supplements to your daily meal planning is not necessary to experience success on Always Eat After 7 PM, doing so may help you see faster and longer-lasting results. There is now so much more research on the science of supplements and weight loss than there was 10 years ago.

For instance, research from U.S. and international universities published in such journals as *Molecules*, *Nutrients*, and *Advances in Nutrition* in recent years has demonstrated that dieters who add certain dietary supplements experience more effective results in losing and managing their weight.

But before you even concern yourself with supplements, make sure that you're following the plan to the letter and that you're getting the majority of your protein, carbs, and fats from whole-food sources, such as Portion Volumizing proteins, Super Carbs, vegetables, and friendly fats.

There are a number of supplements I like. You may not need every single one, but it's good to know which ones can help and why you might want to add them. If you choose to supplement and tweak your progress even more, there are some effective supplements that I recommend.

PROTEIN POWDERS

Why should you use them? As previously mentioned, ounce for ounce, protein is the most fat-loss-friendly food because it burns more calories while being digested than any other macronutrient. In other words, protein increases metabolic rate more than any other food.

The biggest challenge people face when following any type of diet is getting adequate amounts of protein from whole foods each day to reap these benefits. This is when protein powder comes in handy and can help you further accelerate your fat loss.

What are they? Designed to be mixed with a liquid, protein powders are basically dehydrated forms of the protein found in foods. The most common come from milk (whey or casein), egg whites, or plant proteins.

I use a protein powder daily, sometimes twice a day. It's the easiest and most convenient way to get enough fat-burning protein in my diet (and protein drinks are delicious!). And with research showing that higher-protein diets lead to twice as much weight loss, it's important you're getting enough.

What should you look for? Reading labels is essential with any type of dietary supplement. Purchase protein powders that are made from grass-fed protein from pasture-raised cows, are cold-pressed, and contain no more than 4 grams of net carbs (total carbs minus the fiber). I prefer products that are formulated with gut-friendly prebiotics and protein-digesting enzymes for better digestion and absorption. It is also important to choose a product that is free from hormones, antibiotics, GMOs, pesticides, gluten, soy, and artificial sweeteners, flavors, colors, and preservatives.

The best type of protein powder is one formulated with two components of milk protein, whey and casein.

How do they help? Whey is a constituent of milk that is separated from milk to make cheese and other dairy products. It is easily digested and rapidly absorbed, and it is the most concentrated source of essential amino acids, including leucine, which is vital for fat burning and for muscle recovery and growth. Whey protein provides the following benefits:

- **It manages appetite.** Whey protein has been shown to reduce appetite more than other sources of protein (like fish, turkey, and eggs). It stimulates the release of key satiety hormones and decreases levels of the "hunger hormone" ghrelin.
- **It supports weight loss.** As an added bonus, whey protein not only helps accelerate fat loss but also helps maintain and build calorie-burning lean muscle. This means whey protein enhances quality weight loss and supports long-term weight maintenance.
- **It promotes healthy aging.** One of the biggest concerns as you get older is holding on to lean muscle, which keeps you youthful and active and promotes overall quality of life. Supplementing with a low-carb protein powder containing whey is a great choice to promote healthy aging.

The protein casein, found in many protein powders, is an anti-aging standout. It helps prevent muscle breakdown even better than whey. The best form of casein in protein powders is micellar casein (MC). MC is usually made by filtering the casein portion of milk from the lactose, fat, and whey through a special process that does not damage the casein protein. Micellar casein is the slowest-digesting of the casein proteins. (Look for this form of casein when you check the labels of protein powders.)

When you use a protein powder that contains both whey and casein, you're getting the best of both worlds. Studies indicate that consuming fast-digesting whey with slow-digesting casein triggers a stronger anabolic (growth-inducing) effect and thus greater muscle growth.

What I recommend: To get all these benefits, **BioTrust Low Carb Protein Powder Blend** is a good choice. It meets all the criteria I listed above.

How to use it: You can take it any time of day to help you optimize your protein intake, supplement your diet, and help you achieve your health and fitness goals. BioTrust Low Carb Protein Powder Blend can be used as a meal replacement, between meals when your appetite for junk food comes calling, before or after exercise, as a nighttime snack to fend off cravings for sweets, or in protein powder recipes (see pages 199–204 for ideas).

PLANT PROTEIN POWDERS

Why should you use them? If you are a vegan, vegetarian, or flexitarian, are sensitive to dairy, are looking to lower your carbon footprint, or simply desire to increase plant-based foods in your diet, it can be very challenging to consume an optimal amount of protein through whole-food sources alone. Among the best solutions is to supplement with a vegan protein powder.

What are they? Formulated from pea protein, brown rice protein, hemp protein, or various other plant proteins (or a combination), these supplements are rich in amino acids and free of both gluten and known allergens.

What should you look for? Not all vegan protein powders are created equal. In fact, many of today's top-selling plant-based protein powders are riddled with cheap, inferior, and potentially dangerous ingredients, additives, and chemicals.

Many plant-based protein powders contain soy protein, for example. In general, soy underperforms compared to other sources of protein when it comes to fat loss, muscle gain, and appetite control. There are also concerns over phytoestrogens and goitrogens, which may negatively affect reproductive hormones and thyroid production, respectively. Further, many vegan protein powders contain GMOs, including soy- and corn-derived ingredients, which typically come from GMO crops. Also, some are contaminated with herbicide and pesticide residues, which are associated with various health concerns, including cancer, inflammation, hormone disruption, and organ damage.

Watch out for products that are formulated with artificial sweeteners, which are linked to various health problems, including impaired carbohydrate tolerance.

How do they help? Based on my research, the most desirable supplemental plant proteins are pea, hemp, and pumpkin seed. As a nutritional source, pea protein offers several advantages: It is highly digestible and offers a favorable amino acid profile. According to scientific analyses, about 18 percent of the protein consists of branched-chain amino acids (BCAAs), which are responsible for muscle growth. Pea protein also contains significant amounts of glutamine (17 percent), which helps sustain immune function; arginine (8.7 percent), which has been shown to promote antioxidant defenses; and lysine (7.3 percent), which has been shown to promote gut uptake of calcium for improved bone health. When tested alongside whey and casein, pea protein showed an intermediate to fast digestion pattern. This suggests a combination of whey and pea protein could be ideal for supporting long endurance-type workouts. Another nutritional plus is satiety. Proteins have long been known for their impact on fullness.

Hemp protein is loaded with both omega-3 and omega-6 fatty acids, in an ideal ratio. It's also rich in gamma linolenic acid (GLA), a fatty acid that supports brain and heart health. Pumpkin seed powder is 70 percent protein and offers a nice, nutty flavor.

What I recommend: One product, in particular, helps you avoid problems connected with many plant protein powders: **BioTrust Harvest Complete Vegan Plant Protein Powder Blend**. It contains 20 grams of complete plant-based protein from pea, pumpkin, and hemp; 4 grams of net carbs from plants; no added sugar; and 6 grams of fiber, including gut-friendly prebiotics.

How to use it: Use it as you would protein powder: as a meal replacement, between meals, or as a nighttime snack. You can also use this vegan protein powder in many great-tasting recipes (see pages 199–204 for examples).

COLLAGEN PROTEIN POWDERS

Why should you use them? As we get older, the body loses its ability to make collagen, one of the primary structural proteins in joints, bones, cartilage, ligaments, tendons, hair, fingernails, blood vessels, spinal disks, the intestinal wall, the blood-brain barrier, and more. Collagen is the glue—the word actually comes from the Greek word for glue—that supports, connects, and holds everything together.

This explains, at least in part, why over time our skin sags and wrinkles, our hair thins out, our nails lose their strength, our joints get stiff and less flexible, and other age-related effects occur. Fortunately, though, you can ramp up your body's collagen production—and reverse these effects—by supplementing with collagen protein powder.

What are they? Collagen protein powders are made from the connective tissue, skin, and bones of animals. They are similar to bone broth or gelatin used for cooking and they contain a substantial amount of protein.

What should you look for? Please understand that not all collagen powders are created equal. For starters, most collagen protein powders come from a single source, such as chicken or cattle. This is important because different parts of the body are supported by different *types* of collagen. For example, collagen types I and III, which come from cattle and fish, are found in our skin, bones, and tendons. Type II collagen, which comes from chicken, is almost exclusively present in the cartilage between bones. While at least 28 different types of collagen have been identified, the three most common are types I, II, and III, which account for 80–90 percent of the collagen in the body.

Even though it can be confusing, try not to get too caught up in the Roman numeral soup. The point here is that if you want to reap the broad range of benefits associated with collagen protein, then you'll want a collagen powder that contains multiple types of collagen from various sources.

In addition to the problem of coming from only a single source, here are some of the other drawbacks of many collagen powders, including bone broth and gelatin supplements:

- They are not broken down into smaller collagen peptides, also known as collagen hydrolysate or hydrolyzed collagen, which are bioactive collagen building blocks that are more easily and readily absorbed than whole collagen protein.
- They are not complete proteins. Collagen protein is typically considered a "low-quality" protein because it is missing one of the essential amino acids (tryptophan), and this means those conventional collagen supplements can't be used to replace dietary protein.
- They taste and/or smell bad—which limits how you can use them and can ruin the taste of whatever you mix them in.
- They don't dissolve well in cold or room-temperature liquids, often leaving a sticky, clumpy mess at the bottom of your glass that's unpleasant to drink.

How does it help? Research shows you can increase your body's collagen levels again by consuming more collagen in your diet, primarily through supplementation. This is true regardless of your age, and that means—in terms of skin, hair, nails, joints, and more—you really can renew and revitalize the way you look and feel and once again enjoy the benefits of healthy collagen levels. These benefits were confirmed in a 2019 review published in the *Journal of Drugs in Dermatology*. After looking into eight studies, the researchers concluded: "Oral collagen supplements also increase skin elasticity, hydration, and dermal collagen density. Collagen supplementation is generally safe with no reported adverse events."

What I recommend: One collagen protein powder, **Ageless Multi-Collagen Protein Powder**, avoids all the above drawbacks of many products on the market. It contains all five key hydrolyzed collagen types (I, II, III, V, and X) from four different food sources: grass-fed, pasture-raised cattle (types I and III); sustainable fish (types I and III); eggshell membrane (types I, V, and X); and undenatured collagen naturally sourced from chicken (type II). While collagen types I, II, and III are extremely critical, type V works hand in hand with types I and III for optimal skin health, and type X is a rare type of collagen that is especially important for bone health.

How to use it: Take 1–2 scoops daily. It is tasteless, and you can add it to coffee, tea, water, protein shakes, soups, oatmeal, yogurt, salad dressings, and more.

KETO SUPPLEMENTS

Why should you use them? Many people have tried a ketogenic diet, in which the body goes into a fat-burning state called ketosis in the absence of carbohydrates. However, they find it extremely hard to stick to because they don't get to eat their favorite carbs—like breads, pasta, rice, desserts, or even fruits. This is one big reason almost everyone gives up on it. Not to mention that there's a laundry list of unfavorable side effects common with the keto diet, such as the dreaded "keto flu," "keto bad breath," constipation, insomnia, reduced physical performance, and more.

That's the bad news; here's the good: you can reap the fat-burning benefits of a keto-type diet by taking a ketosis-stimulating supplement on my plan—*without* having to follow the strict, complicated rules that go along with a true keto diet. This type of supplement is important because it can accelerate your results.

What are they? The keto supplements I'm talking about are generally formulated with medium-chain triglycerides, or MCTs, a type of fat. (Some products are made with exogenous ketone bodies—chemicals that are really not effective. They are cost prohibitive and can lead to digestive distress.)

Most people know there are different types of fats, such as saturated, monounsaturated, and polyunsaturated, which are classifications based on the presence and number of double bonds in a fatty acid's carbon chains. In addition, fatty acids can vary in length and the number of carbon atoms they contain, ranging from 4 to 22 carbons (or more).

Most fats we eat are long-chain fatty acids, containing 16–18 carbon atoms. Found in coconut oil, palm kernel oil, butter, milk, yogurt, and cheese, MCTs are fats with 6–10 carbons. Caprylic acid (C8) and capric acid (C10) are the two most prominent MCTs. But C8 is the most ketogenic MCT. It has been shown to be up to 3 times more ketogenic than C10 and 4 times higher than coconut oil.

Because of their shorter length, MCTs are metabolized and transported differently in the body than the more common long-chain fatty acids. For example, they are transported directly to the liver, where they are quickly and efficiently burned for energy. Because they are transported directly to the liver, they bypass adipose (fat) tissue, which makes them less likely to be stored as body fat.

What's more, MCTs are known to have a high ketogenicity, which means they are readily converted to ketone bodies. This also means MCTs quickly switch your metabolism into fat-burning mode. In other words, with MCTs, you can induce ketosis without cutting carbs.

What should you look for? You want to find a supplement that is formulated with only C8—and preferably in a powdered form as opposed to an oil (which can be hard on the digestive system). MCT oils, even some powders, almost always contain both C8 *and* C10. To make matters worse, many MCT oils are diluted even further with the addition of C12 (lauric acid), which many don't even consider a true MCT. C10 and C12 are less powerful MCTs that do not provide the same fast, powerful benefits as C8. MCT supplements that contain only C8 will specify "C8 caprylic acid" somewhere on the supplement facts panel and/or in the ingredients listing.

How do they help? When your ketone levels are elevated with help from supplementation, you can experience increased energy levels, mental clarity, and focus. Plus, your metabolism runs more efficiently and you feel less hungry, with fewer cravings. Then of course there's the benefit of fat loss—which we're all interested in. British researchers studied the benefits of ketone supplementation and concluded that it is a practical and effective way to achieve the fat-burning state of ketosis. They published their report in 2017 in *Frontiers in Physiology.*

What I recommend: Your best bet is **Keto Elevate** from BioTrust. Unlike other MCT oils and MCT oil powders, this supplement is pure C8. It is not watered down with less powerful MCTs (it contains no C10 and no C12) or other additives and artificial sweeteners that you find in a lot of these products.

How to use it: Take 1–2 scoops daily, added to coffee or tea (it makes a great creamer), protein shakes, yogurt, baked goods, and more.

SUPER GREENS POWDERS

Why should you use them? If plant foods are in short supply in your diet, not only are you missing out on crucial vitamins, minerals, and fiber, but you may also be lacking in powerful compounds called polyphenols. These natural compounds give plants their vibrant color and contribute to their unique taste and smell. But more than that, they are highly regarded for their powerful antioxidant properties. And considering that excessive oxidative stress is one of the main drivers of human health issues and aging, it's no surprise that consuming both copious amounts and varieties of polyphenols plays a huge role in keeping your body healthy, your appetite under control, and your digestive system running smoothly, among many other benefits. One of the best ways to ensure that you're getting the benefits of polyphenols is to supplement with a super greens powder.

What are they? These supplements are easy-to-digest, concentrated, pulverized vegetables and fruits. They are an efficient way to make up for any deficits you might have if you're not meeting the minimum daily recommendations for fruit (1½–2 cups per day) and vegetables (2–3 cups per day).

What should you look for? As with protein powders, be careful about super greens powder products. It's very important to make sure they are organic. Many are not, and they are therefore laced with GMOs, pesticides, herbicides, and artificial sweeteners. Also, look for products made from many different plants. The more plant components included, the better. Some contain only a few plant foods ground together and are therefore lower in polyphenols and other nutrients. The more polyphenols in a supplement, the healthier the product will be.

How do they help? Super greens powdered supplements are being widely studied for their health benefits. Case in point: In a study published in the *International Journal of Molecular Science* in 2011, 10 healthy adults consumed either 3 or 6 teaspoons of powdered greens a day for four weeks. At the end of the experimental period, there was a significant spike in their antioxidants, polyphenols, and other nutrients. Based on this observation, the researchers concluded that supplementation with powdered greens could help fend off chronic diseases. That's a pretty powerful benefit from a few teaspoons!

What I recommend: BioTrust manufactures a product called **MetaboGreens**, a blend of 45 polyphenol-rich super greens, vegetables, fruits, herbs, and spices. It is made from organic ingredients and free from GMOs, pesticides, herbicides, gluten, dairy, soy, and artificial sweeteners.

This supplement features over 5 grams of prebiotic fiber (see page 103) from organic acacia gum, organic inulin, and beta glucan. These prebiotic fibers are like fuel for healthy gut bacteria. They help increase the body's level of probiotics while helping reduce the number of unhealthy bacteria, which are harmful to health.

MetaboGreens super greens powder also provides an energizing blend of adaptogenic mushrooms. Adaptogens are herbs that help keep you mentally and physically in the "optimal zone" by promoting energy, focus, adaptation to stress, stress resilience, and improved physical performance.

How to use it: Mix 1 scoop of MetaboGreens super greens formula with 8 ounces of water or your favorite beverage. MetaboGreens mixed with water makes a perfect 3-Minute Fat-Burning Morning Ritual when you are doing intermittent fasting and get tired of lemon water or citrus water. Or you can add it to your protein powder shakes.

You can also use it in the afternoon for a natural, caffeine-free pick-me-up. Or you can whip up a serving of MetaboGreens before or between meals to help reduce cravings and promote appetite management. Also, try it before, during, or after exercise to help you hydrate and replenish.

OMEGA 3 FATS (FISH AND KRILL OIL)

Why should you use them? The body requires polyunsaturated essential fatty acids (EFAs), omega-3 fats and omega-6 fats. However, it cannot produce them on its own. So you *must* get them through food, supplementation, or a combination of the two. (This is why these fats are called "essential," just like essential vitamins and minerals—the body needs them, but they must be obtained through diet. Nonessential nutrients, on the other hand, are those that the body needs but produces on its own.)

What are they? The omega-3s are found primarily in marine sources (cold-water fish and ocean-dwelling microalgae), as well as in plants such as flaxseed, hemp, and pumpkin seeds. All forms of omega-3s are high in EPA (eicosapentaenoic acid) and DHA (docosahexaenoic acid). Omega-6 fats come from mostly seed oils and nuts.

Experts estimate that throughout human history, the optimal ratio for consumption of omega-6 to omega-3 fatty acids was about 1:1 or 2:1. With the contemporary diet, the average ratio consumed has shifted dramatically in favor of omega-6 fatty acids to 20:1.

Consuming too many omega-6 and not enough omega-3 fatty acids may lead to an "exaggerated" inflammatory response. In fact, this imbalance has been tied to virtually all negative health outcomes and accelerated aging. According to researchers, there are three main explanations for this heavy imbalance of omega fatty acids:

1. a decrease in consumption of omega-3 fatty acids from natural food sources
2. the widespread presence of refined vegetable oils (such as soybean, safflower, sunflower, corn, canola, and cottonseed oils) in the Western diet
3. the consumption of meat from farm animals raised on oil seeds rich in omega-6 fats (such as corn and soy)

Obviously, reducing consumption of processed foods (which are rife with omega-6-rich oils) and low-quality products from farm-raised animals is a key step to resolving the problematic omega imbalance. On the flip side, the other crucial piece of the puzzle is making sure you're getting plenty of omega-3 fatty acids, particularly EPA and DHA, the two most prominent omega-3 fatty acids.

Along these lines, the American Heart Association recommends adults consume a minimum of 500 milligrams a day of EPA and DHA, and often more is better. Unfortunately, the average person consumes only about a quarter of that recommended amount (around 135 milligrams a day). With this in mind, it's just plain smart to use an omega-3 supplement containing DHA and EPA.

What should you look for? Taking an omega-3 supplement is one of the smartest supplement choices you can make. But when it comes to choosing an omega-3 supplement, buyer beware. Many omega-3 supplements are contaminated with heavy metals or other dangerous toxins (such as PCBs, dioxins, and furans). These can be harmful to your health and can lead to endocrine, neurobehavioral, and developmental disruption. Also, make sure the supplement is certified by the International Fish Oil Standards (IFOS) program, the only third-party testing and certification program for fish oils that sets standards for purity, potency, and freshness. Finally, a good omega-3 supplement should contain five times as much DHA as EPA.

How do they help? Omega-3 supplementation is important on Always Eat After 7 PM. One reason is that omega-3s have been shown to help the body lose weight and improve body composition. Plus, they support muscle building by improving muscle fiber integrity and increasing insulin sensitivity. In addition, they help reduce inflammation and support joint health, both critical for effective athletic performance. Omega-3 fatty acids lower cholesterol, inhibit the tendency of blood cells to form dangerous clots, and reduce the formation of fatty plaques.

What I recommend: Try **BioTrust OmegaKrill 5X**. It is packed with DHA and received a five-star rating from the IFOS program. Its oils are processed from sardines, anchovies, and krill—three superior sources of omega-3 fatty acids. It is formulated with astaxanthin—one of nature's most powerful antioxidants.

How to use it: Take just 3 small soft gels daily, one with each meal or snack.

PROBIOTIC AND PREBIOTIC SUPPLEMENTS FOR DIGESTIVE AND GUT HEALTH

Why should you use them? Probiotic supplements have so many benefits that it might be considered reckless to not take them! Although research is ongoing, there's good evidence that probiotics, by guarding the gut, may prove to be a protector against all types of diseases.

What are they? Probiotics are friendly, living microbes in the gut that help us stay healthy. In fact, you carry about four pounds of microbes (bacteria, yeasts, fungi, and so forth) in your gut—that's about 100 trillion microbes. Considering there are over 30 trillion cells in the human body, this means you are made up of over three times more microbes than cells.

Most (but not all) probiotics are bacteria (such as lactic acid bacteria and bifidobacteria), so you'll often hear people refer to probiotics and probiotic supplements as "good bacteria."

PREBIOTICS VERSUS PROBIOTICS: WHAT'S THE DIFFERENCE?

In addition to hearing about probiotics, you may have also heard the term *prebiotics*. What's the difference between a prebiotic and a probiotic? In simple terms, prebiotics are like fuel for healthy gut bacteria and serve as food for probiotics. Prebiotics help increase levels of "good" bacteria while helping reduce the number of "bad" bacteria, which promotes a healthy balance of gut bacteria.

But that may not be the only set of tricks up the sleeve of prebiotics. Probiotics "feed" on prebiotics via fermentation, and a by-product of this process is the production of short-chain fatty acids (such as butyrate, acetate, and propionate), which fuel the immune system, stimulate the production of appetite-suppressing hormones, support healthy mitochondria, and offer neuroenhancing effects.

So, when it comes to a prebiotic versus a probiotic supplement, which is more important? They both are! In fact, when you combine prebiotics with probiotics that work synergistically with one another, your probiotic supplement becomes what's referred to as a symbiotic. Some researchers have gone so far as to describe the combination as a "fountain of life."

What should you look for? When you purchase a probiotic supplement, the probiotics must be alive when you take them. Unfortunately, a substantial number of conventional probiotics are dead before you take them due to poor manufacturing practices and storage conditions. On top of that, because probiotics are extremely sensitive to stomach acid and bile, research shows that, on average, as little as 10–25 percent of probiotics may actually reach the gut—which is where they need to be to flex their figurative muscle.

Also, you want a product that contains probiotics that are protected by acid-resistant technology (to protect them from stomach and bile acids). An example is microencapsulation technology. It wraps probiotics in an acid-resistant coating that increases their viability and activity. Also, certain probiotics (such as strains from the *Bacillus* genus) are naturally heat stable and acid resistant, making them great options as well.

Look for a multi-strain probiotic that has a variety of friendly bacteria in it. This way, you help ensure a healthy balance of gut bacteria, a healthy digestive tract, and a healthy immune system. The probiotic should contain prebiotics too. Also, the total number of probiotics matters (measured in colony-forming units, or CFUs). According to the International Scientific Association for Probiotics and Prebiotics, a minimum of 1 billion CFUs (per probiotic) is a good starting point, and generally speaking, more is typically considered better

How do they help? Science has begun unraveling many potential benefits of probiotics, such as boosting mood, strengthening the immune system, helping with stress and anxiety, improving cognitive function, supporting weight management, improving appetite control, enhancing recovery and sports performance, and more.

What I recommend: The probiotic I helped develop, **BioTrust Pro-X10**, is an excellent choice. It provides 10 billion CFUs daily of six "super strains" of probiotics for a broad spectrum effect:

- *Bacillus subtilis*
- *Bifidobacterium breve*
- *Bifidobacterium lactis*
- *Lactobacillus acidophilus*
- *Lactobacillus plantarum*
- *Lactobacillus rhamnosus*

It is manufactured using microencapsulation technology, and it contains PreforPro®, a next-generation prebiotic that is unlike other prebiotics that require large servings and several days to begin working.

How to use it: Take 1 capsule, twice daily.

SAMPLE DAILY SUPPLEMENT SCHEDULE

Timeline	Meal Schedule	Supplement Plan
30–60 minutes after waking up	Breakfast Smart Snack (week 1 only) OR 3-Minute Fat-Burning Morning Ritual Drink	2–3 scoops of BioTrust Low Carb Protein Powder Blend shake (week 1 only) OR 1 scoop of MetaboGreens
8 AM to noon	Optional 1 or 2 cups of coffee	Add 1 scoop of Ageless Multi-Collagen Protein Powder OR 1 scoop of Keto Elevate to a cup of coffee or protein shake
Noon to 3 PM	Energizing Lunch	Take 1 Pro-X10 capsule AND 3 OmegaKrill 5X softgel capsules
5 PM to 7 PM	Huge Evening Dinner	Take 1 Pro-X10 capsule
Pre-bedtime	Pre-bedtime Fat-Burning Snack	2–3 scoops of BioTrust Low Carb Protein Powder Blend shake OR 2 scoops of Harvest Complete Vegan Plant Protein Powder Blend shake Feel free to add 1 scoop of Ageless Multi-Collagen Protein Powder OR 1 scoop of Keto Elevate

Note: Protein powders and smoothie recipes can be used as meal replacements whenever necessary.

GET 25 PERCENT OFF ALL BIOTRUST SUPPLEMENTS AS AN ALWAYS EAT AFTER 7 PM VIP

As a VIP owner of the *Always Eat After* 7 PM book, you are entitled to a very special 25 percent discount on any and all supplements at BioTrust.com. There you can find BioTrust Low Carb Protein Powder Blend, MetaboGreens 45X super greens, OmegaKrill 5X fish oil, Pro-X10 probiotics, Ageless Core daily multivitamins, Protein Brownies, and more.

To secure your savings, just use the VIP code **ALWAYSVIP** at checkout. The code can be used only once, so be sure to stock up, as there are no quantity or product restrictions. Enjoy the perks of being a VIP!

PART III
HIT THE KITCHEN

CHAPTER 11
PREPPING YOUR KITCHEN

Planning for each phase of Always Eat After 7 PM is one of the keys to success. It's been said that nobody ever plans to fail—they just fail to plan! Additionally, you're much more likely to make great food choices when you plan and cover your bases ahead of time. Proper planning requires three easy actions: mapping out weekly menus, shopping, and food prep—in that order.

PLAN YOUR WEEKLY MENUS

In each phase of the plan, I've shown you how to structure your meals and your nighttime snack. There is a template you can use, especially if you want to customize your meals. Otherwise, I provide 14 days of sample menus for each phase. You can certainly follow these menus to the letter if you wish, but they are equally useful as a starting place to develop your own meal plans.

SHOP FOR APPROVED FOOD

Once you have your meal plan for the week in place, you'll need to go grocery shopping for anything that's currently not in your pantry or fridge. Buying your groceries ahead of time will let you prep and cook in advance for additional convenience.

Making healthy choices at the grocery store keeps you on track through every phase of the plan. Look over the recipes and the meal choices, and decide what you need to purchase. You may already have many items in your kitchen now; what you buy depends on what you have on hand and what you intend to prepare.

PREP FOR CONVENIENCE

Instead of panicking about what to put on the table or frantically trying to throw something together, get in the habit of meal prepping. It involves taking a couple of hours on the weekend or during the week to prep your food for the upcoming week. It ensures that you have your meals ready quickly, no matter how busy your days get.

Another huge benefit of meal prepping is portion control. We're often seduced to eat a little more, go for seconds, or stop at a restaurant that serves you an entire cow on a plate. But when you prep meals at home in advance, you can give yourself just the right amount of food—exactly as prescribed on the Always Eat After 7 PM plan.

There are several ways to prep and cook in advance, including weekly, twice weekly, daily, and long term (which involves freezing). Personally, I prefer going with the twice-weekly approach, but let's quickly review all four.

With the weekly option, you might spend time on Sunday (or a day when you have lots of spare time) doing all your major cooking for the week—cutting veggies for salads and placing them in containers, cooking Super Carbs so they can be reheated, hard-boiling eggs, baking or roasting proteins, and/or making desserts. You'd then store the prepped food in the fridge to be quickly assembled into meals and reheated.

The twice-weekly option is very similar, with the exception that you prep and cook twice a week (once at the beginning of the week and then again midweek). I like this option best because it's still highly convenient and you can enjoy fresher food from Thursday to Saturday.

The third option is to cook all your food for the day each morning, but this may not be realistic if you're getting kids to school or rushing off to work. But if you're home all day or have a flexible schedule, this is a great approach. You can also try prepping the ingredients in the morning, then cooking them in the evening.

Finally, the long-term option is something you can do anytime. With many dishes, you can prepare all the ingredients needed for a meal, place them in ziplock freezer bags, and toss them in the freezer. They can then be thawed when needed. The meals are not cooked the day they are prepared—just the ingredients that go in them. If you are going to slow-cook your dinner, put the frozen ingredients in the slow cooker in the morning and the entrée will be cooked by dinnertime. Then just make a salad and some sides to accompany the meal. You can also freeze certain leftovers, such as soups and casseroles, and dishes like lasagna.

It's really up to you as long as the approach you select doesn't leave you unprepared.

Now, here are several meal prep hacks that help too:

- So that you can see the contents, use containers that are clear plastic or glass to store produce in the refrigerator that you have already washed, cut up, and pre-portioned for snacks or meal ingredients. I like to use clear glass containers rather than plastic because they are more environmentally friendly, but clear plastic containers or sealable bags also work.
- Cook protein in bulk at the beginning of the week. For me, this means cooking several days' worth of chicken breasts or thighs, extra-lean ground beef,

and fish. These are staple sources of protein I eat weekly, and having them ready to go makes eating these favorites easy. (If you're cooking fish, though, eat it within 48 hours of cooking because it has a shorter refrigerator life than other proteins.)

- Keep healthy, highly versatile ingredients on hand. One example is beans, which are not only a great source of plant protein and a wonderful Super Carb but also an ingredient in lots of dishes, including salads, soups, and chili. Another example is grains such as quinoa or rice. They store easily in airtight containers and can serve as a side dish to any meal. I also recommend frozen steam-in-bag veggies. Frozen vegetables offer the same nutritional value as fresh ones, but with the convenience of microwave cooking in less than five minutes. What's more, they make great side dishes.
- Love your leftovers. Don't stress out by thinking you have to cook a new meal when you still have some food left from the last one. The meal plans in this book call for leftovers on some days so that no food goes to waste. You can also repurpose leftovers by combining them with other foods to make new meals. Try slicing leftover chicken and tossing it into black bean pasta for a great pasta salad. Or use leftover potatoes for lunch (or a cheat day breakfast). Roasted veggies from dinner are delicious on salads for lunch. There's no end to how creative you can get with leftovers.
- Cook wisely for a crowd of one. If you are single, you probably don't need to cook that much food. To make sure no food goes to waste, purchase food in smaller portions—a Cornish hen instead of a big chicken, a single pork chop rather than a large pork roast, a single fish fillet instead of a family pack. Then prep and cook only what you're going to eat.

GO!

As we get ready to turn to the recipes, remember the importance of proteins, Super Carbs, non-starchy vegetables, fruits, and friendly fats—which all form the foundation of Always Eat After 7 PM. These are the foods designed to change your metabolism, regulate key hormones, and get you to your ideal weight.

Day by day, over the upcoming weeks, you will begin losing the weight you want to lose, and living the empowered, energized lifestyle you want to live. Once you get started cycling through the phases, once you begin eating all these delicious foods—even after 7 PM!—it gets easier and easier.

CHAPTER 12
MOUTHWATERING FAT-BURNING RECIPES

My friend and colleague Diana Keuilian has provided delicious recipes for breakfasts, lunches, dinners, desserts, pre-bedtime snacks, and even some healthier cheat day treats to enjoy on the Always Eat After 7 PM plan—along with my favorite smoothies for quick and convenient meals or snacks. As you browse through the recipes, please keep the following in mind:

- The Acceleration Phase is lower in carbohydrates than the other two phases. I have thus added the icon to the recipes that have strict carb limits, contain no Super Carbs, and can be enjoyed in the Acceleration Phase. This icon helps you select recipes for this phase.
- Some of the recipes use natural sweeteners such as erythritol, molasses, honey, coconut sugar, or fruit sources like apples or juice. The amount of sweetener is so tiny that it barely affects calorie or carbohydrate counts and adds amazing flavor.
- The recipe portions are not universal. Just remember that, as I've mentioned, men and women of different sizes require different amounts of food, and your needs will vary slightly depending on phase. So the number of "servings" in any given dish may be different for you; this is the reasoning behind the use of the hand/fist portion method (see page 70).

I have designated on the meal plans where you should increase or decrease your serving size in certain recipes. Before preparing a recipe, check its calorie count per serving. Sometimes you can double up on a serving if you are a man, and sometimes women have to cut a serving in half. You should also pay attention to fullness cues and adjust accordingly. It is always better to underestimate portion sizes than to overestimate.

INSTANT POT EGG WHITE BITES

PREP: 10 MINUTES | COOK: 23 MINUTES | MAKES: 7 SERVINGS

6 egg whites
2 eggs
¼ cup low-fat cottage cheese
¼ teaspoon sea salt
Coconut oil spray
¼ cup chopped roasted red bell pepper
½ cup finely chopped fresh spinach

1. Combine the egg whites, eggs, cottage cheese, and salt in a blender. Blend on high until smooth.
2. Grease a silicone egg bite mold with a small amount of coconut oil spray. Evenly divide the bell pepper and spinach in the wells. Pour the egg mixture over the top, dividing it evenly among the wells.
3. Place a cup of water in an Instant Pot along with a handled trivet. Carefully position the filled silicone mold on top of the trivet. Secure the lid, position the steam release valve to "sealing," and cook at high pressure for 8 minutes.
4. Once the cooking cycle is complete, allow the pressure to release for 5 minutes, then move the steam release to venting. After the floating valve in the lid drops, it's safe to open.
5. Use oven mitts to remove the trivet from the pot. Allow the egg bites to cool for 5 to 10 minutes.

Quick Tip: You'll need a silicone egg bite mold to make this recipe—look on Amazon if you don't have one already. Don't have an Instant Pot? No worries! Simply place the mold on a baking sheet and bake at 350 degrees F for 40 minutes.

NUTRITION
Calories: 43
Fat: 2 g
Carbohydrates: 1 g
Sodium: 162 mg
Fiber: 1 g
Protein: 6 g
Sugar: 1 g

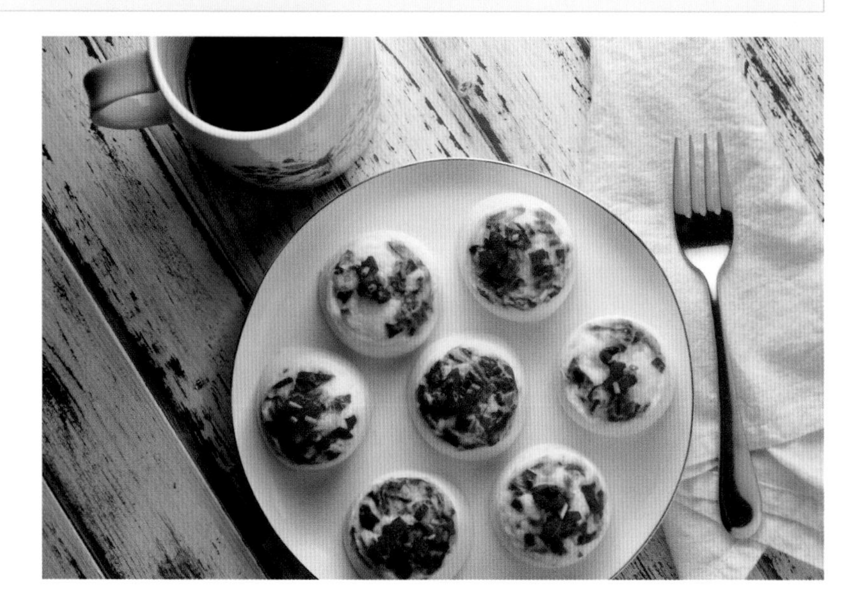

PUMPKIN PIE EGG MUFFINS

PREP: 15 MINUTES | COOK: 22 MINUTES | MAKES: 6 SERVINGS

Coconut oil for greasing, optional
1 banana
2 tablespoons pumpkin puree
6 eggs
½ teaspoon ground cinnamon, plus more for sprinkling
Pinch of sea salt
Cinnamon
Granular erythritol (such as Swerve)

1. Preheat the oven to 350 degrees F. Line 6 muffin tin cups with silicone muffin liners or grease with coconut oil.
2. In a medium bowl, mash the banana until smooth. Mix in the pumpkin. Add the eggs, cinnamon, and salt. Whisk until fully combined. Fill the muffin cups.
3. Bake for 22 to 24 minutes, until the eggs are fully set. Sprinkle with cinnamon and granular erythritol.

Quick Tip: It's a great idea to use reusable silicone muffin liners when making egg muffins because they tend to stick to pans and paper liners. Silicone liners are virtually stick-free.

NUTRITION

Calories: 82 | Fat: 4 g | Carbohydrates: 5 g | Sodium: 62 mg | Fiber: 1 g | Protein: 6 g | Sugar: 3 g

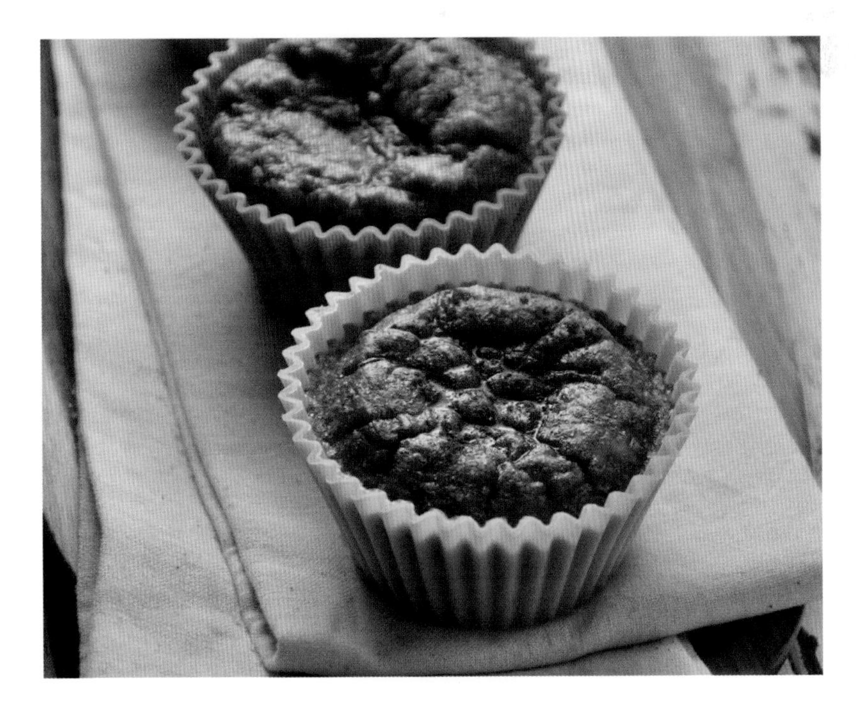

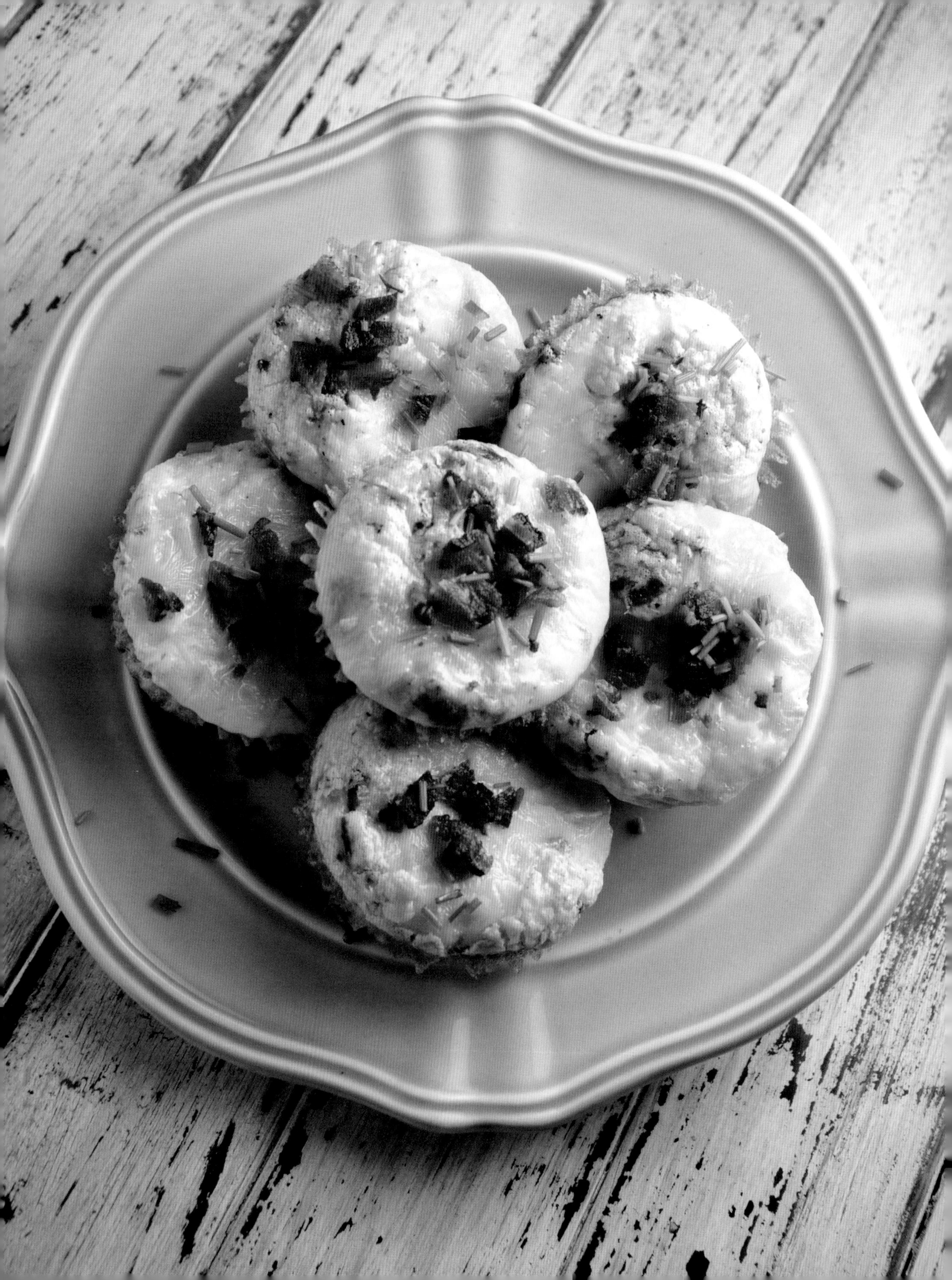

BACON AND CARAMELIZED ONION EGG MUFFINS

PREP: 20 MINUTES | COOK: 20 MINUTES | MAKES: 6 SERVINGS

Coconut oil for greasing, optional
2 strips nitrate-free bacon
⅓ cup finely chopped yellow onion
6 eggs
Sea salt and black pepper, to taste
1 tablespoon minced fresh chives, for garnish

1. Preheat the oven to 350 degrees F. Line 6 muffin tin cups with paper muffin liners or lightly grease with coconut oil.
2. Cook the bacon in a skillet over medium-high heat until crispy. Remove the strips from the skillet; let them cool and then crumble the strips. Reduce the heat to medium. Add the onion to the skillet and sauté for 7 to 8 minutes, until soft and caramelized.
3. In a medium bowl, combine the crumbled bacon and caramelized onion. Add the eggs and season with salt and pepper. Whisk until fully combined. Fill the muffin cups two-thirds full with the egg mixture.
4. Bake for 20 to 22 minutes, until the eggs are fully set. Sprinkle the chives on the muffins.

Quick Tip: Think of these egg muffins as a blank backdrop against which you can add any array of flavors. Using the egg base, add whatever meats, veggies, spices, or fresh herbs you love and have available. And you don't even have to confine yourself to savory items. Try adding ground cinnamon and sautéed apples to egg muffins for a healthy spin on apple fritters!

NUTRITION

Calories: 109 | Fat: 7 g | Carbohydrates: 3 g | Sodium: 251 mg | Fiber: 3 g | Protein: 9 g | Sugar: 1 g

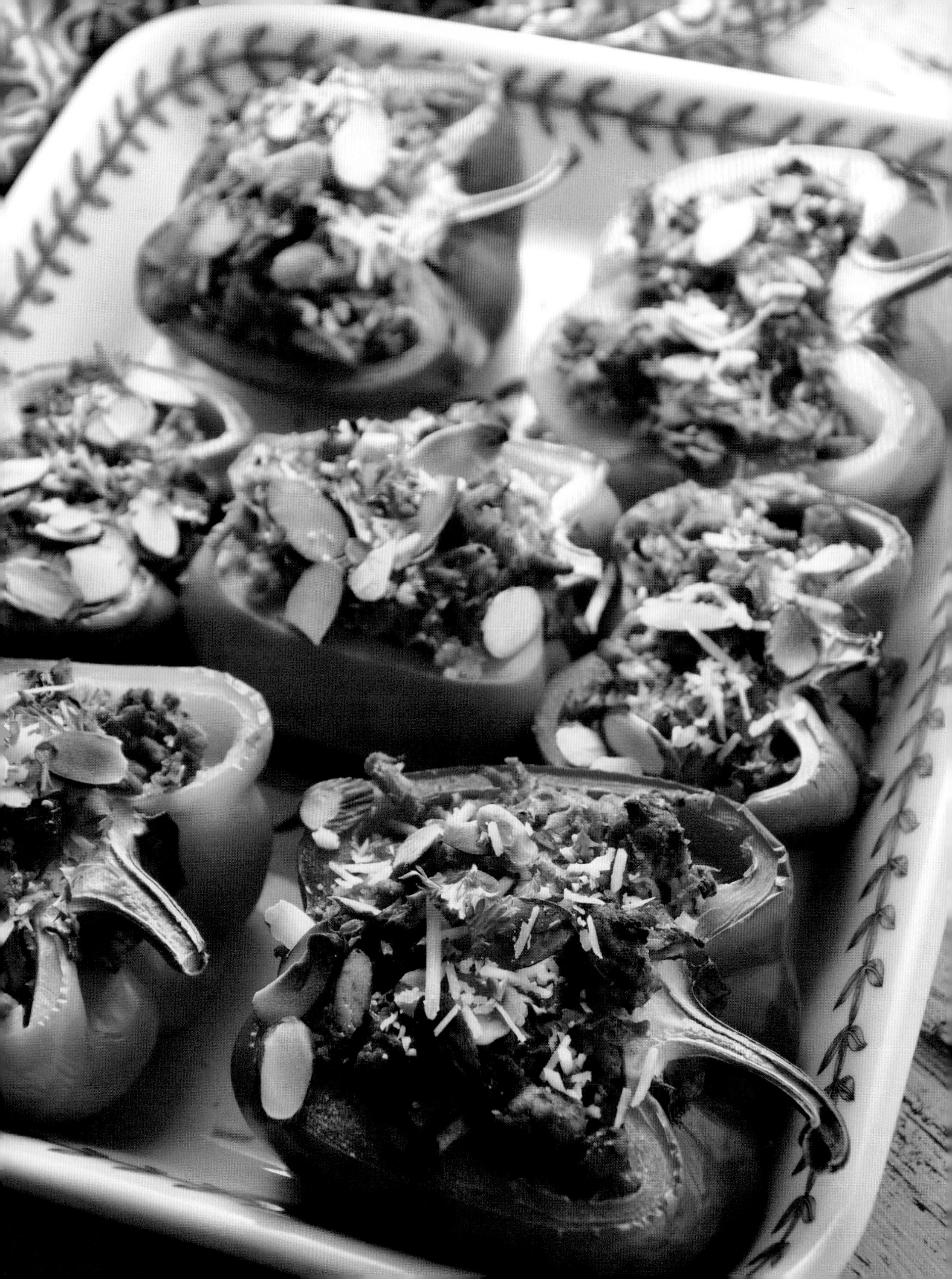

STUFFED BELL PEPPERS

PREP: 25 MINUTES | COOK: 16 MINUTES | MAKES: 8 STUFFED PEPPER HALVES

1 tablespoon olive oil
2 carrots, shredded
½ yellow onion, shredded
Pinch of sea salt
½ teaspoon ground cinnamon
1 pound lean ground turkey
1 head cauliflower, shredded
⅓ cup golden raisins
1 cup chicken broth
Pinch of black pepper
4 bell peppers (1 each of green, red, yellow, and orange)
2 tablespoons sliced almonds
Grated Parmesan cheese (optional)
Minced fresh parsley (optional)

1. Preheat the oven to 400 degrees F.
2. Warm the olive oil over medium-high heat in a large skillet. Add the carrots and onion. Cook for about 3 minutes, until slightly softened. Add the salt, cinnamon, and ground turkey. Cook until the meat is browned and the onions are soft, about 15 minutes. Add the cauliflower, raisins, broth, and black pepper. Cook for about 5 minutes, until the liquid is absorbed.
3. Halve the bell peppers lengthwise, removing the seeds and membranes. Divide the turkey mixture among the bell pepper halves. Place the stuffed bell pepper halves in a 13 × 9-inch baking dish. Add enough water to reach the midpoint on the peppers, being careful not to get the water into the peppers.
4. Cover the pan with foil and bake for 10 minutes. Remove the foil, sprinkle each pepper with sliced almonds, and return to the oven for 5 minutes. Turn on the broiler and broil until the almonds are toasted, about 1 minute. Sprinkle with Parmesan cheese and parsley, if desired.

Quick Tip: This recipe produces crisp-tender bell peppers. If you prefer your bell peppers to be softer, take a few moments to blanch the peppers before stuffing. To do so, drop the seeded bell peppers in a pot of boiling water for 3 minutes, then transfer to a bowl of ice water.

NUTRITION

Calories: 155 | Fat: 6 g | Carbohydrates: 13 g | Sodium: 120 mg | Fiber: 4 g | Protein: 14 g | Sugar: 5 g

CLASSIC CHICKEN STEW

PREP: 15 MINUTES | COOK: 90 MINUTES | MAKES: 8 SERVINGS

1½ pounds boneless, skinless chicken thighs, cut into 1-inch pieces
Sea salt and black pepper, to taste
2 tablespoons plus 1 teaspoon olive oil, divided
1 yellow onion, diced
1½ teaspoons minced fresh garlic
1 teaspoon minced fresh thyme
1 tablespoon coconut flour
4 cups broth (any type)
½ cup dry white wine
½ sweet potato, peeled and diced
¾ cup peeled and diced celery root
½ cup chopped zucchini
1½ carrots, cut into ½-inch slices
1 dried bay leaf
2 tablespoons minced fresh parsley

1. Preheat the oven to 300 degrees F and move a rack to the lowest position. Generously season the chicken with salt and pepper.
2. Heat 1 tablespoon of the olive oil in a large soup pot over medium-high heat. Add half of the chicken and cook until browned, about 5 minutes per side. Transfer the cooked chicken to a plate. Repeat with another 1 tablespoon of the olive oil and the other half of the chicken.
3. Add the remaining 1 teaspoon olive oil to the pot over medium-high heat. Add the onion. Cook, stirring often, for 5 minutes. Add the garlic and thyme and cook for 3 minutes. Add the coconut flour and brown for 2 minutes.
4. Stir in the broth and wine. Add the sweet potato, celery root, zucchini, carrots, and bay leaf. Add the chicken to the pot and bring to a simmer. Cover and transfer to the preheated oven. Bake for 1 hour. Remove the bay leaf, garnish with the fresh parsley, and serve warm.

NUTRITION

Calories: 125 | Fat: 5 g | Carbohydrates: 4 g | Sodium: 256 mg | Fiber: 1 g | Protein: 14 g | Sugar: 1.5 g

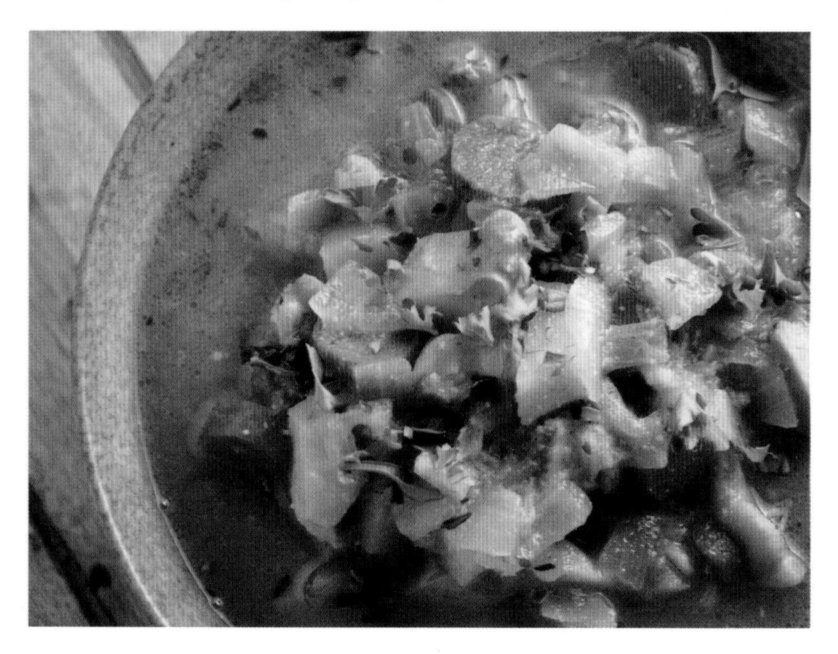

CURRIED PUMPKIN SOUP WITH CHICKEN AND QUINOA

PREP: 5 MINUTES | COOK: 20 MINUTES | MAKES: 12 SERVINGS

1 tablespoon coconut oil
1 yellow onion, diced
1 teaspoon minced fresh garlic
1 tablespoon minced fresh ginger
2 teaspoons curry powder
1 teaspoon ground cumin
½ teaspoon sea salt
1 (15-ounce) can pumpkin puree
1 (13.66-ounce) can full-fat unsweetened coconut milk
3 cups chicken broth
Black pepper, to taste
1 cup cooked quinoa
2 cups shredded cooked chicken
2 tablespoons roasted pumpkin seeds (pepitas)
¼ cup minced red bell pepper, for garnish (optional)

1. In a large soup pot, heat the coconut oil over medium-high heat. Add the onion. Cook, stirring often, until soft, about 5 minutes. Add the garlic and ginger and cook for another 3 minutes. Add the curry, cumin, and salt. Continue cooking for 2 minutes.
2. Stir in the pumpkin, coconut milk, and broth. Increase the heat to high in order to bring the soup to a boil. Reduce the heat to low and simmer for 10 minutes. Remove from the heat.
3. Use an immersion blender to puree the soup until smooth. Season with pepper. Divide the quinoa and shredded chicken between the bowls. Garnish with the pepitas and, if desired, bell pepper.

Quick Tip: This recipe calls for cooked quinoa. This Super Carb is great to pre-cook as part of your meal prepping and have on hand to throw into salads and soups or serve as a quick side dish. To cook quinoa, add 1 cup of uncooked quinoa to 2 cups of water with a pinch of salt in a medium pot. Bring to a boil. Cover, reduce the heat to medium-low, and simmer for 15 to 20 minutes. Remove from the heat and set aside for 5 minutes. Uncover and fluff with a fork.

NUTRITION
Calories: 199
Fat: 11 g
Carbohydrates: 13 g
Sodium: 360 mg
Fiber: 1 g
Protein: 12 g
Sugar: 1 g

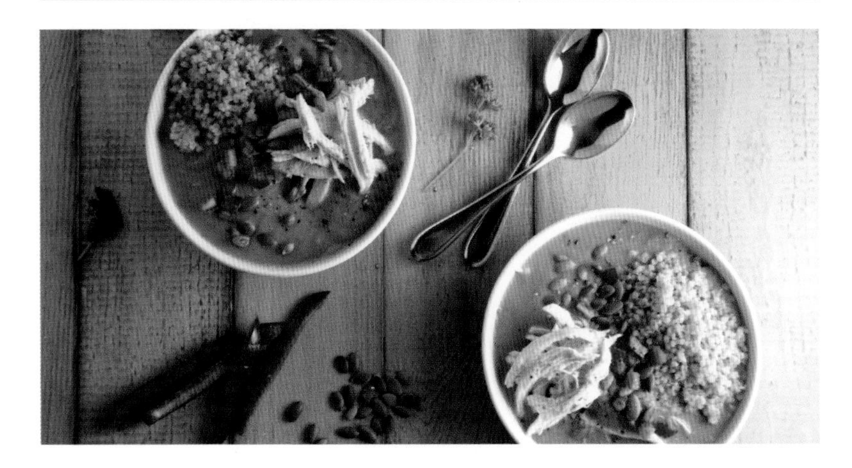

THAI COCONUT SHRIMP SOUP

PREP: 20 MINUTES | COOK: 17 MINUTES | MAKES: 8 SERVINGS

For the Cauliflower Rice

1 head cauliflower
1 teaspoon olive oil
Sea salt and black pepper, to taste

For the Soup

1 teaspoon coconut oil
1 large shallot, sliced
1 tablespoon minced fresh garlic
1 tablespoon minced fresh ginger
1 tablespoon minced lemongrass
4 cups chicken or vegetable broth
2 (13.66-ounce) cans full-fat unsweetened coconut milk
¼ cup fish sauce
2 tablespoons lime juice, plus 1 lime, cut into wedges, for garnish
⅛ teaspoon liquid stevia
½ pound uncooked large shrimp, peeled and deveined
1 Thai chile, thinly sliced into rings with seeds
1 cucumber, halved lengthwise, seeded, and sliced into half-moons
1 red bell pepper, seeded and diced
¼ cup fresh basil leaves, for garnish

1. For the cauliflower rice: Wash the cauliflower, discard the leaves, and chop into small pieces. Process the cauliflower in a food processor until the size of rice grains. In a large skillet, heat the olive oil over medium heat. Add the riced cauliflower. Sauté for about 5 minutes, until tender. Season with salt and pepper.
2. For the soup: Heat the coconut oil in a large saucepan over medium heat. Add the shallot, garlic, ginger, and lemongrass. Sauté, stirring often, for about 5 minutes, until soft. Avoid browning to keep your soup color bright white; if the ingredients are cooking too fast, reduce the heat slightly.
3. Add the broth, coconut milk, fish sauce, lime juice, and stevia. Bring to a simmer and cook for 5 minutes.
4. Stir in the shrimp and chile rings and simmer until the shrimp are just cooked, about 2 minutes. Avoid overcooking the shrimp, to prevent them from becoming tough. Remove the soup from the heat.
5. Off the heat, add the cucumber and bell pepper. Place a scoop of cauliflower rice in each serving bowl and ladle soup over it. Garnish with the fresh basil and lime wedges.

Quick Tip: A few helpful tips for making the very best Thai Coconut Shrimp Soup:

- Be careful not to brown any of the ingredients, in order to preserve the white color of your soup.
- Add the cucumber and bell pepper off the heat, in order to maintain their color and allow them to keep their crunch.
- Watch the shrimp cooking time—2 minutes—like a hawk. Overcooked shrimp is tough and not as tasty.
- The flavors, textures, and colors of this soup are best right off the stove! Plan to enjoy it in one sitting, as it doesn't reheat well.

NUTRITION

Calories: 306 | Fat: 25 g | Carbohydrates: 14 g | Sodium: 1,139 mg | Fiber: 4 g | Protein: 12 g | Sugar: 6 g

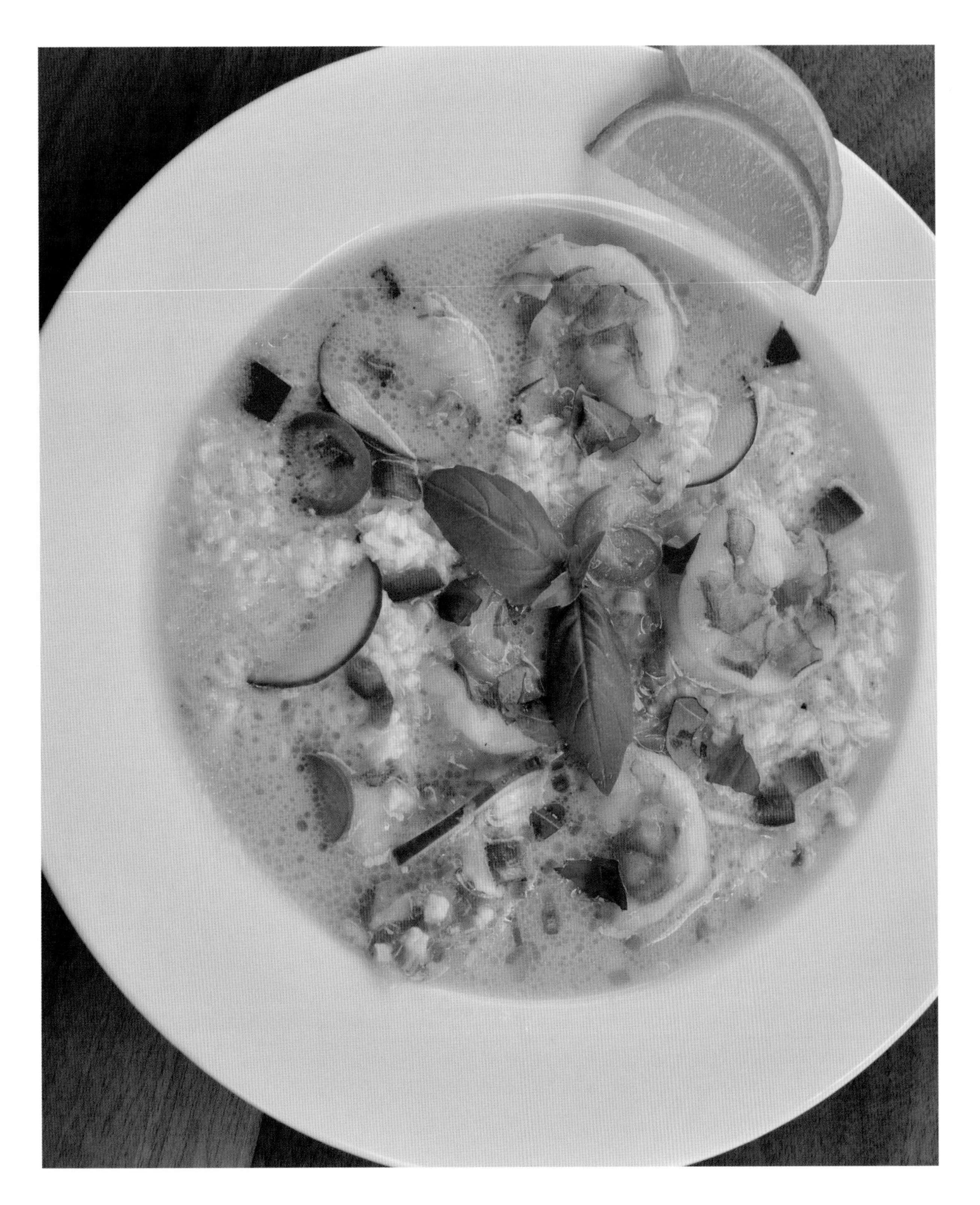

ORANGE SHRIMP AND "NOODLES" EN PAPILLOTE

PREP: 15 MINUTES | COOK: 15 MINUTES | MAKES: 4 SERVINGS

2 teaspoons minced fresh ginger
2 teaspoons minced fresh garlic
2 tablespoons coconut aminos
1 tablespoon freshly squeezed orange juice
1 teaspoon olive oil
1 teaspoon chili paste (or more to taste)
1 medium butternut squash, peeled, seeded, and spiralized or cut into noodle-like strands
1½ pounds uncooked large shrimp, peeled and deveined
Sea salt and black pepper, to taste
¼ cup minced fresh cilantro

1. Preheat the oven to 400 degrees F.
2. Make the marinade: In a small bowl, add the ginger, garlic, coconut aminos, orange juice, olive oil, and chili paste and whisk to combine.
3. In a large bowl, toss the butternut squash noodles and shrimp with the marinade.
4. Cut four 16 × 12-inch pieces of parchment paper and fold each in half. Open the parchment paper and arrange one-quarter of the noodles and shrimp in the center of the top half of each parchment. Generously season with salt and pepper. Sprinkle the cilantro on top.
5. Fold the bottom half of the parchment paper over the shrimp and noodles. Start folding and crimping the parchment paper ends together from one end all the way around to the other end, creating a sealed envelope. Fold the end under the packet. The packet should be fully encased, with no breaks in the parchment paper for steam to escape. Place the packets on a baking sheet.
6. Bake the shrimp and noodle packets for 15 minutes and remove from the oven. Serve the packets on plates, tearing them open just before serving.

Quick Tip: *En papillote* is a French way of saying "cooked in paper." The sky is the limit when it comes to cooking en papillote. Combine chicken or fish with veggies, top with some fresh herbs or marinade, then simply wrap in parchment paper and bake in the oven!

NUTRITION

Calories: 198 | Fat: 2 g | Carbohydrates: 17 g | Sodium: 265 mg | Fiber: 2 g | Protein: 33 g | Sugar: 2 g

STEAMED WHITE FISH EN PAPILLOTE

PREP: 20 MINUTES | COOK: 18 MINUTES | MAKES: 4 SERVINGS

½ cup thinly sliced red onion
1 medium zucchini, cut into matchsticks
1 carrot, cut into matchsticks
1 teaspoon olive oil
1 teaspoon minced fresh garlic
4 (6-ounce) halibut fillets, or other white fish
Sea salt and black pepper, to taste
1 lemon, halved and thinly sliced into half-moons
8 sprigs fresh thyme
¼ cup dry white wine

1. Preheat the oven to 375 degrees F.
2. In a large bowl, toss together the onion, zucchini, and carrot with the olive oil and garlic.
3. Cut four 16 × 12-inch pieces of parchment paper and fold each in half. Open the parchment paper and arrange each fish fillet in the center of the top half of each parchment. Generously season with salt and pepper. Top each fillet with one-quarter of the veggies, 2 slices of lemon, 2 sprigs of thyme, and 1 tablespoon of the wine.
4. Fold the bottom half of the parchment paper over the fish. Start folding and crimping the parchment paper ends together from one end all the way around the fish to the other end, creating a sealed envelope. Fold the end under the fish. The fish and veggies should be fully encased, with no breaks in the parchment paper for steam to escape. Place the packets on a baking sheet.
5. Bake the fish packets for 12 to 18 minutes, depending on the thickness of the fish, and remove from the oven. Serve the packets on plates, tearing them open just before serving.

Quick Tip: The key to a delicious fish dish is making sure your fish is very fresh. Your dish is going to turn out only as tasty as the freshness and quality of the fish fillet used. How do you know if your fish is fresh? Do the sniff test before you buy: raw fillets should smell faintly of the ocean but never overly fishy, and the flesh should be translucent and resilient.

NUTRITION

Calories: 231 | Fat: 4 g | Carbohydrates: 8 g | Sodium: 166 mg | Fiber: 2 g | Protein: 36 g | Sugar: 3 g

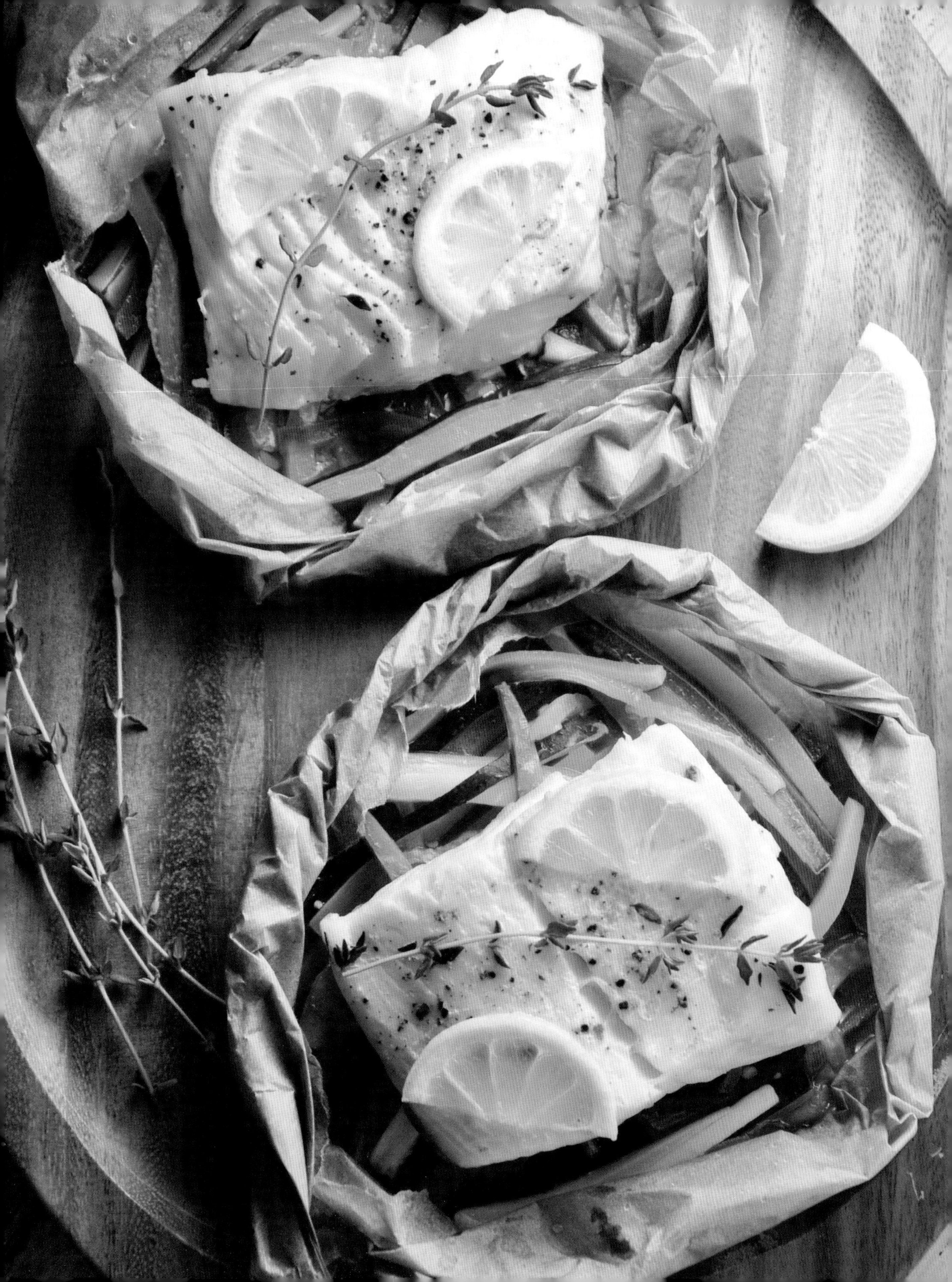

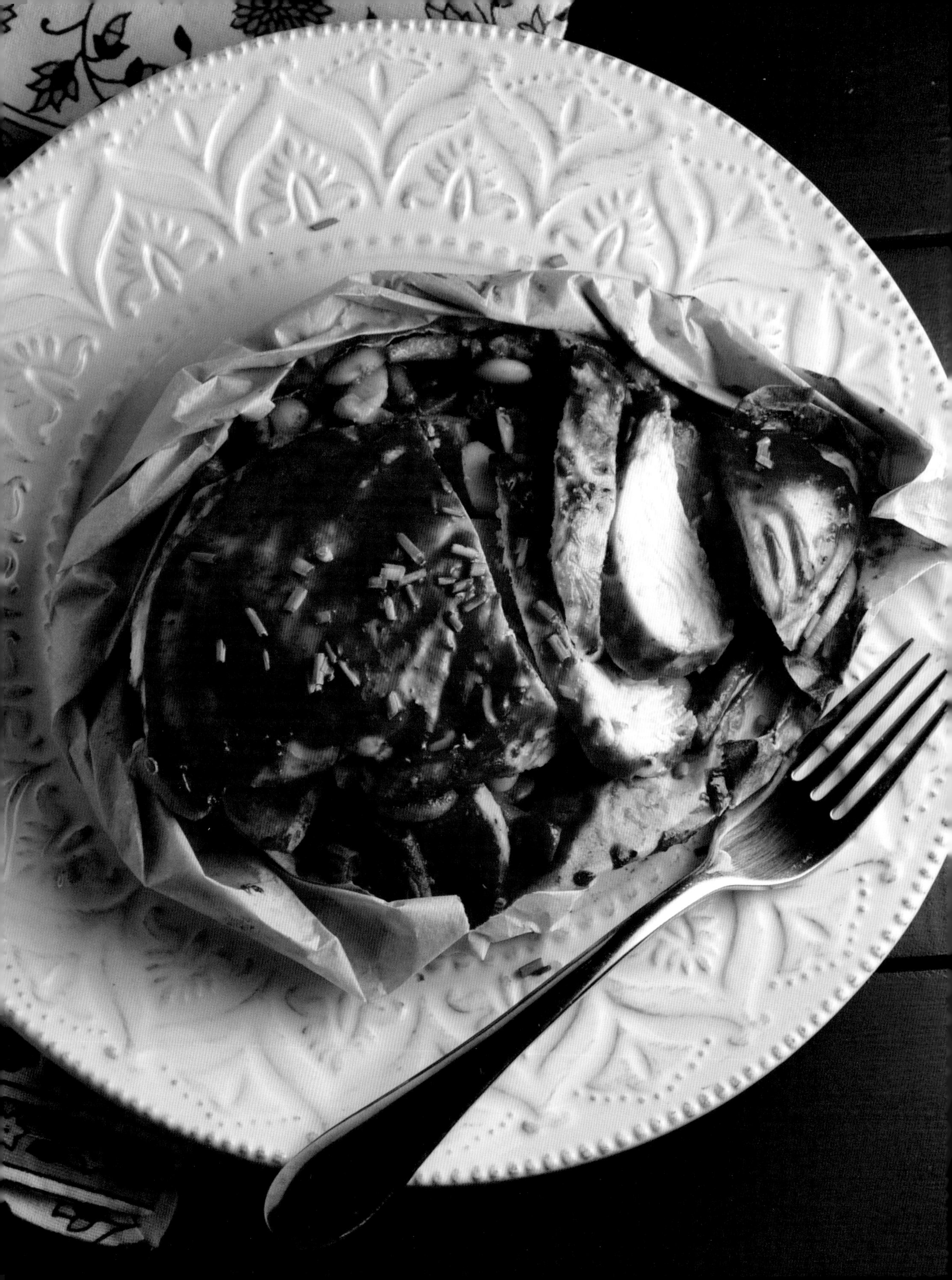

BBQ CHICKEN EN PAPILLOTE

PREP: 20 MINUTES | COOK: 30 MINUTES | MAKES: 4 SERVINGS

- 2 shallots, thinly sliced
- 1 sweet potato, peeled, halved, and thinly sliced into half-moons
- 1 cup green beans, trimmed and cut into 1-inch pieces
- 1 (15-ounce) can butter beans, drained and rinsed
- ½ cup natural barbecue sauce (no added sugar)
- 4 boneless, skinless chicken breasts, sliced lengthwise into thin cutlets
- Sea salt and black pepper, to taste
- 2 tablespoons minced fresh chives

1. Preheat the oven to 400 degrees F.
2. In a large bowl, toss together the shallots, sweet potato, green beans, and butter beans with half of the barbecue sauce. Rub the remaining sauce over the chicken breasts.
3. Cut four 16 × 12-inch pieces of parchment paper and fold each in half. Open the parchment paper and arrange one-quarter of the sweet potato and green beans and a chicken breast in the center of the top half of each parchment. Generously season with salt and pepper. Sprinkle the chives on top.
4. Fold the bottom half of the parchment paper over the chicken and veggies. Start folding and crimping the parchment paper ends together from one end all the way around to the other end, creating a sealed envelope. Fold the end under the packet. The packet should be fully encased, with no breaks in the parchment paper for steam to escape. Place the packets on a baking sheet.
5. Bake the chicken and veggie packets for 30 minutes and remove from the oven. Serve the packets on plates, tearing them open just before serving.

Quick Tip: Be sure to slice the sweet potato very thin, as you want it to be tender at the end of the 30-minute baking time. This is also why the recipe calls for thinly sliced chicken breast: you want to be sure that the meat is cooked through.

NUTRITION

Calories: 268 | Fat: 4 g | Carbohydrates: 22 g | Sodium: 625 mg | Fiber: 5 g | Protein: 35 g | Sugar: 3 g

SALMON AND LENTILS EN PAPILLOTE

PREP: 20 MINUTES | COOK: 25 MINUTES | MAKES: 4 SERVINGS

2 tablespoons dry sherry (or white grape juice)
1 tablespoon olive oil
1 teaspoon ground cumin
1 teaspoon sweet paprika
½ cup fresh cilantro, plus more for (optional) garnish
1 lemon, zested and juiced, plus more zest for (optional) garnish
1 teaspoon minced fresh garlic
4 (6-ounce) salmon fillets
½ teaspoon sea salt
¼ teaspoon black pepper
1 cup cooked or canned lentils
4 cups chopped and steamed kale
20 cherry tomatoes, halved (various colors), plus more for (optional) garnish

1. Preheat the oven to 400 degrees F.
2. In a blender, combine the sherry, olive oil, cumin, paprika, cilantro, lemon zest, lemon juice, and garlic to make the dressing.
3. Season the salmon fillets with the salt and pepper.
4. Cut four 16 × 12-inch pieces of parchment paper and fold each in half. Open the parchment paper and arrange one-quarter of the lentils and kale in the center of the top half of each parchment. Top with a salmon fillet, 10 tomato halves, and one-quarter of the dressing.
5. Fold the bottom half of the parchment paper over the salmon and veggies. Start folding and crimping the parchment paper ends together from one end all the way around to the other end, creating a sealed envelope. Fold the end under the packet. The packet should be fully encased, with no breaks in the parchment paper for steam to escape. Place the packets on a baking sheet.
6. Bake the salmon packets for 25 minutes and remove from the oven. Serve the packets on plates, tearing them open just before serving. If desired, garnish with additional cilantro, lemon zest, and cherry tomatoes.

Quick Tip: Take care not to confuse wax paper with parchment paper. Wax paper cannot be used for cooking en papillote, as it is not heat resistant and can melt or even ignite. Parchment paper, on the other hand, can be used for most any nonstick application of wax paper.

NUTRITION

Calories: 535 | Fat: 26 g | Carbohydrates: 25 g | Sodium: 389 mg | Fiber: 7 g | Protein: 46 g | Sugar: 5 g

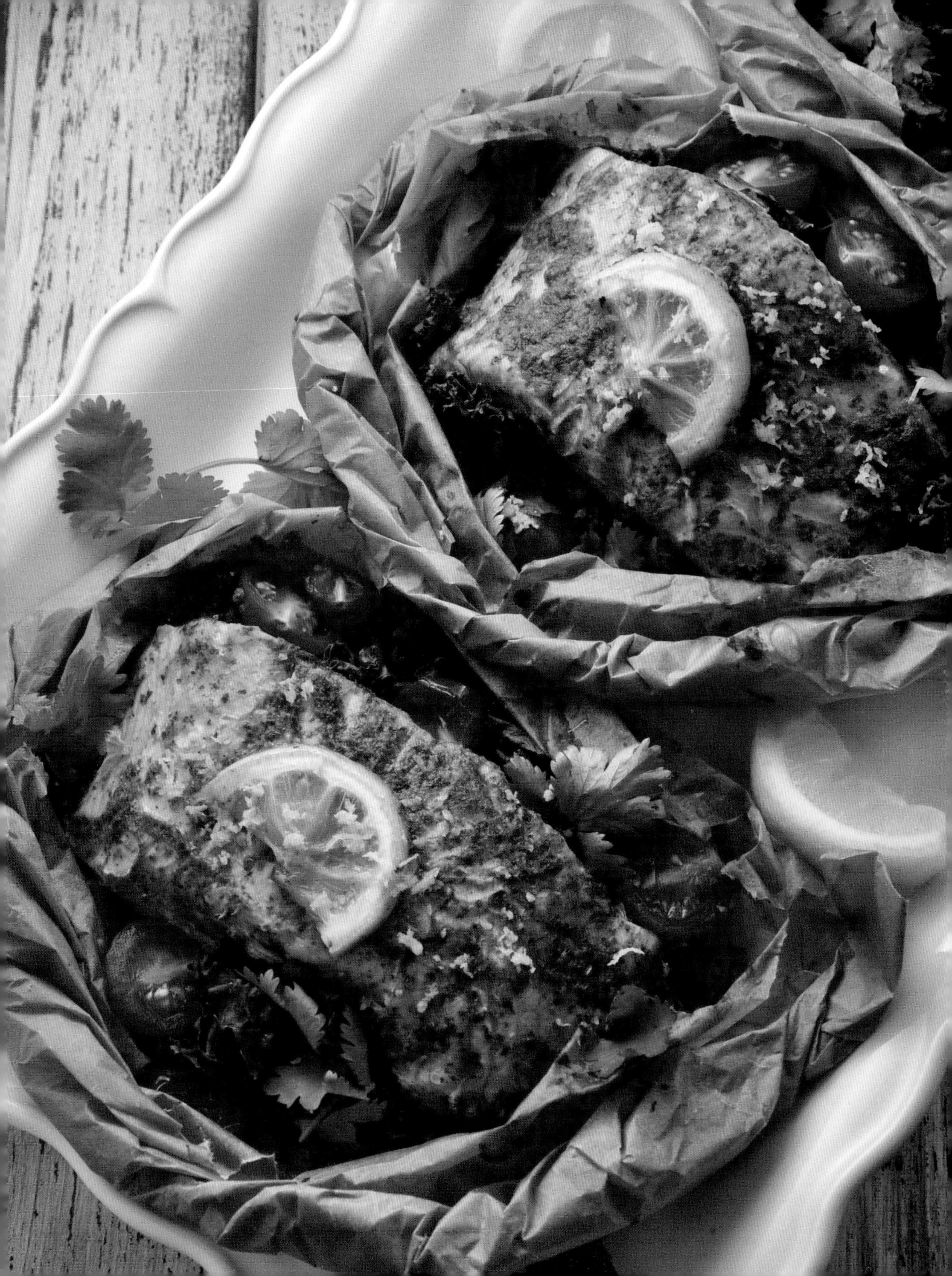

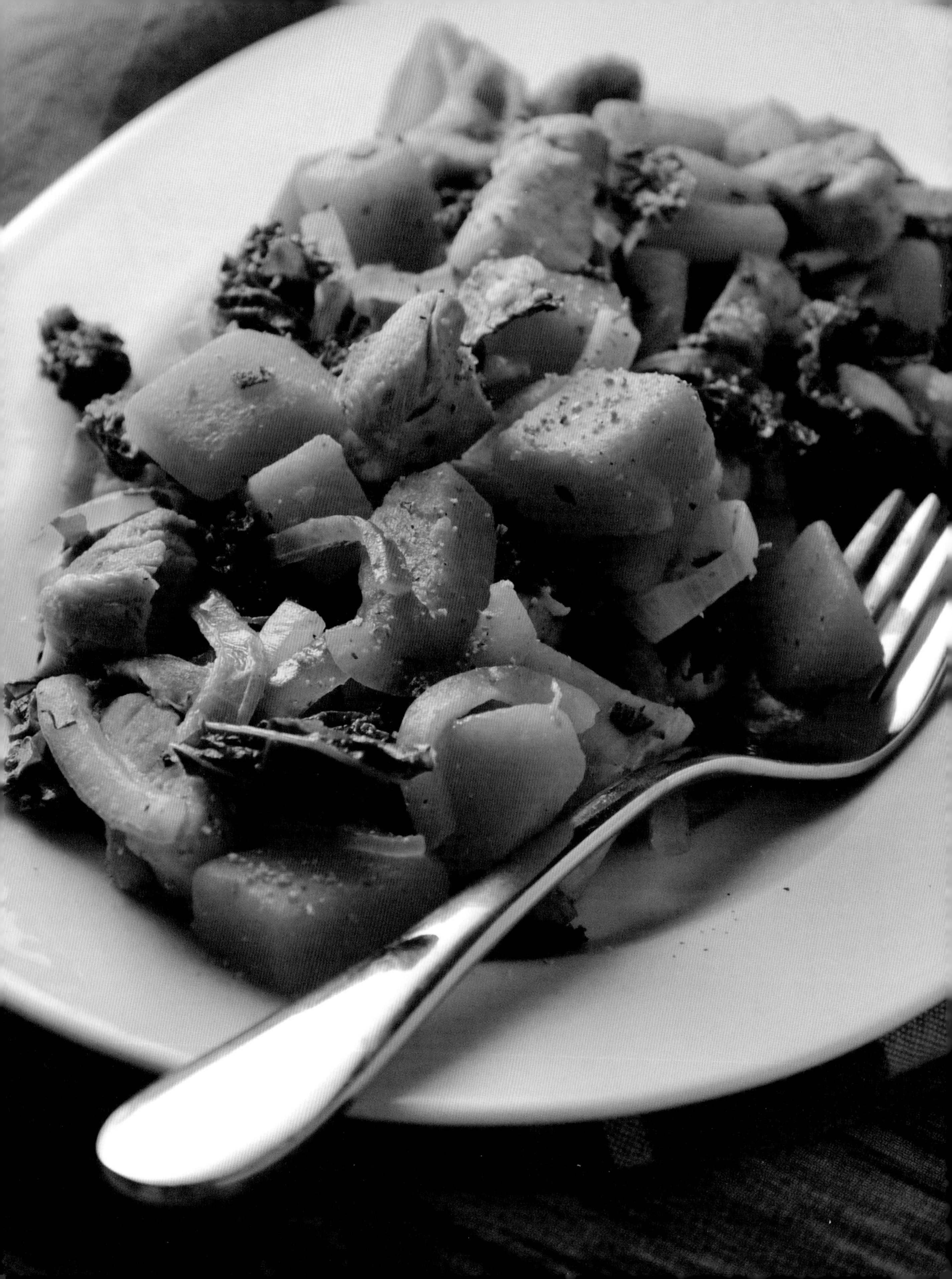

CHICKEN HASH WITH KALE AND BUTTERNUT SQUASH

PREP: 10 MINUTES | COOK: 30 MINUTES | MAKES: 6 SERVINGS

1 medium butternut squash, peeled, seeded, and cubed
1 bunch curly kale, stemmed and roughly chopped
1 pound boneless, skinless chicken thighs, cut into 2-inch pieces
Sea salt and black pepper, to taste
1 tablespoon olive oil
1 red onion, sliced
1 tablespoon chopped fresh sage
½ cup chicken broth
¼ teaspoon liquid stevia
1 tablespoon Dijon mustard

1. Bring a large pot of salted water to a boil. Add the butternut squash and blanch for 3 minutes, until almost cooked through.
2. Remove from the heat and stir in the kale. Let stand, uncovered, for 3 minutes. Drain the pot and set the veggies aside.
3. Season the chicken with salt and pepper. Return the emptied pot to medium-high heat and add the olive oil and chicken. Sauté until the chicken is browned on all sides, 3 to 5 minutes per side.
4. Add the onion and sauté for 2 minutes. Mix in the butternut squash and kale mixture and the sage. Sauté for another 2 minutes.
5. In a small bowl, combine the broth, stevia, and mustard. Pour the mixture over the hash and simmer for 8 to 10 minutes, until the liquid is reduced. Season with salt and pepper.

Quick Tip: This dish is great for meal prep, as it holds up well for several days in the fridge and can be easily packed in individual containers to eat on the go.

NUTRITION

Calories: 217 | Fat: 8 g | Carbohydrates: 12 g | Sodium: 208 mg | Fiber: 2 g | Protein: 24 g | Sugar: 3 g

TURKEY AND BACON GOULASH

PREP: 15 MINUTES | COOK: 35 MINUTES | MAKES: 8 SERVINGS

3 strips nitrate-free bacon, chopped
2 pounds ground turkey
Sea salt and black pepper, to taste
2 apples, cored and diced
2 yellow onions, diced
1 red bell pepper, seeded and diced
2 tablespoons minced fresh thyme
1 dried bay leaf
3 tablespoons sweet paprika
1 tablespoon ground cumin
1 lemon, juiced
2½ cups chicken or bone broth
5 medium zucchinis
1 tablespoon olive oil
2 tablespoons minced fresh parsley
2 tablespoons minced fresh dill
Coconut sour cream (optional; see Quick Tip)

1. Place a Dutch oven over medium-high heat. Add the bacon and cook until crispy. Using a slotted spoon, transfer the bacon to a plate.
2. Add the ground turkey to the pot with the bacon drippings. Cook the turkey, breaking it into smaller pieces, for 10 to 15 minutes, until brown. Season with salt and pepper.
3. Add the apples, onions, bell pepper, thyme, and bay leaf. Cook until the onions soften, about 5 minutes. Mix in the paprika and cumin.
4. Return the bacon to the pot, along with the lemon juice and broth. Bring to a boil, reduce the heat to a simmer, and cook until the goulash thickens, 7 to 10 minutes. Remove the bay leaf.
5. Meanwhile, use a veggie peeler to peel the zucchinis into wide, flat noodles in a large bowl. Toss with the olive oil and season with salt. Mix in the parsley and dill.
6. Serve the goulash warm with the zucchini noodles and topped with a dollop of coconut sour cream, if desired.

Quick Tip: Coconut sour cream is very simple to make! Simply combine a (13.66-ounce) can of full-fat unsweetened coconut cream with 1 tablespoon of lemon juice, ¼ teaspoon of apple cider vinegar, and ⅛ teaspoon of sea salt. Whisk together with a fork until fully combined. Keep chilled and serve by the tablespoon.

NUTRITION

Calories: 360 (with optional 1 tablespoon coconut cream, 410 calories) | Fat: 18 g (with optional 1 tablespoon coconut cream, 23 g fat) | Carbohydrates: 19 g | Sodium: 359 mg | Fiber: 5 g | Protein: 37 g | Sugar: 10 g

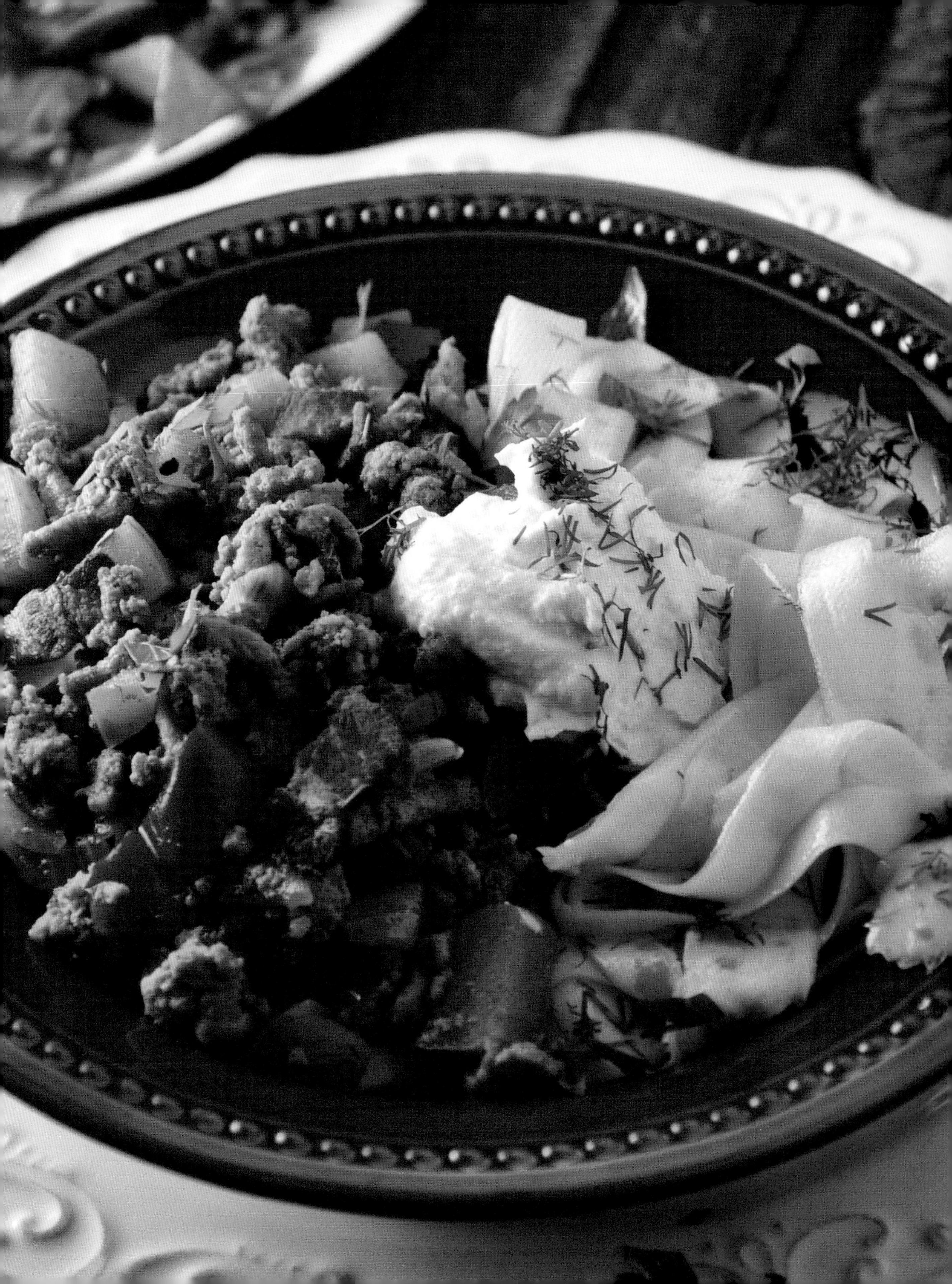

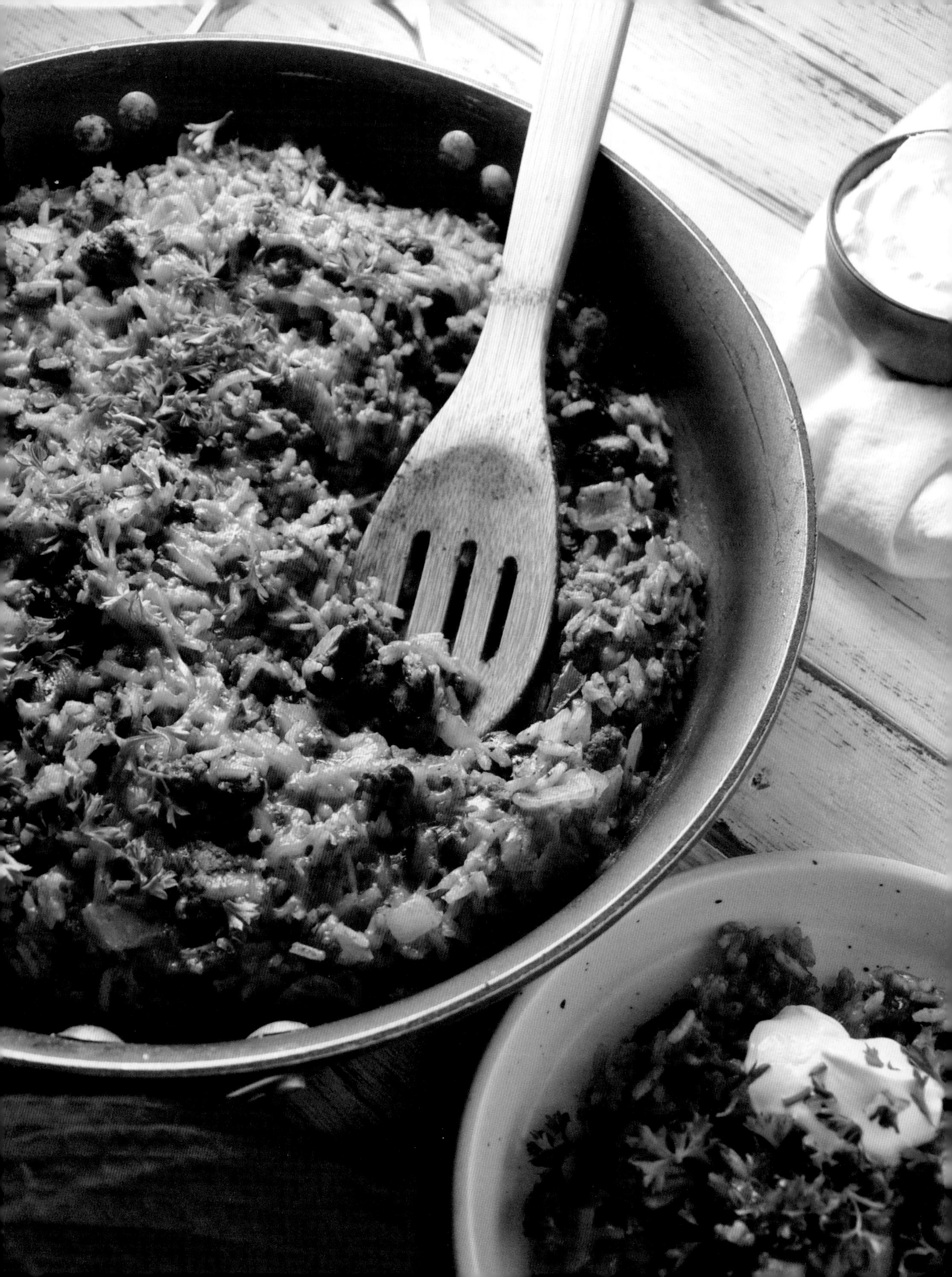

CHEESY GROUND BEEF SKILLET

PREP: 20 MINUTES | COOK: 38 MINUTES | MAKES: 6 SERVINGS

1¾ cups water
1½ teaspoons sea salt, divided
1 cup uncooked white rice
1 tablespoon olive oil
1 pound extra-lean ground beef
1 yellow onion, chopped
1 tablespoon chopped fresh garlic
1 red bell pepper, seeded and chopped
1 teaspoon dried oregano
1 teaspoon dried basil
½ teaspoon crushed red pepper
¼ teaspoon black pepper
½ cup tomato sauce
1 (15-ounce) can kidney beans, drained and rinsed
1 cup shredded cheddar cheese
⅓ cup minced fresh parsley

1. Bring the water to a boil in a saucepan over high heat. Add 1 teaspoon of the salt and the rice. Stir once, then cover the pot and reduce to low heat. Simmer, covered, for 18 minutes.
2. Meanwhile, heat the olive oil in a large skillet over medium-high heat. Add the ground beef. Cook and stir until the beef is crumbly and no longer pink, 10 to 12 minutes. Drain and discard any excess grease. Mix in the onion and garlic. Cook until tender, about 5 minutes. Add the bell pepper, oregano, basil, crushed red pepper, remaining ½ teaspoon salt, and black pepper. Cook and stir until the bell pepper is tender, about 5 minutes.
3. Stir in the cooked rice, tomato sauce, and kidney beans. Reduce the heat and cover the skillet. Cook until the vegetables are tender, about 8 minutes. Remove the pan from the heat, sprinkle the cheese over the top, and garnish with the parsley.

Quick Tip: If you love the flavors of this skillet, try using it as the filling for the *Stuffed Bell Peppers* (page 117). Also, consider doubling the recipe and freezing some of it to enjoy one day when you're too busy to cook. Throw it in a skillet with a bit of water over medium-low heat to reheat.

NUTRITION

Calories: 399 | Fat: 14 g | Carbohydrates: 36 g | Sodium: 816 mg | Fiber: 4 g | Protein: 30 g | Sugar: 3 g

FIESTA CHICKEN SKILLET

PREP: 80 MINUTES | COOK: 35 MINUTES | MAKES: 8 SERVINGS

For the Spice Blend

1 tablespoon garlic powder
1 teaspoon ground cumin
½ teaspoon smoked paprika
½ teaspoon black pepper
1 lime, juiced
1 tablespoon minced fresh cilantro
1 teaspoon minced jalapeño

For the Chicken Skillet

6 boneless, skinless chicken breast halves
1 teaspoon olive oil
1 yellow onion, chopped
2 Roma tomatoes, chopped
1 tablespoon minced fresh garlic
2 teaspoons sea salt
½ teaspoon ground cumin
¼ teaspoon ground cinnamon
¼ teaspoon ground cayenne pepper
1 (15-ounce) can black beans, drained and rinsed
1 (15-ounce) can pinto beans, drained and rinsed
1 (15-ounce) can white beans, drained and rinsed
1 ripe avocado, pitted, peeled, and sliced
½ cup pico de gallo
¼ cup minced fresh cilantro

1. For the spice blend: Combine all the spice blend ingredients in a small bowl.
2. For the chicken skillet: Rub the spice blend over all the chicken pieces. Place in a ziplock bag in the fridge to marinate for 1 hour or up to overnight.
3. Preheat the oven to 425 degrees F. Heat the olive oil in a large, oven-safe skillet over medium-high heat. Add the onion and cook until soft, about 5 minutes.
4. Stir in the tomatoes, garlic, salt, cumin, cinnamon, and cayenne. Sauté for 3 minutes. Add the beans and bring to a simmer, about 4 minutes.
5. Arrange the marinated chicken breasts over the top of the bean mixture. Transfer the skillet to the oven and bake, uncovered, until the chicken is cooked through, 20 to 25 minutes. Top with the avocado, pico de gallo, and cilantro.

Quick Tip: Leftovers from this meal are simply wonderful as packed meals the next day. I like to chop one of the leftover chicken breasts and enjoy it with a handful of fresh arugula and a spoonful of the bean mixture.

NUTRITION

Calories: 322 | Fat: 14 g | Carbohydrates: 14 g | Sodium: 829 mg | Fiber: 6 g | Protein: 35 g | Sugar: 3 g

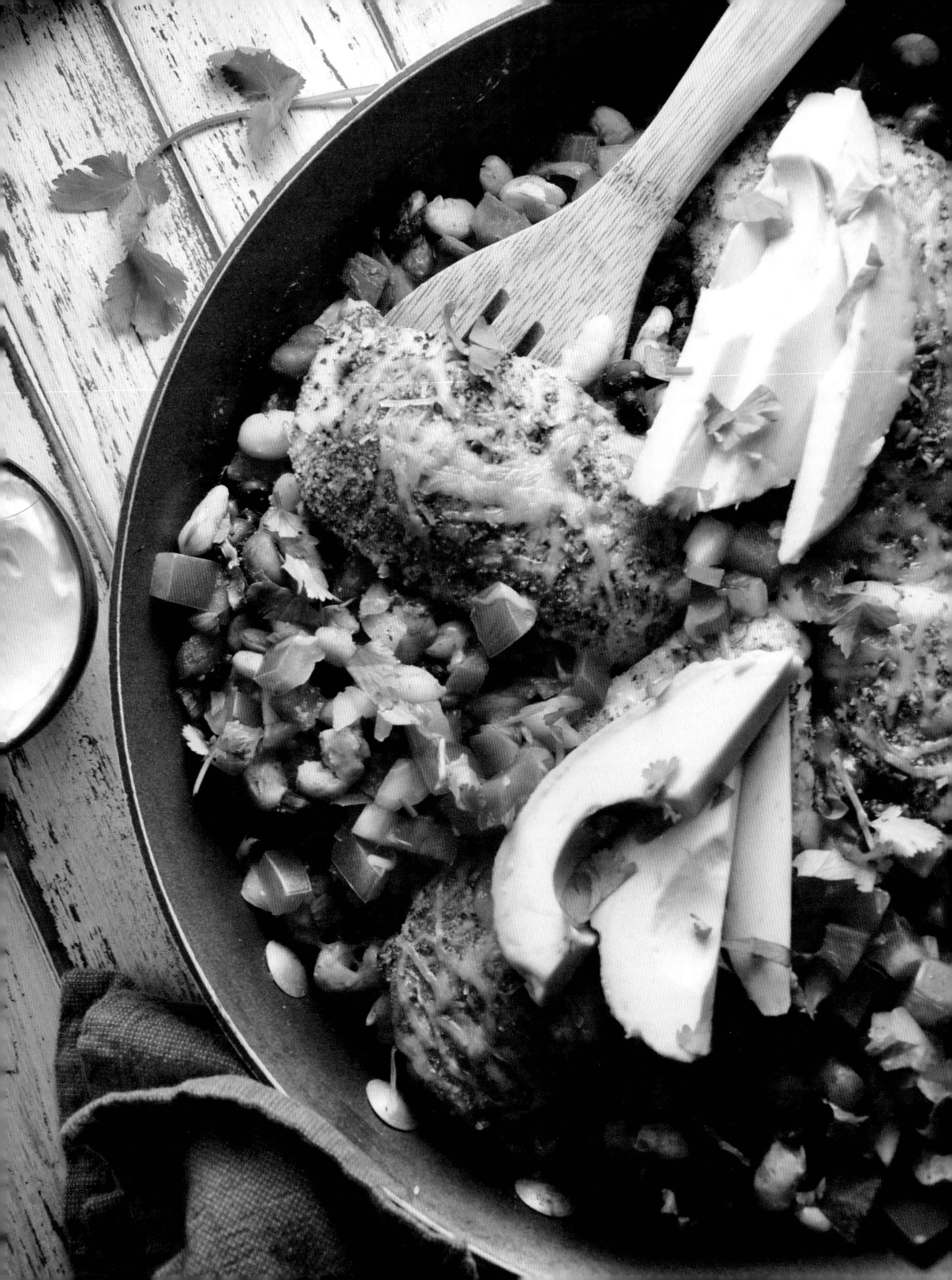

ONE-PAN "SPAGHETTI" AND MEATBALLS

PREP: 15 MINUTES | COOK: 30 MINUTES | MAKES: 6 SERVINGS

Olive oil spray
1 pound extra-lean ground beef
¾ cup grain-free bread crumbs
⅓ cup basil pesto
1 teaspoon sea salt
¼ teaspoon black pepper
6 cups butternut squash noodles
1 (24-ounce) jar marinara sauce (no added sugar)
1 sprig fresh basil

1. Preheat the oven to 425 degrees F and place an oven rack in the middle position. Spray a 13 × 9-inch baking dish with olive oil spray.
2. In a medium bowl, use your hands to combine the beef, bread crumbs, pesto, salt, and pepper. Roll the mixture into about 15 meatballs, about 1 inch in diameter. Place the meatballs in the prepared baking dish and bake for 15 minutes. Remove the meatballs, setting them aside on a plate, and drain off any liquid from the pan.
3. Spread the squash noodles in the baking dish. Pour the marinara sauce over the noodles and toss gently with tongs to coat. Return the meatballs to the pan, gently nestling throughout the noodles. Cover the pan tightly with foil and bake for 7 minutes. Remove the foil and bake for another 3 to 5 minutes, until cooked through.
4. Remove the pan from the oven. Toss to coat the squash noodles and meatballs with the sauce. Season generously with salt and pepper and garnish with the basil.

Quick Tip: Many grocery stores now sell pre-spiralized butternut squash noodles in the refrigerated produce section. While these aren't quite as fresh as homemade squash noodles, they will save you some time and effort.

NUTRITION
Calories: 289
Fat: 10 g
Carbohydrates: 23 g
Sodium: 860 mg
Fiber: 4 g
Protein: 26 g
Sugar: 11 g

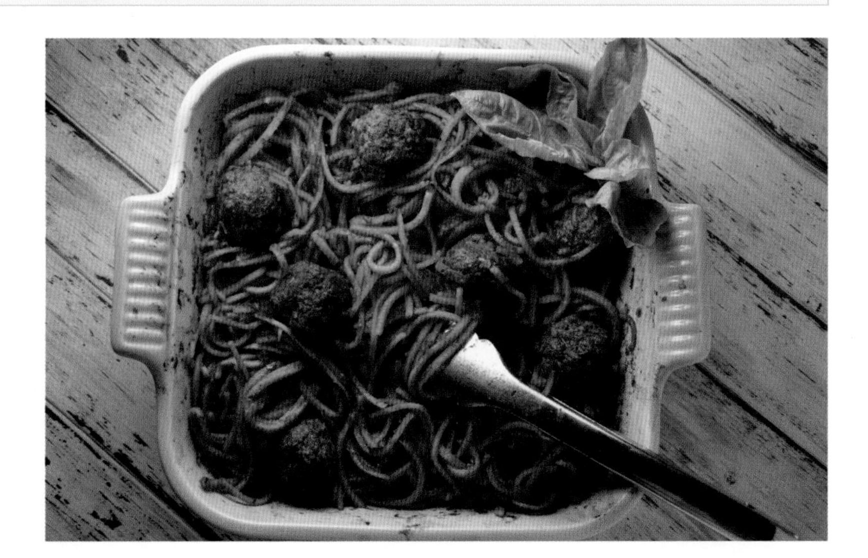

GROUND TURKEY “SPAGHETTI” SAUCE

PREP: 20 MINUTES | COOK: 35 MINUTES | MAKES: 16 SERVINGS

- 1 tablespoon olive oil
- 2 tablespoons minced fresh garlic
- 1 yellow onion, minced
- 1 fennel bulb, minced
- 3 medium zucchinis, diced
- 2 pounds lean ground turkey
- 1 (28-ounce) can crushed tomatoes
- 2 (6-ounce) cans tomato paste
- 2 (8-ounce) cans tomato sauce
- 1 cup water
- 1 tablespoon coconut sugar
- 2 teaspoons dried Italian seasoning blend
- 1 teaspoon dried basil
- ½ teaspoon sea salt
- ¼ teaspoon black pepper

1. Place an extra-large nonstick skillet or medium saucepan over medium heat. Add the olive oil and warm for 3 minutes. Add the garlic, onion, and fennel. Sauté, mixing often, for 5 minutes, until the onion is tender. Add the zucchinis and continue to cook for 5 minutes.
2. Add the ground turkey and cook, stirring and breaking the turkey apart with your spoon or spatula, until all the pink is gone, 10 to 12 minutes. Drain any excess fat from the pan and return to medium heat.
3. Add the crushed tomatoes, tomato paste, and tomato sauce to the pan and mix until well combined. Add the water, coconut sugar, Italian seasoning, basil, salt, and pepper. Decrease the heat to low and simmer for 20 minutes. Season with additional salt and pepper as needed.

Quick Tip: Serve this hearty sauce over cooked cabbage in the Acceleration Phase, and over cooked spaghetti squash in the other phases.

NUTRITION

Calories: 319
Fat: 6 g
Carbohydrates: 12 g
Sodium: 451 mg
Fiber: 4 g
Protein: 56 g
Sugar: 7 g

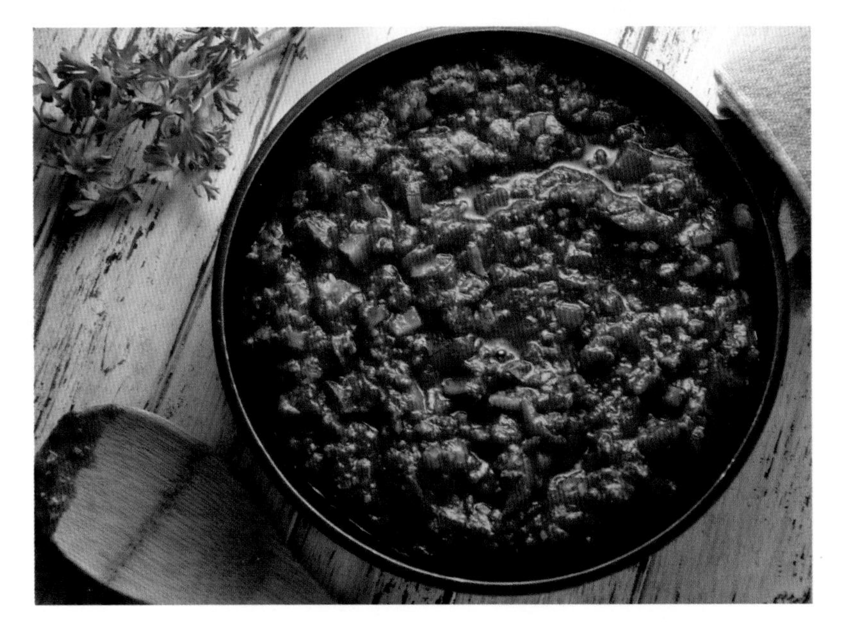

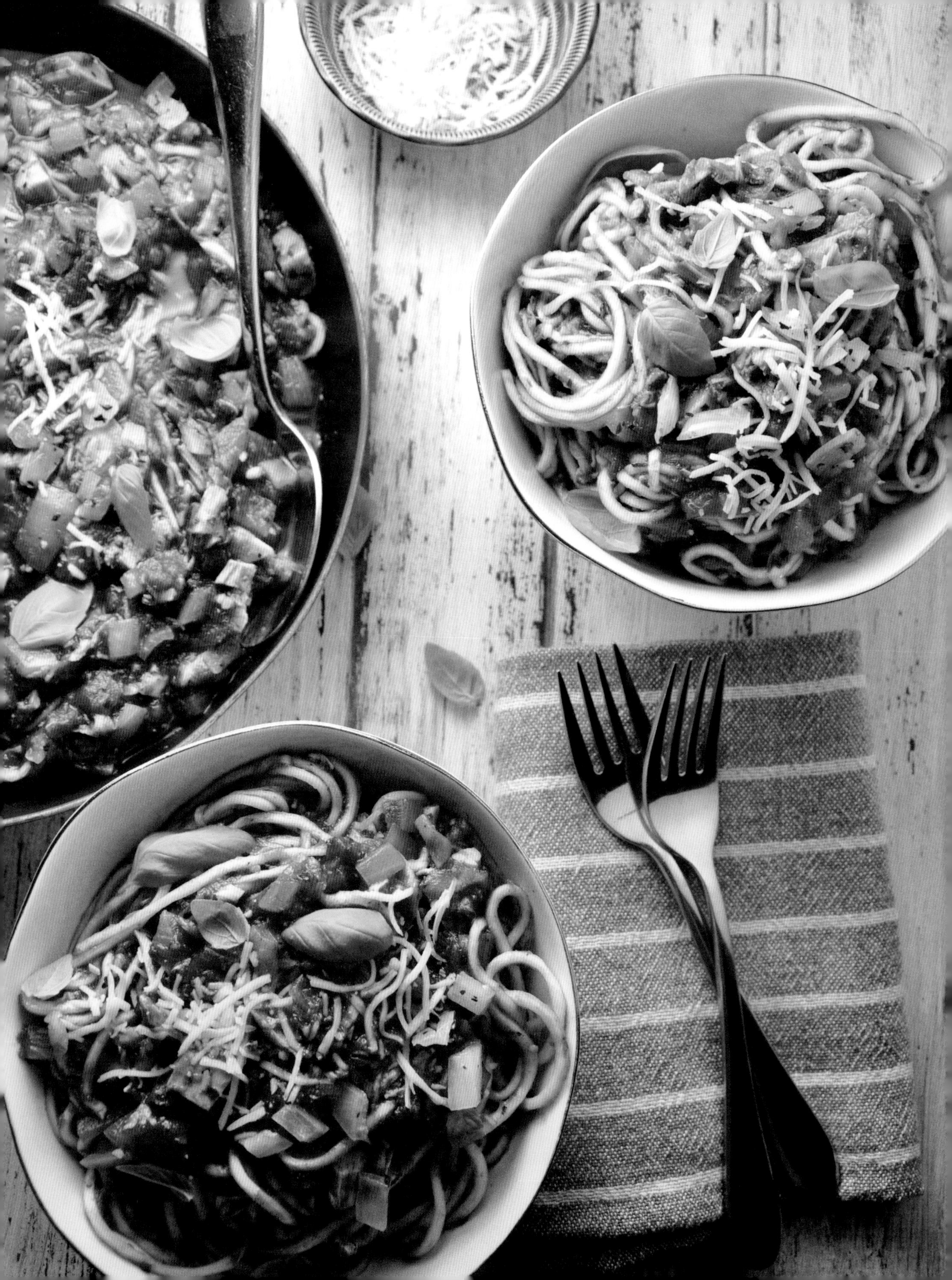

CHICKEN "SPAGHETTI" SKILLET

PREP: 10 MINUTES | COOK: 15 MINUTES | MAKES: 4 SERVINGS

4 large zucchinis, spiralized or cut into noodle-like strands (zoodles)
2 teaspoons olive oil, divided
1 tablespoon minced fresh garlic
1 yellow onion, chopped
2 teaspoons dried Italian seasoning blend
1 (24-ounce) jar marinara sauce (no added sugar)
2 cups chopped cooked chicken
¼ cup fresh basil leaves

NUTRITION

Calories: 263
Fat: 7 g
Carbohydrates: 20 g
Sodium: 193 mg
Fiber: 5 g
Protein: 28 g
Sugar: 15 g

1. Sauté the zoodles in 1 teaspoon of the olive oil in a large skillet over medium-high heat for 3 to 5 minutes, until they are al dente (still a bit crisp). Transfer the zoodles to a bowl.
2. Return the emptied skillet to medium-high heat. Add the remaining 1 teaspoon olive oil, along with the garlic and onion. Sauté for 5 minutes, until the onion is tender.
3. Add the Italian seasoning and continue to cook for another 3 minutes.
4. Add the marinara sauce, chicken, and zoodles. Mix well and cook for 4 minutes.
5. Remove from the heat and garnish with the basil.

Quick Tip: This recipe calls for zoodles—strands of zucchini that sub for regular noodles but without the carbs. A great tool to have on hand for making zoodles is a spiralizer, or you can simply slice the zucchini into thin strips. Use them skin and all, or peel before spiralizing to make them more enticing for picky eaters (as shown).

GROUND BEEF LASAGNA WITH TOMATO BASIL SAUCE

PREP: 15 MINUTES | COOK: 75 MINUTES | MAKES: 6 SERVINGS

Olive oil for greasing
Vegetable oil spray
1 pound extra-lean ground beef
1 tablespoon minced fresh garlic
1 yellow onion, chopped
2 teaspoons dried oregano
1 cup marinara sauce (no added sugar)
½ cup chopped fresh basil, plus more for garnish
2 large butternut squashes
1 cup part-skim ricotta cheese
¼ cup shredded Parmigiano-Reggiano cheese
2 tablespoons chopped fresh parsley
1 egg, beaten
1 cup shredded part-skim mozzarella cheese

1. Preheat the oven to 375 degrees F. Lightly grease a 13 × 9-inch casserole dish with olive oil.
2. Spray a large skillet over medium-high heat with vegetable oil spray. Add the ground beef, garlic, onion, and oregano. Cook, stirring often, until the beef is browned, about 10 minutes. Add the marinara sauce and basil. Cover and simmer on low for 5 minutes.
3. Cut the squashes in half where the neck meets the wider base. With the flat cut ends on your working surface, peel the necks. Then slice the neck of each squash into 12 rounds about ⅛ inch thick. (Use only the neck here. Use the base of the squash in another recipe; peel, cut the fatter part in half, and scoop out the seeds before slicing or cutting into cubes for another dish.)
4. In a medium bowl, combine the ricotta, Parmigiano-Reggiano, parsley, and egg.
5. Spread half of the meat sauce over the bottom of the prepared casserole pan. Top with 12 butternut squash rounds. Spread half of the ricotta mixture over the top of the butternut squash. Repeat with the remaining meat sauce, remaining 12 butternut rounds, and remaining ricotta mixture. Cover with foil and bake for 30 minutes. Uncover, sprinkle with the mozzarella, and bake for another 30 minutes. Let stand for 10 minutes before serving. Sprinkle with additional fresh basil.

Quick Tip: It is possible to use zucchini as a replacement for butternut squash. Slice the zucchini more thickly than the butternut squash, about ¼ inch thick, and tent the foil loosely for the first 30 minutes of the bake time. The zucchini version will inevitably have more liquid released during the baking, so you may want to drain off some of this liquid before serving.

NUTRITION

Calories: 368 | Fat: 12 g | Carbohydrates: 32 g | Sodium: 342 mg | Fiber: 6 g | Protein: 34 g | Sugar: 6 g

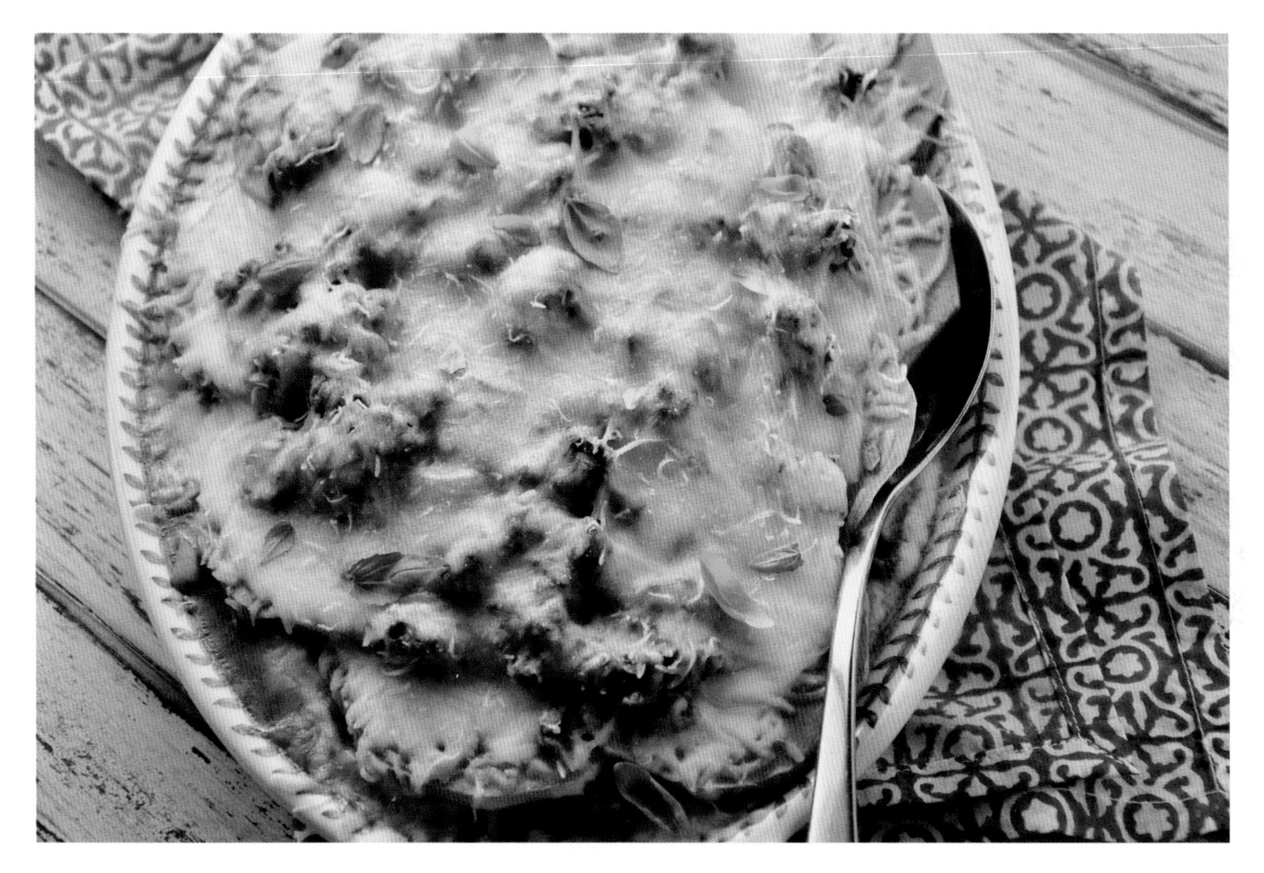

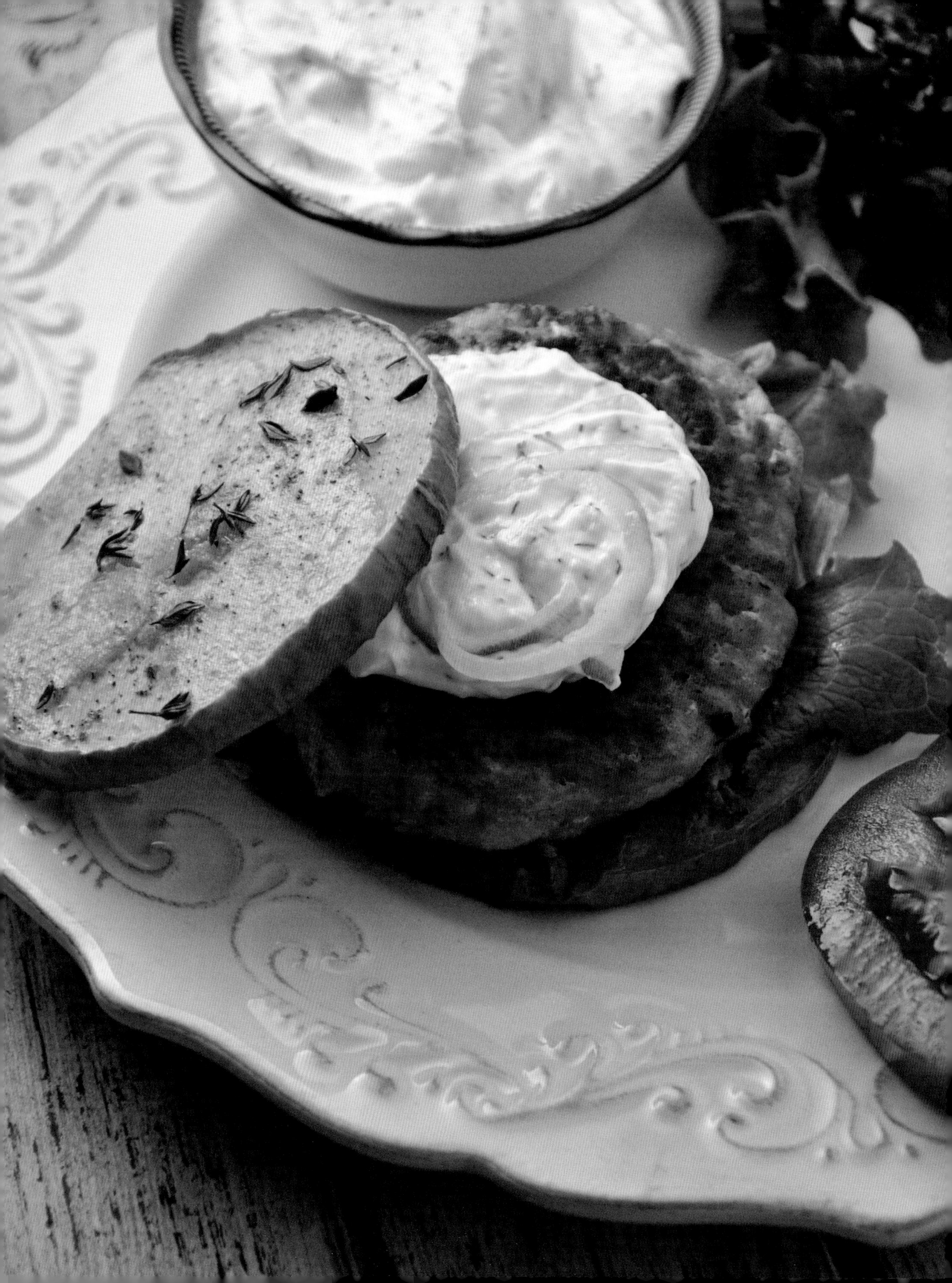

TURKEY BURGERS WITH BUTTERNUT BUNS

PREP: 20 MINUTES | COOK: 35 MINUTES | MAKES: 4 SERVINGS

For the Butternut Buns

1 tablespoon olive oil, plus more for greasing
1 large butternut squash
2 teaspoons fresh thyme leaves
Sea salt and black pepper, to taste

For the Yogurt Sauce

¾ cup plain full-fat Greek yogurt
1 teaspoon lemon juice
¼ teaspoon dried minced garlic
½ teaspoon dried dill
Sea salt and black pepper, to taste

For the Turkey Burgers

1 pound lean ground turkey
1 egg, beaten
1 teaspoon minced fresh garlic
1 tablespoon Worcestershire sauce
2 tablespoons minced fresh cilantro
Sea salt and black pepper, to taste
1 tablespoon olive oil

1. For the butternut buns: Preheat the oven to 400 degrees F. Lightly grease a baking sheet with olive oil. Slice the neck of the butternut squash into 8 rounds about ¼ inch thick. (Reserve the rest of the squash for another use.) Place the rounds on the prepared baking sheet, drizzle with the olive oil, and sprinkle with the thyme, salt, and pepper. Roast for 25 minutes, flipping the rounds once halfway through the roasting time.
2. For the yogurt sauce: In a medium bowl, combine the yogurt, lemon juice, garlic, and dill. Season with salt and pepper.
3. For the turkey burgers: In a large bowl, mix together the ground turkey, egg, garlic, Worcestershire sauce, and cilantro; season with salt and pepper. Form the mixture into 4 patties.
4. In a medium skillet, over medium heat, heat the olive oil. Add the patties and cook until golden and cooked through, 5 minutes per side. Serve each burger between 2 butternut squash rounds, (or, for the Acceleration Phase, wrapped in lettuce leaves) with a dollop of the yogurt sauce.

Quick Tip: You could also serve these tasty burgers wrapped in butter lettuce leaves, rather than the butternut buns. This option makes the dish perfect for the Acceleration Phase. If using lettuce wraps instead of butternut buns, omit the squash and skip step 1.

NUTRITION with the butternut buns

Calories: 455 | Fat: 22 g | Carbohydrates: 16 g | Sodium: 257 mg | Fiber: 8 g | Protein: 35 g | Sugar: 6 g

NUTRITION with the lettuce wrap

Calories: 374 | Fat: 22 g | Carbohydrates: 2 g | Sodium: 247 mg | Fiber: 2 g | Protein: 35 g | Sugar: 2 g

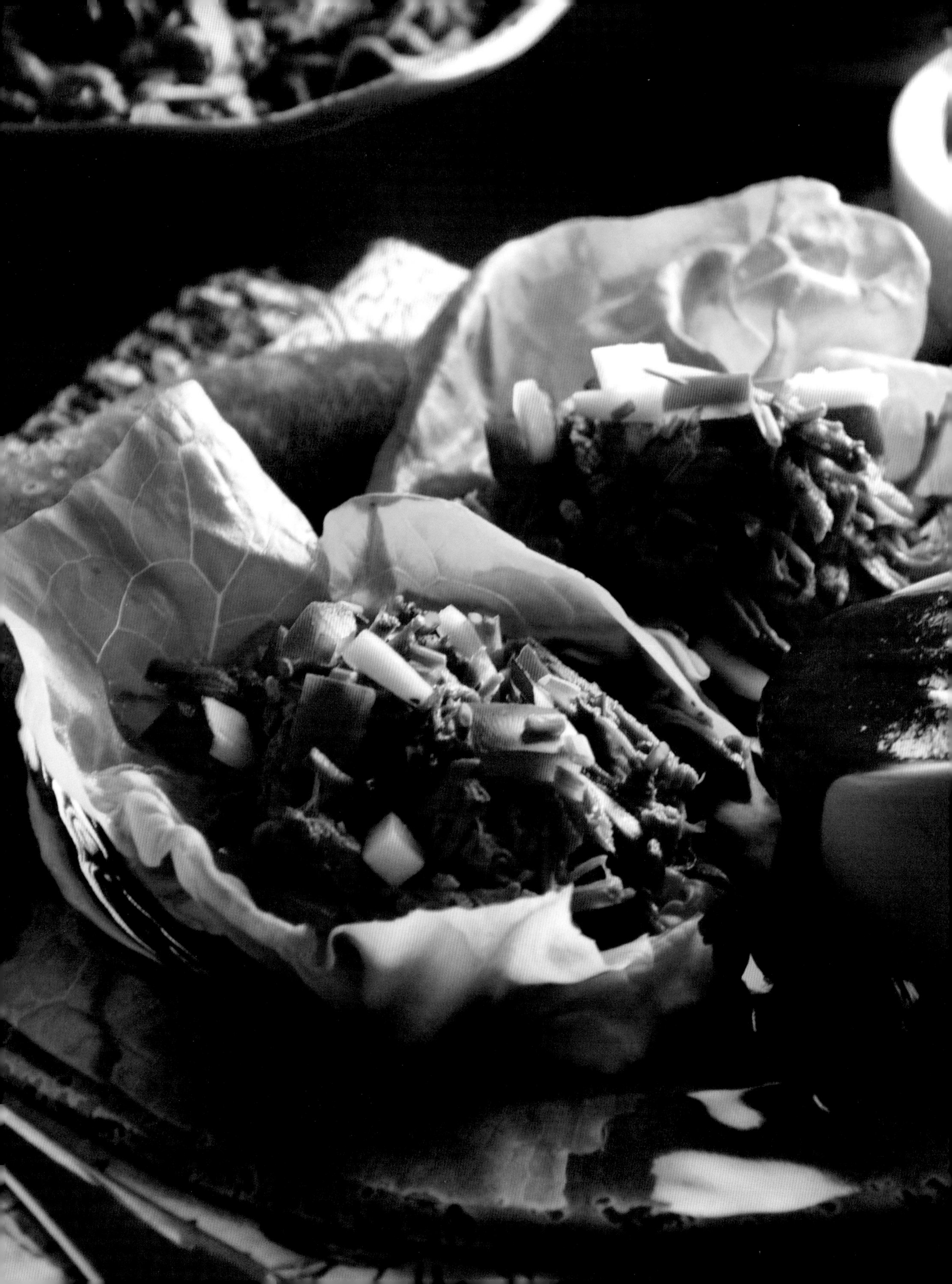

BBQ CARNITAS LETTUCE TACOS

PREP: 15 MINUTES | COOK: 7–9 HOURS | MAKES: 12 SERVINGS

2 tablespoons olive oil, divided
2 (3-pound) boneless pork shoulders
1 yellow onion, sliced
6 sprigs fresh oregano
2 tablespoons minced fresh garlic
1 cup chicken broth, divided
¾ cup apple cider vinegar
2 tablespoons coconut sugar
½ cup natural barbecue sauce (no added sugar)
1 head butter lettuce
2 tablespoons minced fresh chives
¼ cup chopped tomatoes
1 bunch radishes, thinly sliced

1. Heat 1 tablespoon of the olive oil in a large skillet over high heat. Add one of the pork shoulders and brown on all sides, 5 to 7 minutes per side. Transfer the cooked pork to a plate and repeat with the remaining 1 tablespoon olive oil and the second pork shoulder.
2. Place the onion, oregano, and garlic in the bottom of a slow cooker and top with the browned pork. Deglaze the skillet with ½ cup of the broth, scraping up the browned bits, and pour the liquid over the pork.
3. In a bowl, combine the remaining ½ cup broth, vinegar, and coconut sugar. Pour over the pork.
4. Cover and cook on high for 6 hours or on low for 8 hours.
5. Remove the meat and shred. Strain and reserve the drippings. After the liquid has cooled slightly, skim off the fat.
6. Preheat the oven to 400 degrees F. Place the pork on a baking sheet and drizzle with ½ cup of the drippings. Roast until the pork begins to brown, about 20 minutes. Combine the pork with the barbecue sauce.
7. Assemble the tacos by filling large lettuce leaves with a scoop of pork. Sprinkle with the chives, tomatoes, and radishes.

Quick Tip: Deglazing is a cooking technique in which you dilute any sediment left in the pan after browning meat or vegetables in order to make a gravy or sauce. Deglazing agents are typically broth, wine, or other cooking liquids.

NUTRITION

Calories: 375 | Fat: 11 g | Carbohydrates: 6 g | Sodium: 1,054 mg | Fiber: 1 g | Protein: 60 g | Sugar: 2 g

POT ROAST TACOS WITH CHIMICHURRI

PREP: 10 MINUTES | COOK: 5 MINUTES | MAKES: 8 SERVINGS

For the Chimichurri

1½ cups fresh parsley
1 cup fresh cilantro
2 tablespoons chopped scallion
1 tablespoon chopped fresh garlic
¼ cup olive oil
2 tablespoons lemon juice
1 tablespoon water
1 teaspoon sea salt
1 teaspoon crushed red pepper

For the Tacos

3 cups chopped *Slow Cooker Braised Pot Roast* (page 154)
8 (6-inch) yellow corn tortillas
1 ripe avocado, pitted, peeled, and sliced
4 radishes, sliced
¼ cup crumbled queso fresco
1 lime, sliced

1. For the chimichurri: Combine the parsley, cilantro, scallion, and garlic in the bowl of a food processor. Pulse until roughly chopped. Add the olive oil, lemon juice, water, salt, and crushed red pepper and process until fully combined.
2. For the tacos: Place the chopped chuck roast in a medium skillet over medium-high heat and cook for 5 minutes. Remove from the heat and mix in ½ cup of the chimichurri. Char the tortillas in a grill pan for a few seconds, then fill evenly with the meat, avocado, radishes, and queso. Serve with the remaining chimichurri sauce and lime slices.

Quick Tip: There are endless ways to enjoy this chimichurri sauce. Toss it with roasted veggies, serve it over grilled meat, or use it to top off a fried egg.

NUTRITION

Calories: 410 | Fat: 24 g | Carbohydrates: 12 g | Sodium: 366 mg | Fiber: 2 g | Protein: 41 g | Sugar: 1 g

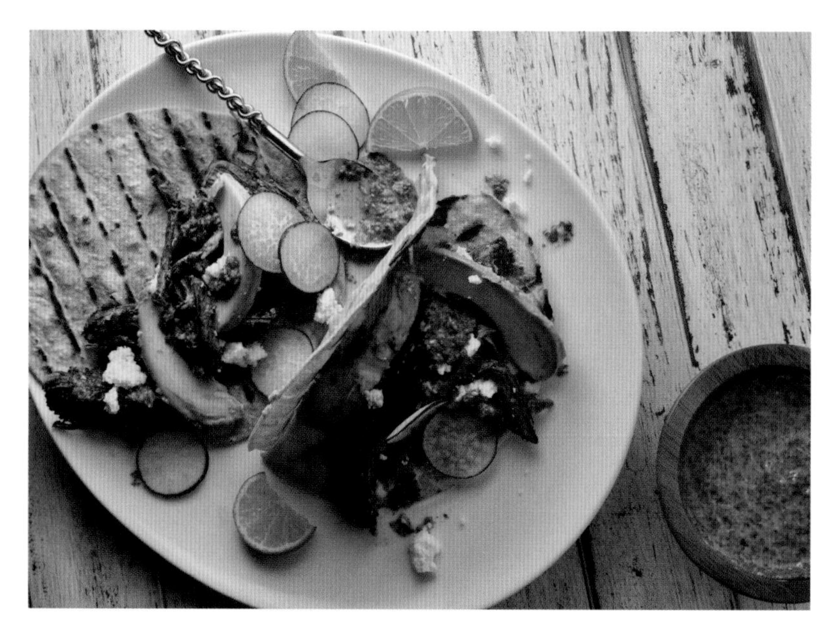

SHRIMP CURRY WITH COCONUT RICE

PREP: 15 MINUTES | COOK: 45 MINUTES | MAKES: 8 SERVINGS

For the Coconut Rice

2 cups uncooked jasmine rice
1½ cups water
1 (13.66-ounce) can full-fat unsweetened coconut milk
1 teaspoon sea salt

For the Shrimp Curry

1 tablespoon olive oil
1 large yellow onion, finely chopped
2 bell peppers of any color, seeded and chopped
1 tablespoon minced fresh garlic
1 (8-ounce) can tomato sauce
½ cup chicken broth
½ cup minced fresh cilantro, plus more for garnish
1 teaspoon curry powder
¼ teaspoon sea salt
¼ teaspoon black pepper
2 pounds uncooked large shrimp, peeled and deveined
Fresh basil leaves and lime wedges, for garnish

NUTRITION

Calories: 320
Fat: 5 g
Carbohydrates: 44 g
Sodium: 579 mg
Fiber: 4 g
Protein: 26 g
Sugar: 4 g

1. For the coconut rice: Combine all the coconut rice ingredients in a medium pot over high heat. Bring to a boil. Stir and cover, reducing the heat to the lowest setting. Cook for 15 minutes, until the rice is tender and the liquid is absorbed. Remove from the heat.
2. For the curry: In a large skillet, heat the olive oil over medium-high heat. Add the onion and bell peppers and sauté until tender, about 5 minutes. Add the garlic and cook for 1 minute more.
3. Stir in the tomato sauce, broth, cilantro, curry, salt, and pepper. Bring to a boil. Reduce the heat, cover, and simmer, stirring occasionally, for 10 minutes.
4. Stir in the shrimp. Cook for 5 to 7 minutes, until the shrimp turns pink. Remove from the heat and serve over the coconut rice. Garnish with additional cilantro, basil leaves, and lime wedges.

Quick Tip: Frozen shrimp works in this flavorful dish. Just be sure to thaw the shrimp completely before adding it to the skillet.

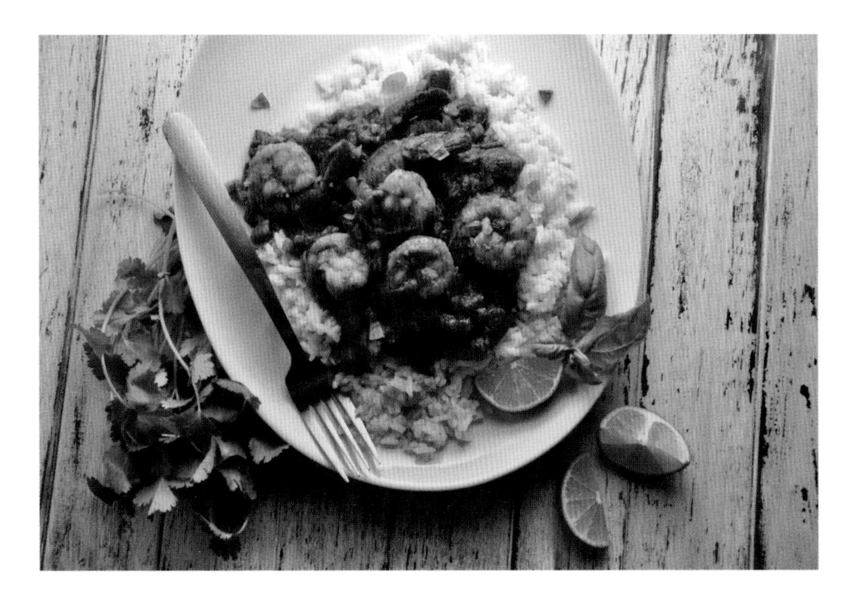

GREEK SALMON QUINOA BOWL

PREP: 20 MINUTES | COOK: 24 MINUTES | MAKES: 4 SERVINGS

For the Bowl

2 cups chicken broth
1 cup uncooked quinoa
1 cup cherry tomatoes, halved
1 cup sliced cucumber
⅓ cup pitted Kalamata olives, halved
¼ cup finely chopped red onion
⅓ cup crumbled feta cheese

For the Dressing

3 tablespoons olive oil
2 tablespoons red wine vinegar
1 tablespoon minced fresh dill
1 tablespoon minced fresh oregano
Sea salt and black pepper, to taste

For the Salmon

1 tablespoon olive oil, plus more for greasing
4 (6-ounce) skin-on salmon fillets
1 tablespoon minced fresh dill, plus more for garnish
1 tablespoon minced fresh oregano, plus more for garnish
1 teaspoon grated lemon zest
Sea salt and black pepper, to taste
Lemon slices, for garnish

1. Preheat the oven to 450 degrees F.
2. For the bowl: Combine the broth and quinoa in a medium pot over medium-high heat and bring to a boil. Reduce the heat to low and cover. Simmer for 12 minutes, until the quinoa is tender and all the liquid is absorbed. Remove from the heat, uncover, and fluff with a fork.
3. In a large bowl, combine the cooked quinoa with the tomatoes, cucumber, olives, onion, and feta.
4. For the dressing: In a small bowl, whisk together the olive oil, vinegar, dill, and oregano. Toss the dressing into the quinoa mixture. Season with salt and pepper.
5. For the salmon: Lightly grease a rimmed baking sheet with olive oil. Place the salmon fillets, skin side down, on the prepared baking sheet. Drizzle the olive oil over the salmon fillets and evenly sprinkle with the dill, oregano, and lemon zest. Season generously with salt and pepper. Bake the salmon for 10 to 12 minutes, until it is flaky and cooked through.
6. Divide the quinoa mixture among four serving bowls. Top each with a fillet of salmon, and garnish with additional fresh dill, oregano, and lemon slices.

NUTRITION

Calories: 599 | Fat: 33 g | Carbohydrates: 34 g | Sodium: 693 mg | Fiber: 5 g | Protein: 41 g | Sugar: 3 g

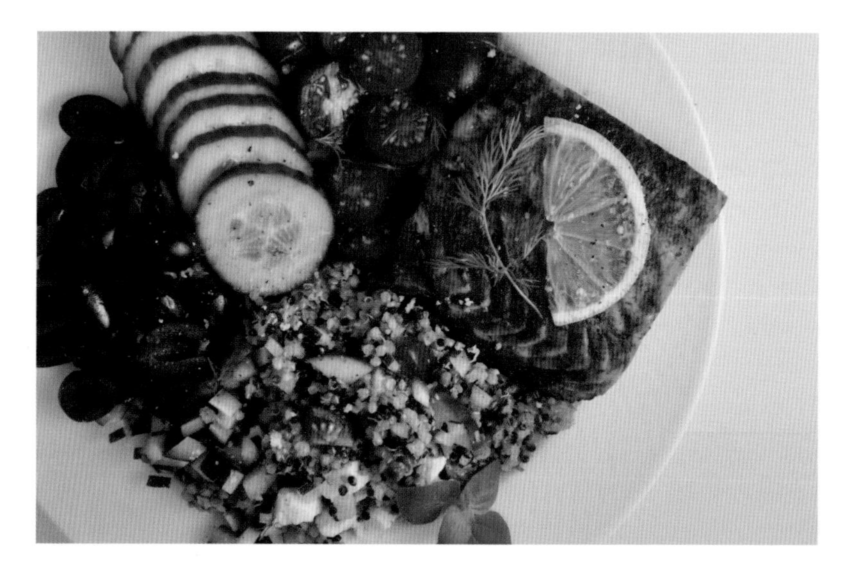

CHILI-LOADED BAKED POTATO

PREP: 15 MINUTES | COOK: 95 MINUTES | MAKES: 6 SERVINGS

- 6 (8-ounce) sweet potatoes
- Olive oil spray
- Sea salt and black pepper, to taste
- 1 tablespoon olive oil
- 2 pounds ground chuck
- 2 yellow onions, diced
- 2 tablespoons minced fresh garlic
- 3 tablespoons chili powder
- 2 tablespoons ground cumin
- 1 tablespoon dried oregano
- 2 teaspoons smoked paprika
- ¼ teaspoon ground cayenne pepper
- 3 cups beef broth
- 1 (28-ounce) can crushed tomatoes
- 1 tablespoon apple cider vinegar
- 1 (15-ounce) can butter beans, drained and rinsed
- ½ cup chopped fresh cilantro, plus ¼ cup cilantro leaves for garnish
- 1 Anaheim chile, minced
- 6 tablespoons shredded cheddar cheese
- ½ cup plain full-fat Greek yogurt
- ¼ cup minced red onion

1. Preheat the oven to 400 degrees F. Line a baking sheet or pan with parchment paper. Rinse and scrub the sweet potatoes. Pat dry with a paper towel and pierce several times with a fork or knife. Place in the prepared pan. Lightly spray the sweet potatoes with olive oil spray and season with salt and pepper. Bake for 45 minutes to 1 hour, until tender when poked with a fork.
2. Heat the olive oil in a skillet over medium-high heat. Add the ground chuck and sauté, breaking up with a spoon, until fully cooked, 7 to 10 minutes. Drain off the fat and return the beef to the pot with the yellow onions, garlic, chili powder, cumin, oregano, paprika, and cayenne. Reduce the heat to medium-low and sauté, stirring often, until the onions are soft, about 10 minutes.
3. Add the broth, crushed tomatoes, and vinegar. Increase the heat to high and bring to a boil. Reduce the heat to medium-low and simmer for 10 minutes. Add the butter beans, cilantro, and Anaheim chile. Cook for another 5 minutes. Season with salt.
4. Split the potatoes lengthwise and fluff the flesh with a fork. Top evenly with the chili, cheddar cheese, a dollop of yogurt, and a sprinkle of cilantro and red onion.

NUTRITION

Calories: 573 | Fat: 10 g | Carbohydrates: 58 g | Sodium: 588 mg | Fiber: 11 g | Protein: 25 g | Sugar: 12 g

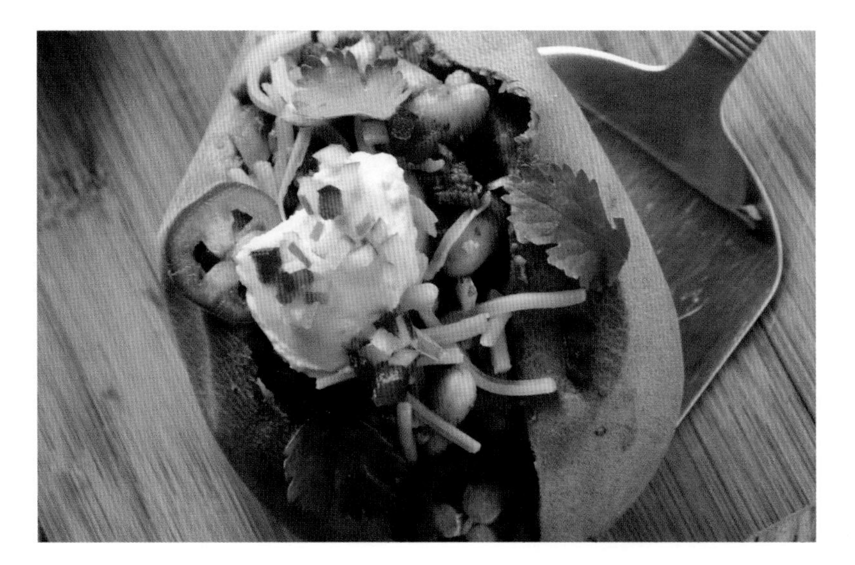

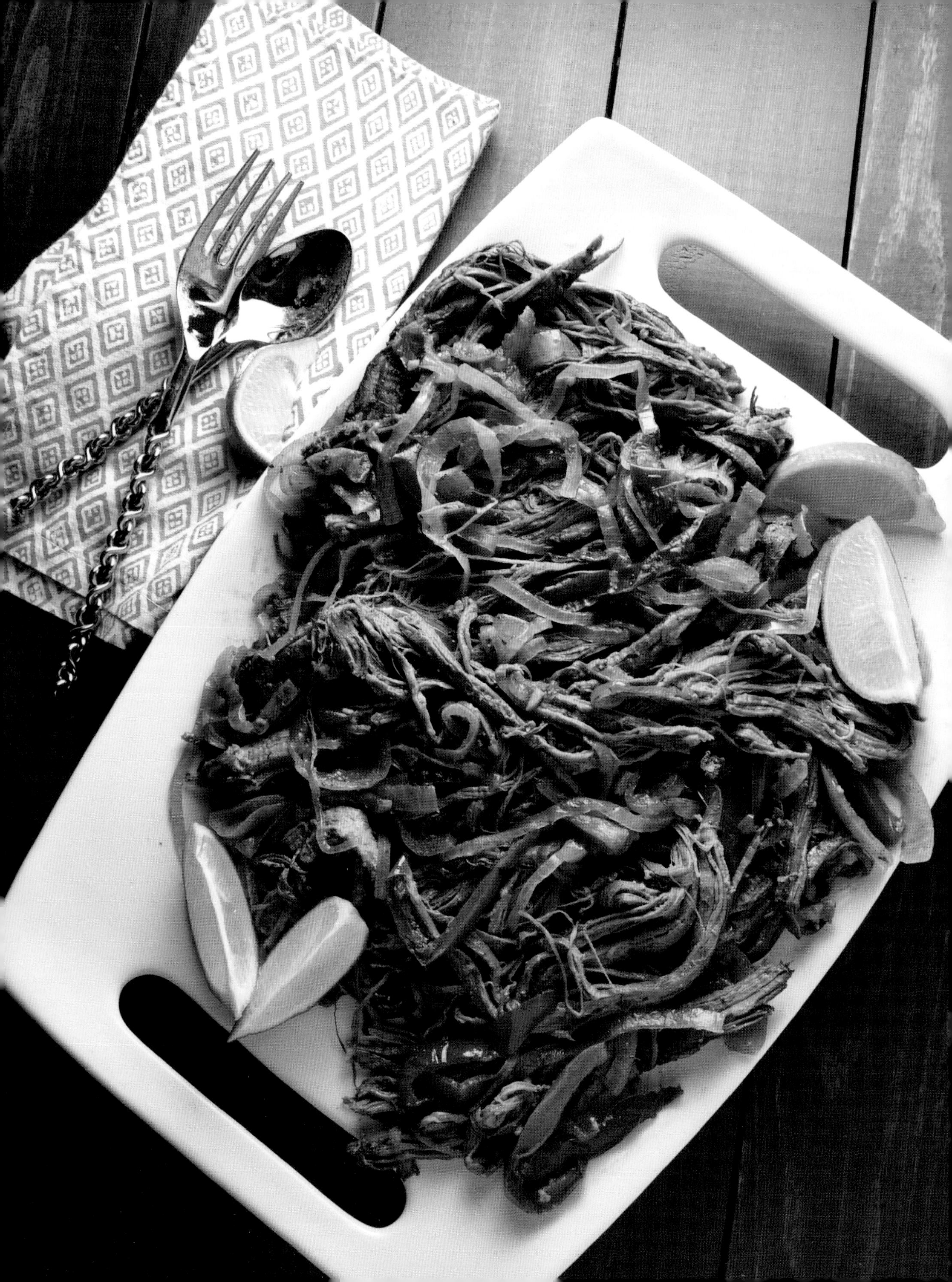

BRAISED CUBAN FLANK STEAK

PREP: 20 MINUTES | COOK: 8 HOURS | MAKES: 8 SERVINGS

Olive oil spray
2 pounds lean flank steak
½ cup chicken broth
2 medium tomatoes, seeded and chopped
2 yellow onions, chopped
1 red bell pepper, seeded and chopped
1 green bell pepper, seeded and chopped
2 tablespoons minced fresh garlic
2 tablespoons dried oregano
1 tablespoon ground cumin
2 teaspoons smoked paprika
1 teaspoon sea salt
½ teaspoon crushed red pepper
1 lime, cut into wedges

1. Place a large skillet over medium-high heat. Lightly coat it with olive oil spray. Add the flank steak and sear on both sides, about 4 minutes per side. Transfer the steak to a plate.
2. Deglaze the pan with the broth, scraping any drippings from the bottom. Set aside.
3. Combine the tomatoes, onions, bell peppers, garlic, oregano, cumin, paprika, salt, and crushed red pepper in the slow cooker. Add the steak and pan drippings. Cover and cook on low for 8 hours, until the steak is fall-apart tender.
4. Transfer the meat to a serving platter and let it rest for 5 minutes. Shred the meat with two forks. Squeeze the juice from one of the lime wedges over the meat. Serve the meat with the tender veggies and the remaining lime wedges.

Quick Tip: Slow cooker recipes, like this one, are a seriously handy tool for preparing nutritious, homemade meals. This is a lifesaver when you have a demanding job and a family to tend to.

NUTRITION

Calories: 258 | Fat: 9 g | Carbohydrates: 7 g | Sodium: 351 mg | Fiber: 2 g | Protein: 34 g | Sugar: 3 g

SLOW COOKER BRAISED POT ROAST

PREP: 40 MINUTES | COOK: 6½ HOURS | MAKES: 4 SERVINGS

- 1 (3- to 4-pound) boneless chuck roast, trimmed
- 2½ teaspoons sea salt
- 1½ teaspoons black pepper
- 2 tablespoons coconut flour
- 2 tablespoons olive oil
- 2 tablespoons minced fresh garlic
- 1 onion, cut into 1-inch wedges
- 2 tablespoons tomato paste
- 1 cup dry red wine
- 3 cups broth (any type)
- 2 carrots, cut in half lengthwise, then cut into 2-inch pieces
- 3 parsnips, cut in half lengthwise, then cut into 2-inch pieces
- 2 sprigs fresh thyme, plus more for garnish
- 3 dried bay leaves

1. Rinse the roast and pat dry. Rub on all sides with the salt, pepper, and coconut flour.
2. Heat the olive oil in a large pot over high heat. Add the roast and sear on all sides, about 10 minutes per side. Transfer the roast to a slow cooker.
3. Add the garlic and onion to the pot over medium heat. Sauté for 3 minutes. Add the tomato paste and cook for 1 minute. Add the wine and cook, occasionally scraping the bottom of the pan, until the mixture has reduced by half. Add the broth and bring to a boil. Remove from the heat.
4. Add the carrots, parsnips, thyme, and bay leaves to the slow cooker. Pour the broth mixture over the roast and veggies. Cover and cook on low for 6 hours. Remove the thyme sprigs and bay leaves before serving. Garnish with additional thyme.

Quick Tip: Use leftovers for the incredible *Pot Roast Tacos with Chimichurri* (page 148).

NUTRITION

Calories: 587 | Fat: 40 g | Carbohydrates: 9 g | Sodium: 557 mg | Fiber: 3 g | Protein: 41 g | Sugar: 2 g

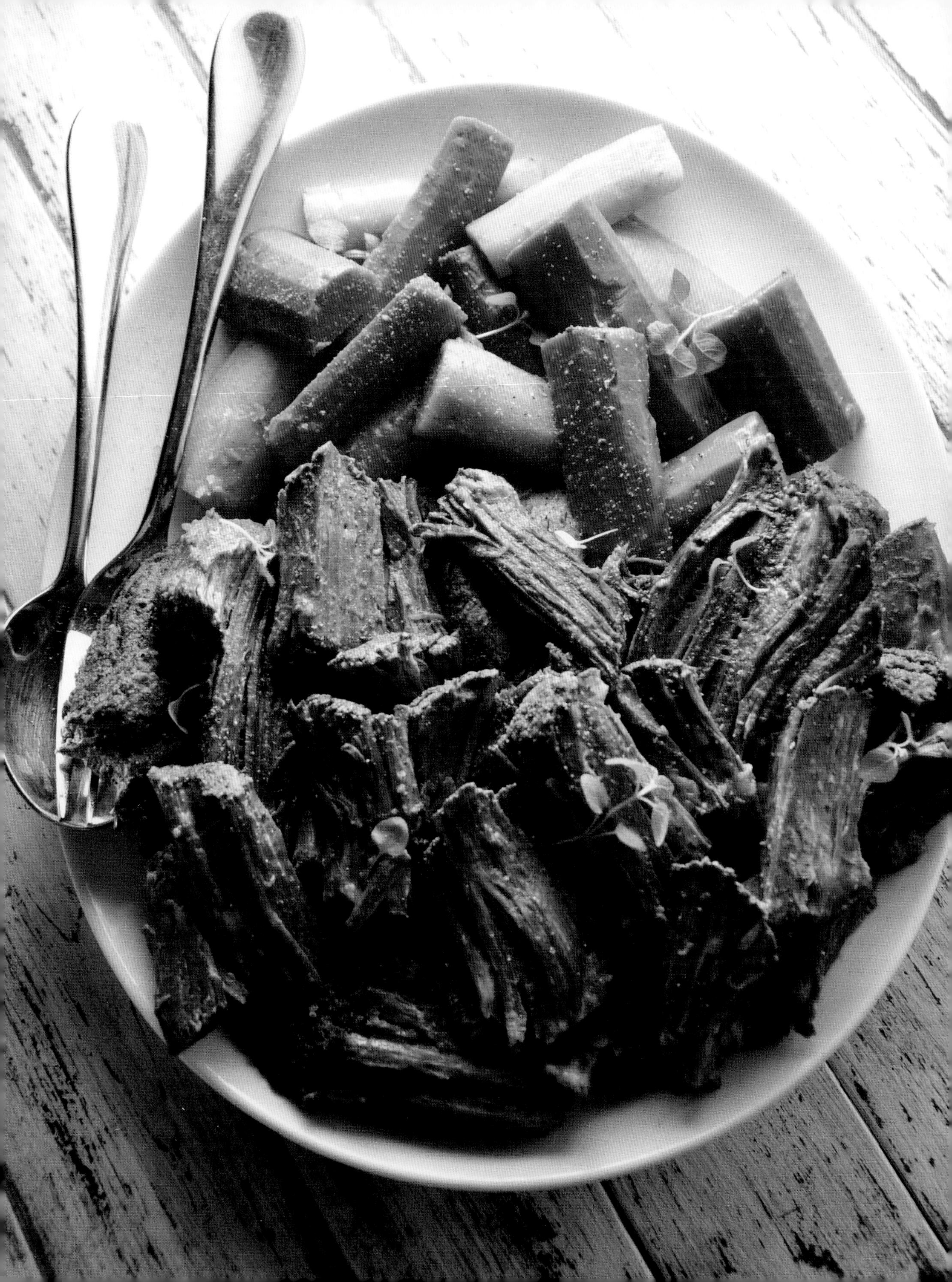

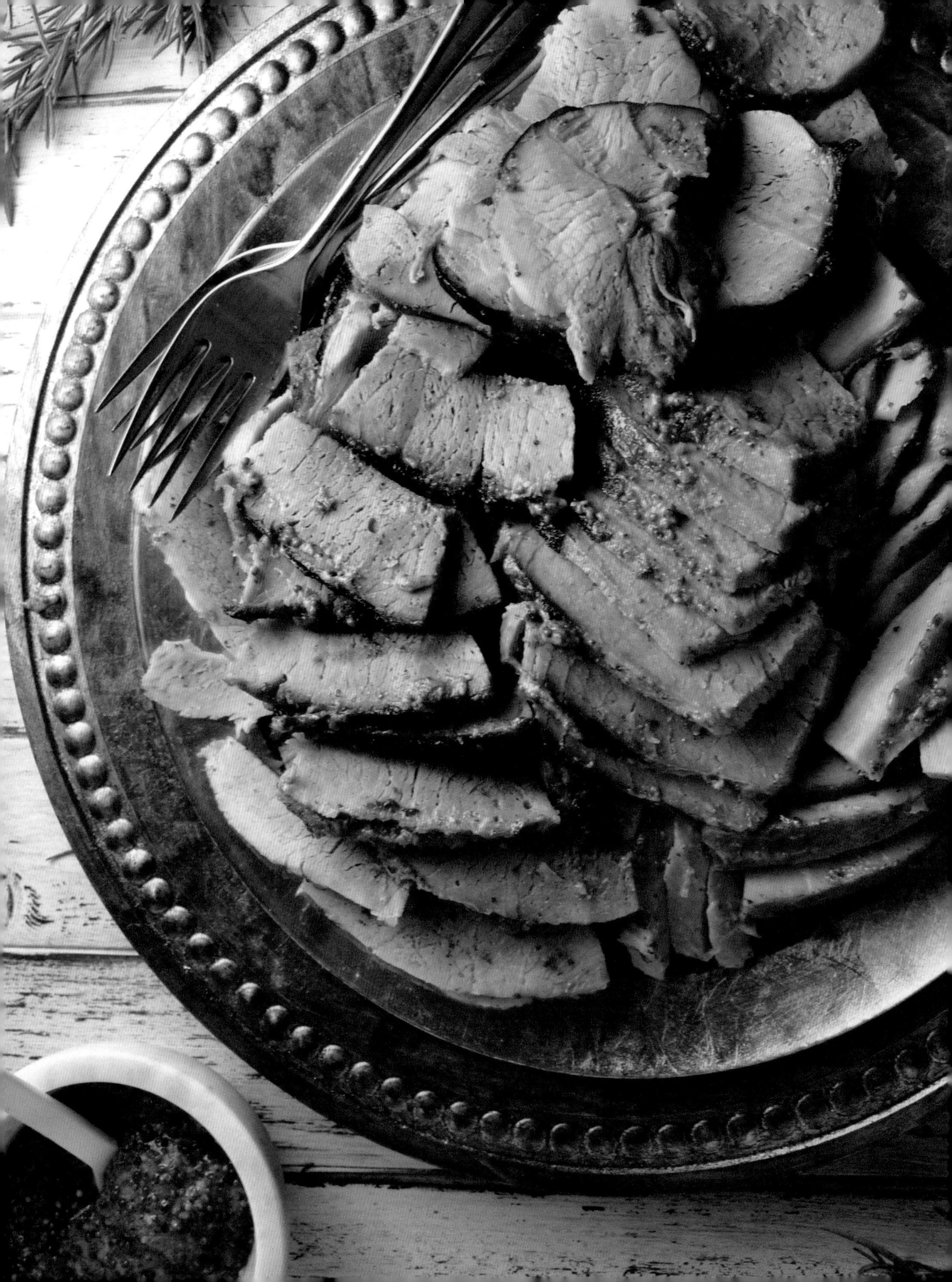

MOSCATO-DIJON HAM ROAST

PREP: 40 MINUTES | COOK: 3½ HOURS | MAKES: 20 SERVINGS (¾ LB PER SERVING FOR BONE-IN)

1 (14- to 16-pound) whole cured, smoked bone-in ham
2 cups Moscato wine, divided
3 cups chicken broth
4 cups water
2 tablespoons coconut oil
½ cup finely chopped shallots
1 tablespoon fresh thyme leaves
½ cup whole-grain Dijon mustard
1 tablespoon honey
½ teaspoon black pepper
¼ teaspoon sea salt

NUTRITION

Calories: 549
Fat: 20 g
Carbohydrates: 5 g
Sodium: 2,042 mg
Fiber: 0 g
Protein: 58 g
Sugar: 2 g

1. Place an oven rack at the lowest level and preheat to 300 degrees F. Remove the outer rind from most of the ham, leaving a band around the end of the bone shank and leaving the fat intact. On the top of the ham, score the fat crosswise, not cutting into the meat, with parallel cuts ½ inch apart. Place the ham in a roasting pan.
2. In a large pot, combine 1 cup of the Moscato with the broth and water. Bring to a boil. Pour into the bottom of the roasting pan.
3. Bake the ham, basting with the pan juices every 20 minutes, until an instant-read thermometer inserted into the center of the ham registers 110 degrees F, 2½ to 3 hours. (As a rule of thumb, roast a minimum of 10 minutes per pound.)
4. While the ham is cooking, in a large skillet, heat the coconut oil over medium heat. Add the shallots and thyme. Cook, stirring often, about 10 minutes, until the shallots are soft. Remove the pan from the heat and add the remaining 1 cup Moscato. Return the pan to medium-high heat and bring the mixture to a simmer. Cook until the mixture has reduced to ¼ cup, about 10 minutes. Transfer the mixture to a blender along with the mustard, honey, pepper, and salt. Blend until smooth.
5. Remove the ham from the oven and increase the oven temperature to 350 degrees F. Brush the mustard mixture over the ham. Bake for 15 to 30 more minutes, until the internal temperature registers 135 degrees F and the crust is golden brown. If the ham is browning too quickly, tent the pan with foil.
6. Transfer the ham to a serving platter. Let it rest for 30 minutes prior to carving. Skim the fat from the pan drippings and heat the drippings in a skillet until reduced. Serve the reduced drippings with the ham.

Quick Tip: If you'd prefer not to cook with wine, you can substitute white grape juice.

PROSCIUTTO-WRAPPED PORK ROAST WITH ROASTED PEPPER STUFFING

PREP: 30 MINUTES | COOK: 2½ HOURS | MAKES: 10 SERVINGS

For the Stuffing

1 tablespoon coconut oil
1 tablespoon olive oil
1 tablespoon minced fresh garlic
1 fennel bulb, chopped, plus ¼ cup chopped fronds
1 yellow onion, chopped
Sea salt and black pepper, to taste
1 cup dry white wine, divided
⅓ cup chopped roasted red bell pepper
2 tablespoons fresh thyme
1 teaspoon grated lemon zest

For the Pork Roast

1 (3-pound) boneless pork loin roast, trimmed
Sea salt and black pepper, to taste
⅓ pound thinly sliced prosciutto di Parma
20 cipollini onions
4 tablespoons olive oil, divided
5 parsnips, peeled, halved lengthwise, and cut into 2-inch pieces
2 tablespoons minced fresh rosemary leaves
1 tablespoon minced fresh garlic
1 cup chicken or bone broth

1. Preheat the oven to 400 degrees F.
2. For the stuffing: In a skillet, heat the coconut oil and olive oil over medium heat. Add the garlic, chopped fennel bulb, and onion. Season with salt and pepper and cook until the veggies soften, about 12 minutes. Deglaze the pan with ½ cup of wine, scraping the browned bits from the bottom. Transfer the veggies to a bowl and cool completely.
3. Add the roasted bell pepper, thyme, and lemon zest to the fennel mixture. Mix to combine.
4. For the pork roast: Butterfly the pork loin for stuffing: Holding your knife so that the blade is parallel with your cutting board, make a horizontal cut lengthwise about one-third of the way from the bottom of the loin. Slice the pork almost through, stopping short of the end so that the two flaps stay attached; open it like a book. Starting in the middle, make another horizontal cut into the thicker side of the loin, again cutting almost through but leaving the sides attached. It should now be butterflied into a single slab. Place a sheet of plastic wrap over the butterflied pork and pound it so that it flattens to ¾ inch thick.
5. Sprinkle the pork with salt and pepper. Spread the stuffing over the meat, leaving a 1-inch border clear. Roll the roast up, cover with overlapping slices of prosciutto, and tie up every 3 inches with kitchen twine.
6. Bring a saucepan of water to a boil and prepare a bowl of ice water. Cook the cipollini in the boiling water for 3 minutes; then drain and immediately plunge into the ice water. Peel and trim.
7. In a large skillet, heat 2 tablespoons of the olive oil over medium-high heat. Brown the pork roast evenly on all sides, 7 to 10 minutes per side. In a roasting pan, combine the parsnips, cipollini, rosemary, garlic, remaining 2 tablespoons olive oil, salt, and pepper. Place the browned roast on top of the parsnip mixture. Deglaze the skillet with the remaining wine, scraping up the browned bits, and pour this liquid over the roast.

8. Roast until the internal temperature reaches 145 degrees F, about 2 hours. Remove the roast from the roasting pan and let it rest on a plate under a foil tent for 30 minutes. Transfer the parsnips and cipollini from the roasting pan to a plate.
9. Place the roasting pan on a burner over medium heat. Deglaze with the broth, scraping up the browned bits. Stir in the fennel fronds. Slice the roast, spoon the roast juices from the pan over the top, and serve with the parsnips and cipollini.

Quick Tip: It helps to arrange the slices of prosciutto on a piece of foil. Then, when you are rolling the prosciutto over the roast, you can use the foil as a lift.

NUTRITION

Calories: 469 | Fat: 28 g | Carbohydrates: 20 g | Sodium: 317 mg | Fiber: 7 g | Protein: 32 g | Sugar: 5 g

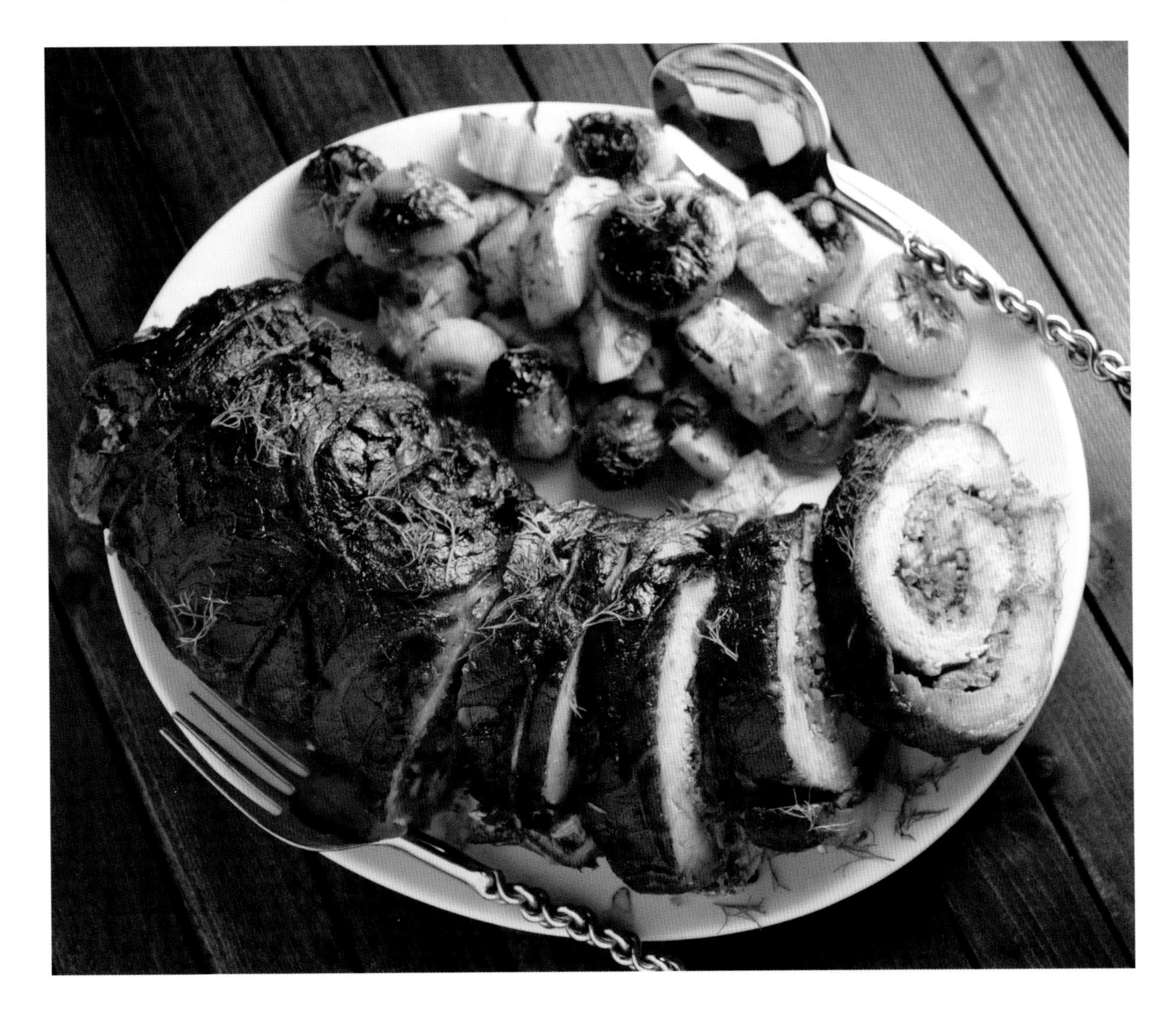

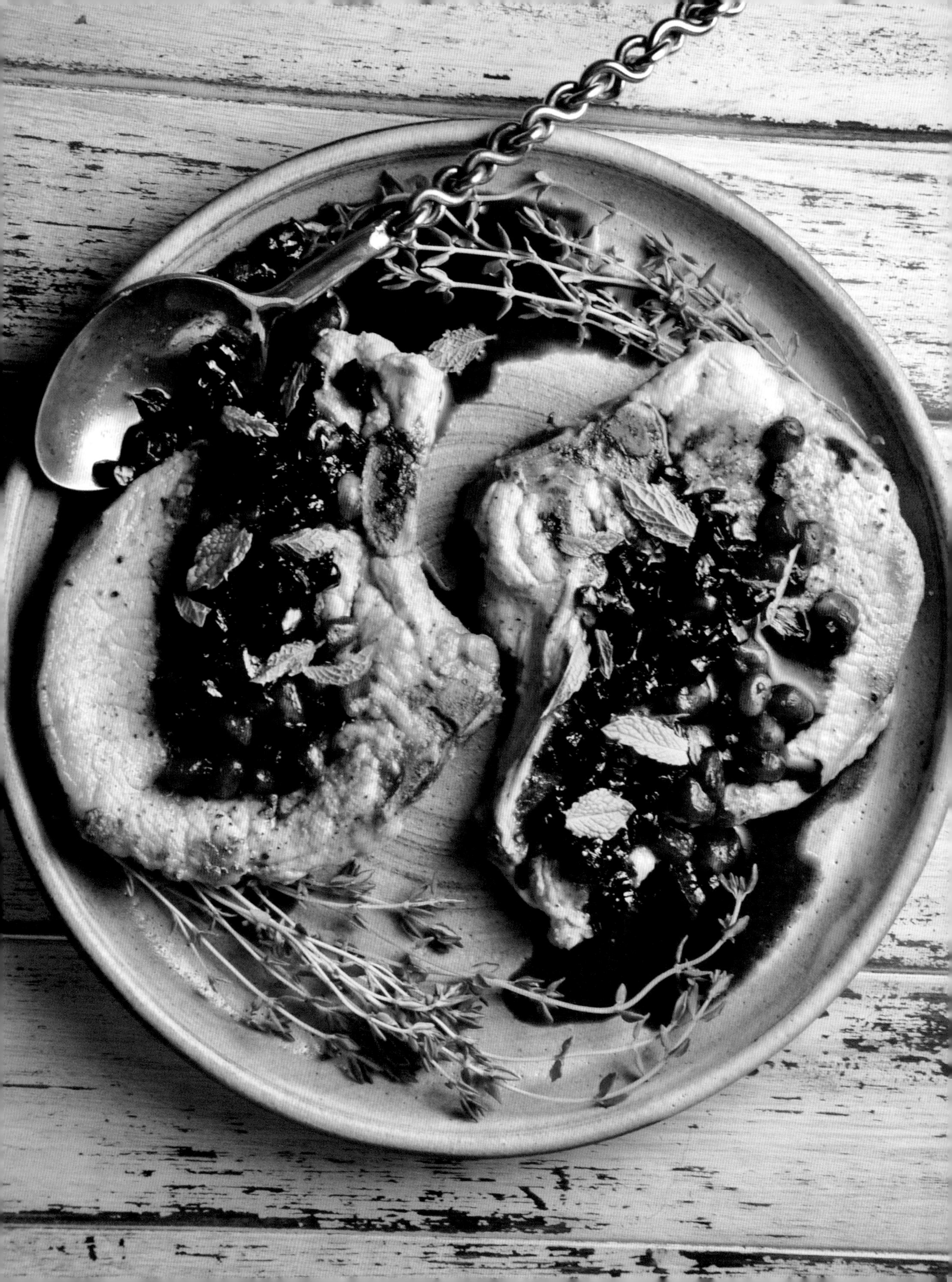

POMEGRANATE-GLAZED PORK CHOPS

PREP: 10 MINUTES | COOK: 15 MINUTES | MAKES: 4 SERVINGS

4 (1-inch-thick) bone-in center-cut pork chops
Sea salt and black pepper, to taste
2 tablespoons olive oil
3 tablespoons finely chopped shallots
1 cup pomegranate juice
2 tablespoons water
1 tablespoon honey
1 tablespoon balsamic vinegar
2 sprigs fresh thyme, plus more for garnish
1 tablespoon coconut oil
2 tablespoons fresh mint leaves
¼ cup pomegranate arils (the juicy sections that surround the white seeds of the pomegranate)

1. Generously season the pork chops with salt and pepper. Heat the olive oil in a large skillet over medium-high heat. Sear the chops for 3 to 5 minutes per side, or until an instant-read thermometer inserted into the center registers 145 degrees F. Transfer to a plate and cover with foil.
2. Pour off all but a thin layer of the oil in the pan and return it to the heat. Add the shallots and cook for 2 minutes, scraping up the browned bits at the bottom of the pan. Add the pomegranate juice, water, honey, vinegar, and thyme and bring to a boil. Reduce to a simmer and cook for 5 minutes, until reduced and thickened. Remove from the heat, remove the thyme, and whisk in the coconut oil.
3. Transfer the chops to plates and garnish with the fresh mint, pomegranate arils, and additional thyme sprigs.

Quick Tip: Bone-in chops have more flavor and don't dry out as easily as boneless ones.

NUTRITION

Calories: 486 | Fat: 20 g | Carbohydrates: 39 g | Sodium: 571 mg | Fiber: 1 g | Protein: 30 g | Sugar: 14 g

HONEY GARLIC PORK LOIN

PREP: 30 MINUTES | COOK: 6½ HOURS | MAKES: 8 SERVINGS

1 (3- to 4-pound) pork loin roast
Sea salt and black pepper, to taste
2 tablespoons olive oil
20 garlic cloves, peeled and smashed
1 yellow onion, chopped
1 tablespoon coconut flour
1 cup chicken or bone broth
2 tablespoons balsamic vinegar
2 tablespoons coconut aminos
2 tablespoons dried Italian seasoning blend
2 tablespoons honey
Fresh thyme, for garnish

1. Generously season the pork loin with salt and pepper. Heat the olive oil in a large skillet over medium-high heat. Sear the pork until browned on all sides, 8 to 10 minutes per side. Transfer to a slow cooker.
2. Add the garlic to the skillet and cook over medium-high heat, stirring often, for 5 minutes, until browned. Add the onion and cook for 3 minutes, until softened. Sprinkle the coconut flour over the garlic and onion and cook for 2 minutes.
3. Deglaze the pan with the broth, scraping up the browned bits. Stir in the vinegar, coconut aminos, and Italian seasoning. Bring to a boil, then pour over the pork in the slow cooker. Drizzle the honey over the pork, cover, and cook on low for 6 hours.
4. Transfer the pork to a plate and let it rest while you make the sauce. Strain the solids from the slow cooker liquid into a saucepan over high heat and bring to a boil. Reduce the heat to medium and simmer until the sauce thickens, about 5 minutes. Slice the pork and serve with the sauce. Garnish with fresh thyme.

Quick Tip: If you don't have 6 hours for slow cooking, then feel free to roast the pork loin in the oven. Follow step 1 for searing the loin, then roast in the oven at 400 degrees F for 12 minutes, or until an instant-read thermometer inserted into the center registers 140 degrees F. Continue with making the sauce in steps 2 and 3, and once you bring the mixture to a boil, return the roasted loin to the skillet. Cover with the honey and continue to simmer. Gently tilt the skillet so that the liquid pools to one side, then continuously spoon the liquid over the loin until it becomes thick and syrupy. Remove from the heat and let the loin rest for 5 minutes before slicing and serving.

NUTRITION

Calories: 357 | Fat: 17 g | Carbohydrates: 10 g | Sodium: 177 mg | Fiber: 1 g | Protein: 38 g | Sugar: 5 g

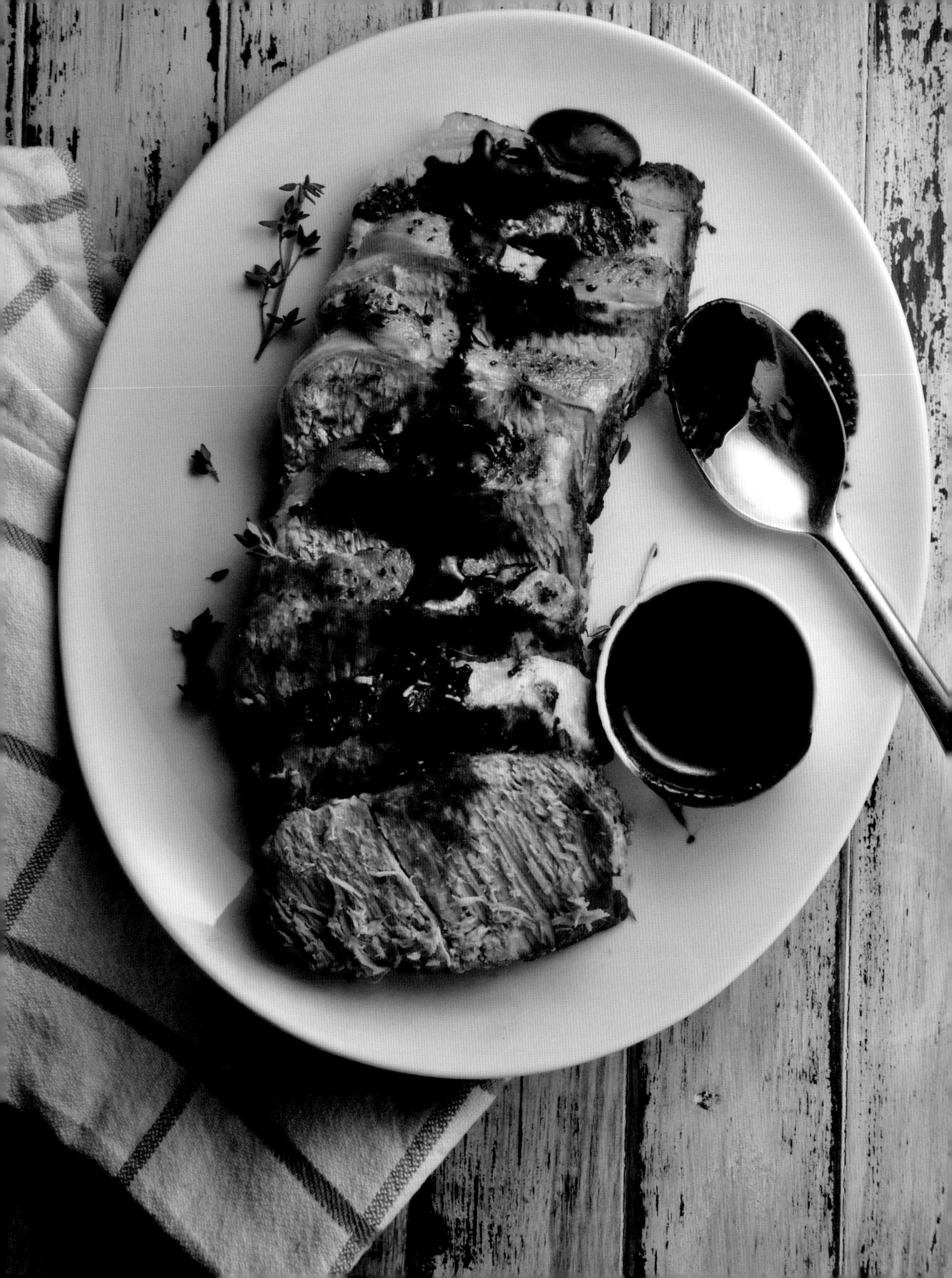

ROASTED TURKEY ROULADE

PREP: 45 MINUTES | COOK: 45 MINUTES | MAKES: 6 SERVINGS

For the Sauce

Olive oil, for greasing
3 Roma tomatoes, chopped
¾ cup pimento-stuffed green olives, chopped
1 fennel bulb, halved and sliced
2 tablespoons minced fresh garlic
1 tablespoon capers
1 tablespoon grated lemon zest
1 tablespoon minced fresh oregano
Black pepper, to taste

For the Stuffing

2 cups chopped thawed frozen spinach
2 teaspoons grated lemon zest
½ teaspoon crushed red pepper
Sea salt and black pepper, to taste
1 (15-ounce) can chickpeas, drained and rinsed, roughly chopped
1 egg, beaten
1 tablespoon minced fresh oregano

For the Turkey

1 (5-pound) boneless turkey breast, butterflied and flattened
Salt and black pepper, to taste

For the Basting Vinaigrette

¼ cup lemon juice
2 tablespoons olive oil
1 teaspoon grated lemon zest
1 teaspoon dried rosemary, crushed

1. Preheat the oven to 425 degrees F.
2. For the sauce: Lightly grease a 13 × 9-inch casserole dish with olive oil. In a medium bowl, combine all the sauce ingredients together. Spread over the bottom of the prepared casserole pan.
3. For the stuffing: In a medium skillet over medium-high heat, sauté the spinach, lemon zest, and crushed red pepper for 3 minutes. Remove from the heat. Use a paper towel to squeeze out any remaining liquid. Transfer to a bowl and mix in the salt, pepper, chickpeas, egg, and oregano.
4. For the turkey: Place the turkey breast flat on a work surface and season with salt and pepper. Spread the stuffing in an even layer, then tightly roll the turkey. Tie the roll with kitchen twine, spaced about every 4 inches. Place the roulade in the casserole pan, on top of the sauce.
5. For the basting vinaigrette: In a small bowl, whisk together all the vinaigrette ingredients.
6. Roast the roulade, basting with the vinaigrette every 10 minutes, for about 45 minutes. The turkey is done when an instant-read thermometer inserted into the center registers 165 degrees F.
7. Let the roulade rest for 10 minutes, then slice and serve with the sauce.

Quick Tip: Here are a few suggestions for rolling your roulade:

- Pound your turkey breast to an even ¾-inch thickness.
- Evenly spread the filling over the pounded breast, leaving a 1-inch border on all sides.
- Securely tie the roulade with kitchen twine every 4 inches along the cylinder.

NUTRITION

Calories: 374 | Fat: 12 g | Carbohydrates: 19 g | Sodium: 976 mg | Fiber: 5 g | Protein: 51 g | Sugar: 3 g

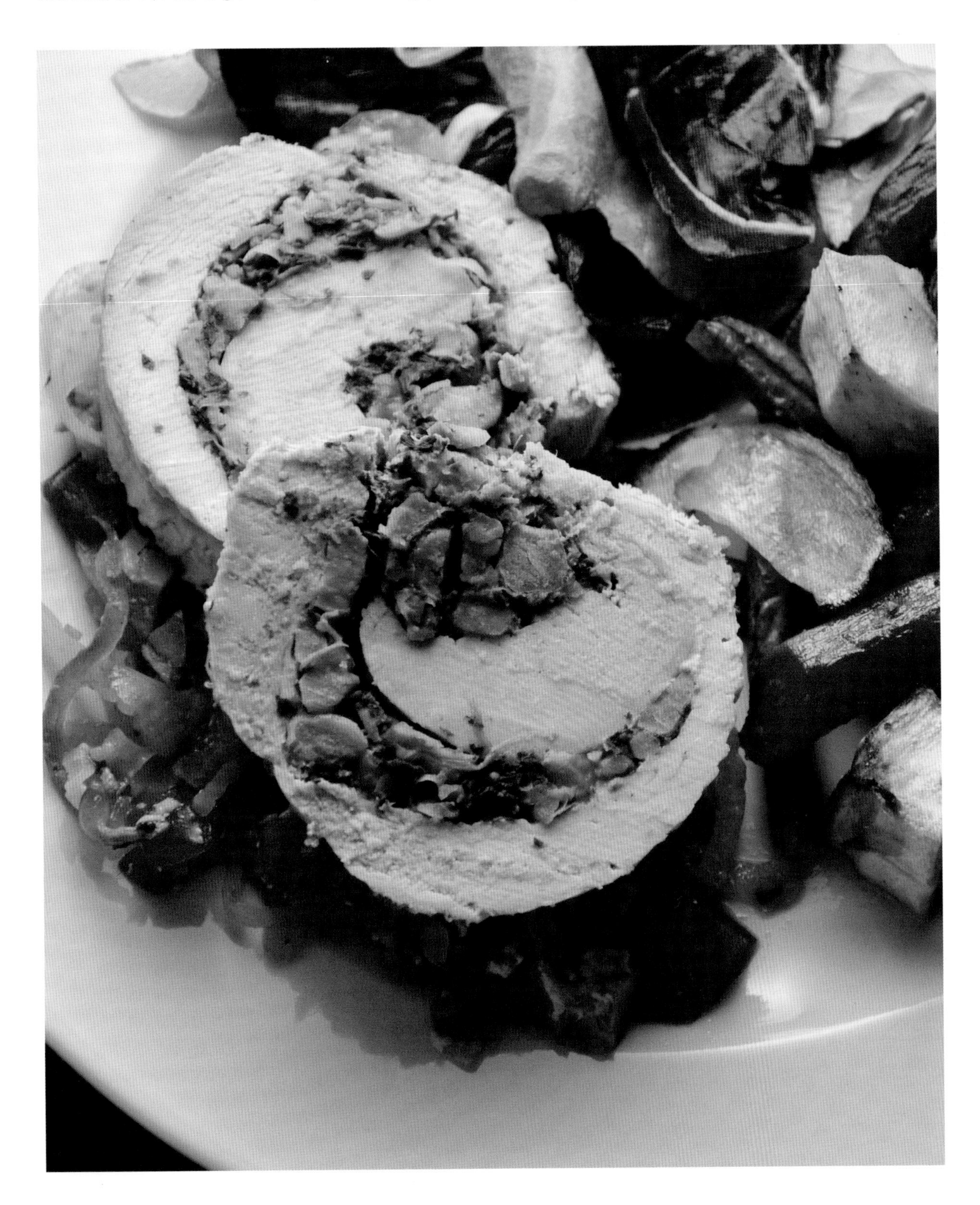

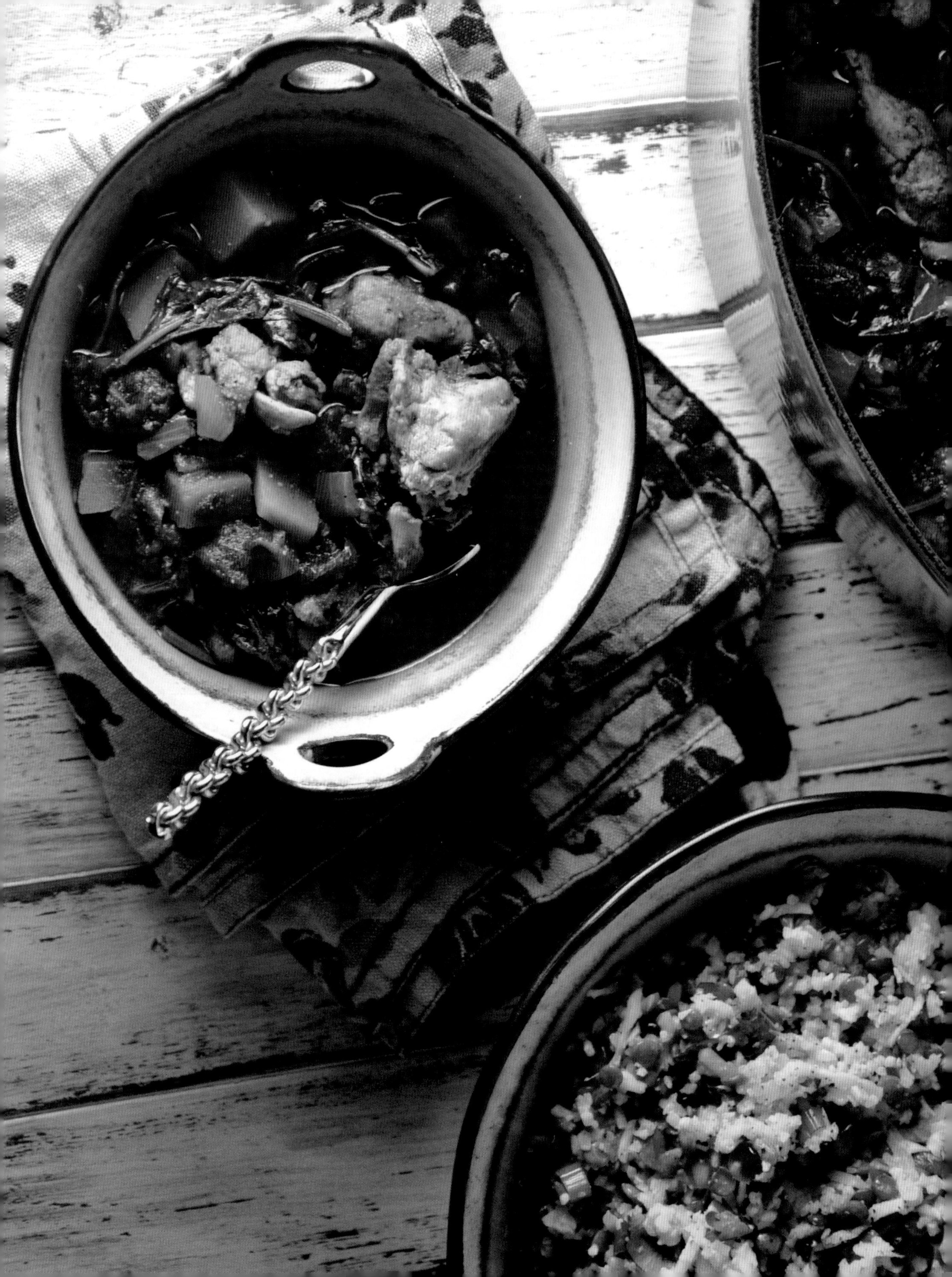

MOROCCAN SPICED CHICKEN AND SQUASH

PREP: 15 MINUTES | COOK: 55 MINUTES | MAKES: 10 SERVINGS

3 pounds boneless, skinless chicken thighs
Sea salt and black pepper, to taste
3 tablespoons coconut flour, for dredging
2 tablespoons coconut oil
1 tablespoon olive oil
2 tablespoons grated fresh ginger
1 tablespoon chopped fresh garlic
2 yellow onions, diced
1 red serrano pepper
3 tablespoons ras el hanout spice blend
2 cups chicken or bone broth
1 medium butternut squash, peeled, seeded, and chopped into 2-inch cubes
1 (28-ounce) can diced tomatoes, undrained
3 cups fresh spinach

1. Season the chicken with salt and pepper. Place the coconut flour on a plate and dredge the chicken in the flour. In a Dutch oven over medium-high heat, heat the coconut oil and olive oil. Working in batches, cook the chicken until browned and crisp on the outside and cooked through, about 7 minutes per side. Transfer to a plate and tent with foil.
2. Add the ginger, garlic, onions, and serrano pepper to the pot. Sprinkle with salt. Add the ras el hanout and cook until the veggies are tender, about 12 minutes.
3. Add the broth, squash, and tomatoes. Simmer for 15 minutes. Return the chicken to the pot and simmer for 10 minutes. Add the spinach and cook until wilted, 2 to 3 minutes.

Quick Tip: It's also possible to make this meal in a slow cooker. Simply transfer the chicken to the bottom of the slow cooker after step 1, and then add all the remaining ingredients, except the fresh spinach. Cover and cook on low heat for 6 hours. Stir in the fresh spinach just before serving.

NUTRITION

Calories: 336 | Fat: 15 g | Carbohydrates: 8 g | Sodium: 302 mg | Fiber: 3 g | Protein: 41 g | Sugar: 1 g

SLOW COOKER HONEY GARLIC CHICKEN

PREP: 5 MINUTES | COOK: 6 HOURS | MAKES: 8 SERVINGS

- 3 pounds boneless, skinless chicken thighs
- Sea salt and black pepper, to taste
- ½ cup coconut aminos
- ½ cup natural ketchup (no added sugar)
- ¼ cup honey
- 1 tablespoon minced fresh garlic
- 1 teaspoon dried basil
- Sesame seeds and sliced scallions, for garnish (optional)

1. Generously season the chicken thighs with salt and pepper. Place in the bottom of a slow cooker.
2. In a small bowl, combine the coconut aminos, ketchup, honey, garlic, and basil. Pour over the chicken. Cover and cook on low for 6 hours. Garnish with sesame seeds and scallions, if desired.

Quick Tip: I like to serve this tender, flavorful chicken with a vibrant green salad and steamed veggies.

NUTRITION

Calories: 372 | Fat: 12 g | Carbohydrates: 12 g | Sodium: 314 mg | Fiber: 0 g | Protein: 50 g | Sugar: 12 g

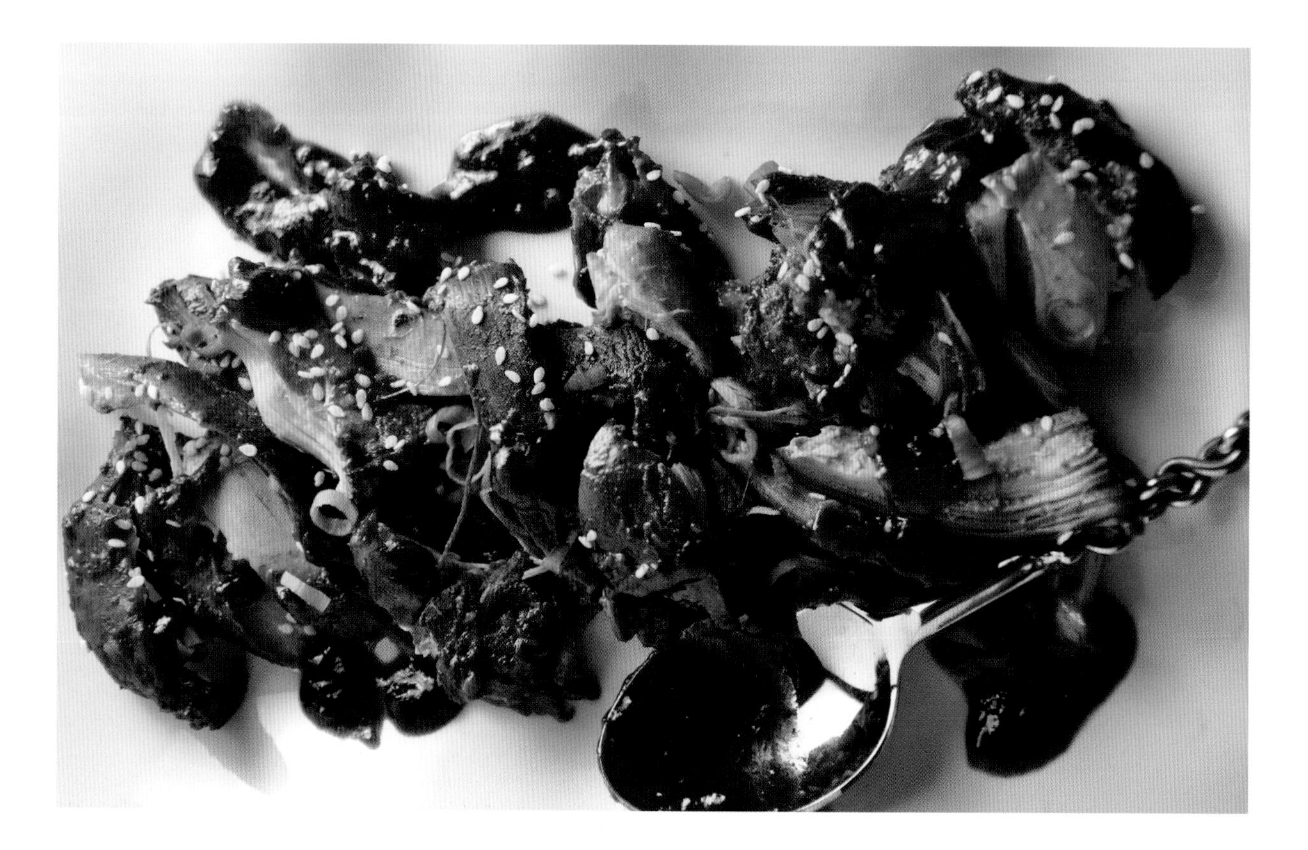

MAPLE CHICKEN AND VEGGIES

PREP: 15 MINUTES | COOK: 40 MINUTES | MAKES: 6 SERVINGS

1 tablespoon minced fresh thyme
1 tablespoon Dijon mustard
1 tablespoon pure maple syrup
4 bone-in, skin-on chicken breasts
4 cups peeled, seeded, and cubed butternut squash
½ acorn squash, seeded and cut crosswise into slices
3 shallots, peeled and quartered
2 cups Brussels sprouts, peeled and halved
2 tablespoons coconut oil, melted
1 tablespoon olive oil
¾ teaspoon sea salt
¼ teaspoon black pepper

1. Place a rimmed baking sheet in the oven and preheat to 425 degrees F.
2. Combine the thyme, mustard, and syrup in a small bowl; brush over the chicken. Remove the hot pan from the oven, place the chicken on the pan, and bake for 20 minutes.
3. Add the squashes, shallots, and Brussels sprouts to the pan with the chicken. Top the veggies with the coconut oil, olive oil, salt, and pepper. Return the pan to the oven for another 20 minutes. Serve immediately.

Quick Tip: Here's an idea: Prepare the chicken and veggies the night before and store them in separate ziplock bags in the fridge, already marinated and seasoned. Then, when you're ready to pop dinner into the oven, simply throw the ready-to-go ingredients on the pan and start roasting.

NUTRITION

Calories: 464
Fat: 11 g
Carbohydrates: 21 g
Sodium: 399 mg
Fiber: 4 g
Protein: 35 g
Sugar: 5 g

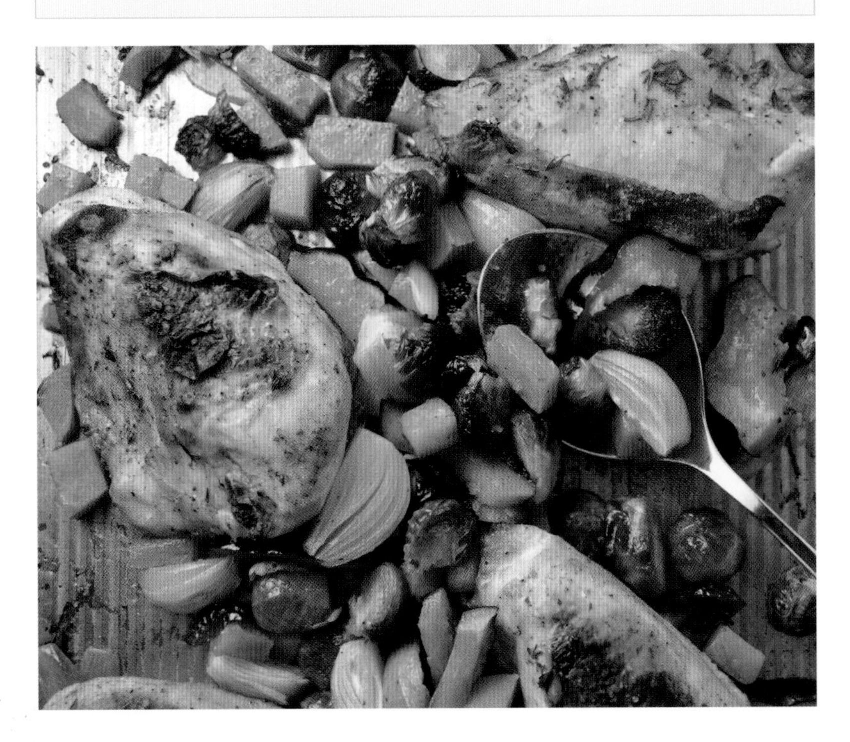

CARAMEL CHICKEN

PREP: 10 MINUTES | COOK: 50 MINUTES | MAKES: 6 SERVINGS

2 tablespoons olive oil
3 pounds bone-in, skin-on chicken legs and thighs
Sea salt, to taste
1 tablespoon minced fresh garlic
½ cup water
3 tablespoons coconut sugar
¼ cup apple cider vinegar
2 tablespoons minced fresh ginger
1 cup broth (any type)
¼ cup coconut aminos
2 scallions, thinly sliced

1. Place a Dutch oven over medium-high heat and add the olive oil. Season the chicken with salt and cook in two batches until golden and crisp, about 7 minutes per side. Transfer the chicken to a plate and pour off most of the fat from the pot.
2. Return the Dutch oven to medium-high heat and add the garlic, stirring until golden. Add the water, scraping up browned bits. Add the coconut sugar and stir to dissolve. Cook, stirring, until the mixture thickens and turns deep amber, about 5 minutes. Add the vinegar and stir.
3. Add the ginger, broth, and coconut aminos; then add the chicken, skin side up. Bring to a boil, reduce the heat, and simmer gently until the chicken is cooked through, 20 to 25 minutes. Transfer the chicken to a plate.
4. Bring the liquid to a boil and cook until thick enough to coat a spoon, about 10 minutes. Return the chicken to the pot and turn to coat. Top with the scallions and serve immediately.

Quick Tip: Having a sweet tooth is no problem when you have an array of sugar substitutes to choose from. Coconut sugar, maple syrup, and honey can be used in moderation, as these still affect your blood sugar and contain calories. Liquid stevia and erythritol don't affect your blood sugar and have zero calories.

NUTRITION
Calories: 521
Fat: 22 g
Carbohydrates: 10 g
Sodium: 411 mg
Fiber: 1 g
Protein: 27 g
Sugar: 6 g

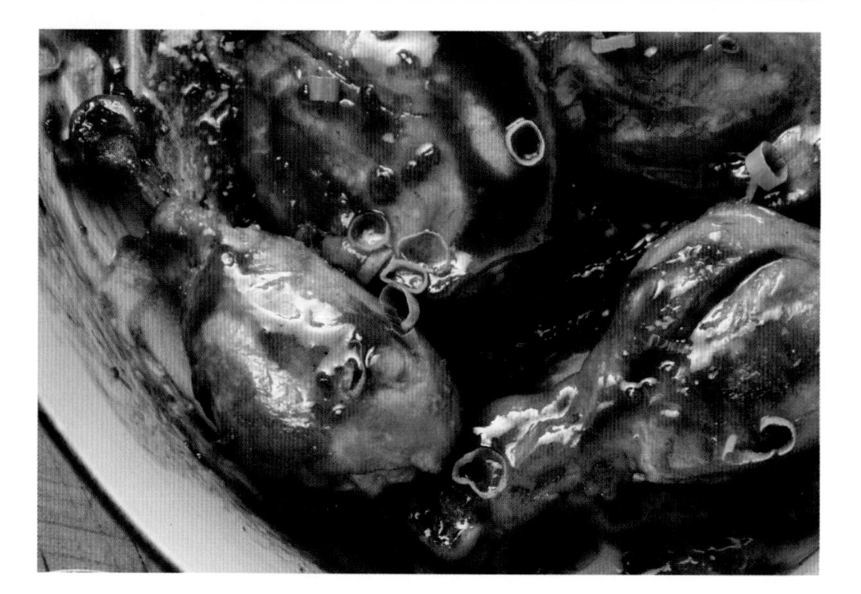

SPICED TILAPIA

PREP: 10 MINUTES | COOK: 12 MINUTES | MAKES: 4 SERVINGS

For the Spice Mixture

1 tablespoon ground turmeric
½ teaspoon ground cinnamon
½ teaspoon ground ginger
Pinch of ground nutmeg
½ teaspoon sea salt
½ teaspoon black pepper

For the Tilapia

4 (6-ounce) tilapia fillets
2 tablespoons coconut oil, divided
¼ cup fresh cilantro leaves
1 red bell pepper, seeded and cut into matchsticks
¼ cup unsweetened flaked coconut, toasted

1. For the spice mixture: Combine all the spice mixture ingredients in a small dish.
2. For the tilapia: Rub the spice mixture all over the tilapia fillets.
3. Heat 1 tablespoon of the coconut oil in a large skillet over medium heat. Cook two of the fillets until golden and flaky, about 3 minutes per side. Remove from the skillet and repeat with the remaining 1 tablespoon coconut oil and the remaining two fillets.
4. Top with the cilantro, bell pepper, and coconut.

Quick Tip: You can easily toast your own coconut flakes. Preheat your oven to 325 degrees F. Spread the flakes on a baking sheet and bake for 5 to 7 minutes, until golden brown. They toast quickly, so be sure to watch them.

NUTRITION

Calories: 291 | Fat: 11 g | Carbohydrates: 4 g | Sodium: 447 mg | Fiber: 2 g | Protein: 21 g | Sugar: 2g

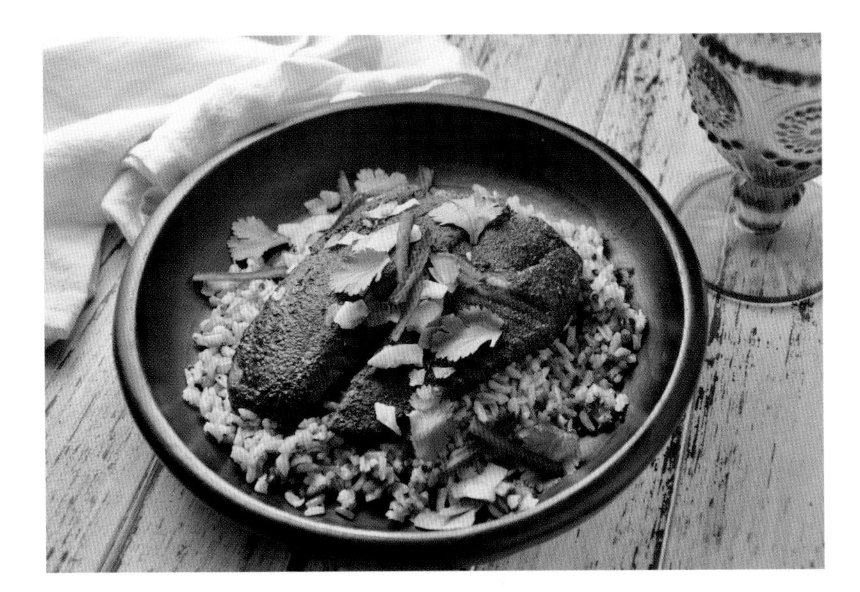

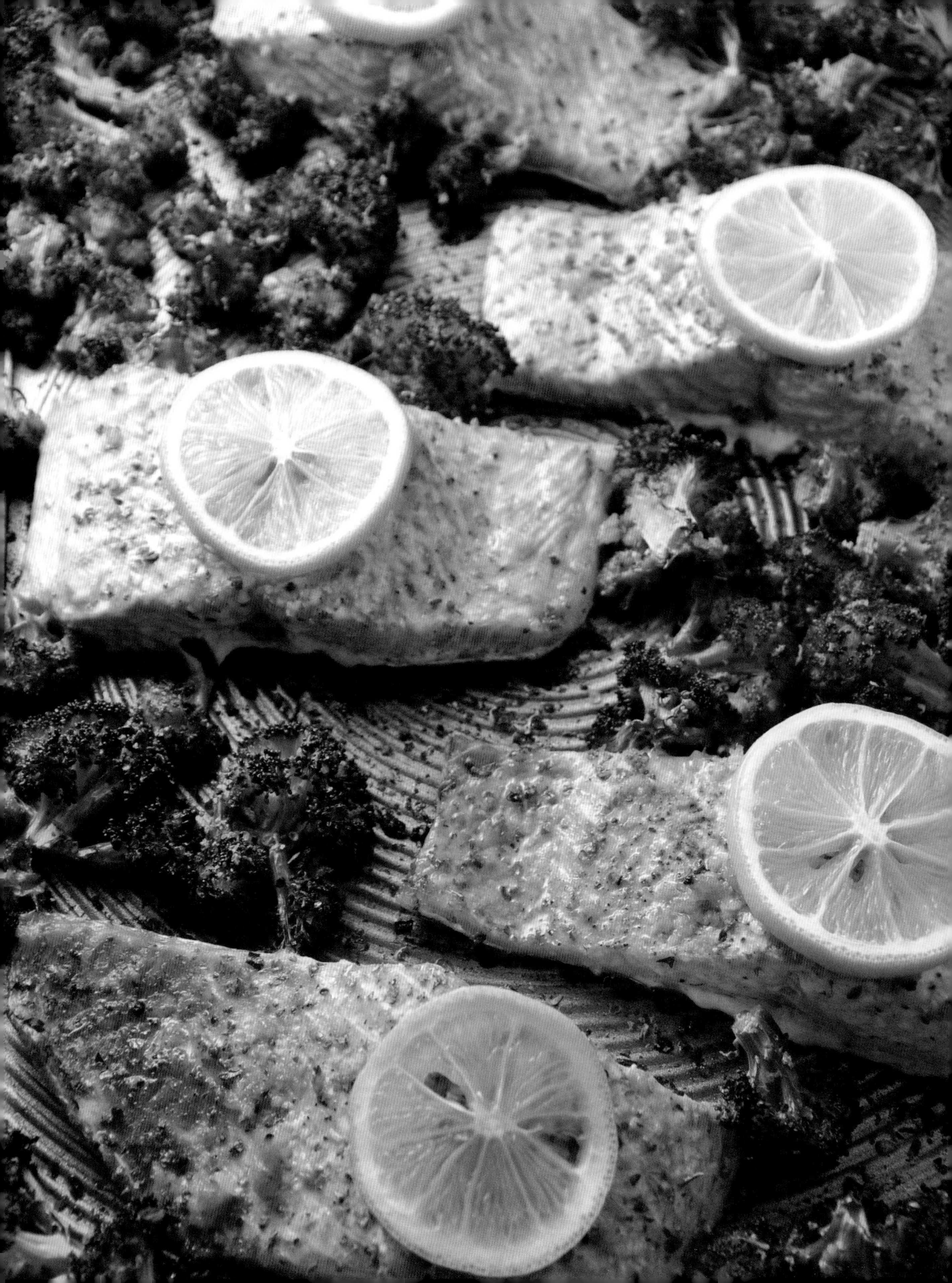

ONE-PAN GARLIC ROASTED SALMON AND BROCCOLI

PREP: 10 MINUTES | COOK: 23 MINUTES | MAKES: 5 SERVINGS

For the Broccoli

2 tablespoons olive oil, plus more for greasing
2 heads broccoli, cut into florets
1 tablespoon minced fresh garlic
Sea salt and black pepper, to taste

For the Salmon

5 (6-ounce) skin-on salmon fillets
1 tablespoon olive oil
2 teaspoons minced fresh garlic
1 teaspoon grated lemon zest
2 teaspoons dried marjoram
Sea salt and black pepper, to taste
1 lemon, cut into 5 slices

1. For the broccoli: Preheat the oven to 450 degrees F. Lightly grease a rimmed baking sheet with olive oil.
2. In a large bowl, toss together the broccoli, olive oil, and garlic. Season generously with salt and pepper. Mix until well combined.
3. Spread the seasoned broccoli in a single layer over the prepared baking sheet and roast for 10 minutes.
4. For the salmon: While the broccoli is cooking, place the salmon fillets on a plate. Drizzle the salmon with the olive oil and evenly sprinkle with the minced garlic, lemon zest, and marjoram. Season generously with salt and pepper.
5. Remove the baking sheet from the oven, and move the broccoli to create open spaces for the fillets. Place the salmon in the empty spaces and put back in the oven for 10 to 12 minutes, until the salmon is flaky and cooked through. Turn on the broiler. Top each fillet with a slice of lemon and place under the broiler for 1 minute.

Quick Tip: I have a list in the back of my mind of dinner recipes that are fast and simple enough to be made with just a quick stop at the store on my way home from the office and a few minutes in the kitchen. This *One-Pan Garlic Roasted Salmon and Broccoli* lives at the top of my fast and simple list.

NUTRITION

Calories: 401 | Fat: 19 g | Carbohydrates: 12 g | Sodium: 356 mg | Fiber: 8 g | Protein: 42 g | Sugar: 3 g

CHOCOLATE SUPER-SEED BARK

PREP: 30 MINUTES | COOK: 25 MINUTES | MAKES: 24 SERVINGS

¼ cup pure maple syrup
4 tablespoons coconut oil, melted, divided
1 tablespoon vanilla extract
1 tablespoon instant espresso powder
Pinch of flake sea salt, plus more for garnish
1 cup uncooked quinoa
½ cup raw cashews, roughly chopped
½ cup raw walnuts, roughly chopped
2 tablespoons hemp seeds
2 tablespoons chia seeds
2 tablespoons flaxseeds
2 tablespoons sesame seeds
5 ounces stevia-sweetened dark chocolate chips (such as Lily's brand)

NUTRITION
Calories: 143
Fat: 10 g
Carbohydrates: 14 g
Sodium: 25 mg
Fiber: 3 g
Protein: 4 g
Sugar: 2 g

1. Preheat the oven to 350 degrees F. Line a baking sheet with parchment paper.
2. In a large bowl, combine the syrup, 3 tablespoons of the coconut oil, the vanilla, espresso powder, sea salt, quinoa, cashews, walnuts, and all the seeds. Mix until fully combined and then spread the mixture over the prepared baking sheet in a thin layer. Bake for 20 minutes, until golden and crisp.
3. In a double boiler, melt the chocolate chips and remaining 1 tablespoon coconut oil, about 5 minutes. Drizzle the chocolate over the seed bark in an even layer, smoothing it with a spatula. Sprinkle with sea salt and place in the fridge to set for 30 minutes. Remove and cut or break into pieces. Store in an airtight container in the fridge or freezer.

Quick Tip: Keep a bag of these tasty morsels in the freezer and reward yourself with a delightful bite of omega-3s for dessert or as a bedtime snack.

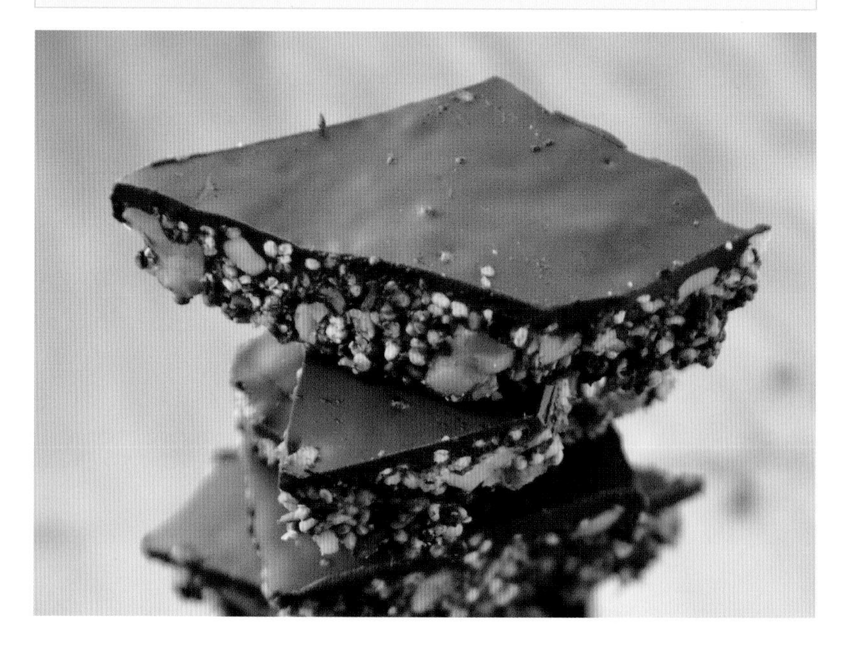

CHOCOLATE CHUNK COOKIES

PREP: 15 MINUTES | COOK: 10 MINUTES | MAKES: 24 SERVINGS (1 COOKIE EQUALS 1 SERVING)

⅓ cup palm shortening
¼ cup coconut oil, softened
⅔ cup coconut sugar
½ teaspoon baking soda
½ teaspoon sea salt
1 egg
1 tablespoon vanilla extract
2 cups blanched almond flour
1 cup chopped stevia-sweetened dark chocolate caramel bar (such as Lily's brand)
Flake sea salt

1. Preheat the oven to 350 degrees F. Line 2 or 3 baking sheets with parchment paper.
2. In the bowl of an electric mixer, beat the palm shortening and coconut oil on high for 30 seconds. Add the coconut sugar, baking soda, and sea salt. Beat on medium for 2 minutes, scraping down the sides of the bowl as needed. Beat in the egg and vanilla. Beat in the almond flour until well incorporated. Stir in the chocolate pieces.
3. Drop the dough by rounded tablespoons 2 inches apart on the prepared baking sheets. Sprinkle with flake sea salt. Bake for 8 to 10 minutes, until the edges are lightly browned. Transfer the parchment paper with the cookies onto a wire rack to cool.

Quick Tip: Save a cookie to use in the tasty *Cookie Butter Protein Smoothie* recipe (page 199).

NUTRITION
Calories: 82
Fat: 7 g
Carbohydrates: 5 g
Sodium: 90 mg
Fiber: 0 g
Protein: 1 g
Sugar: 4 g

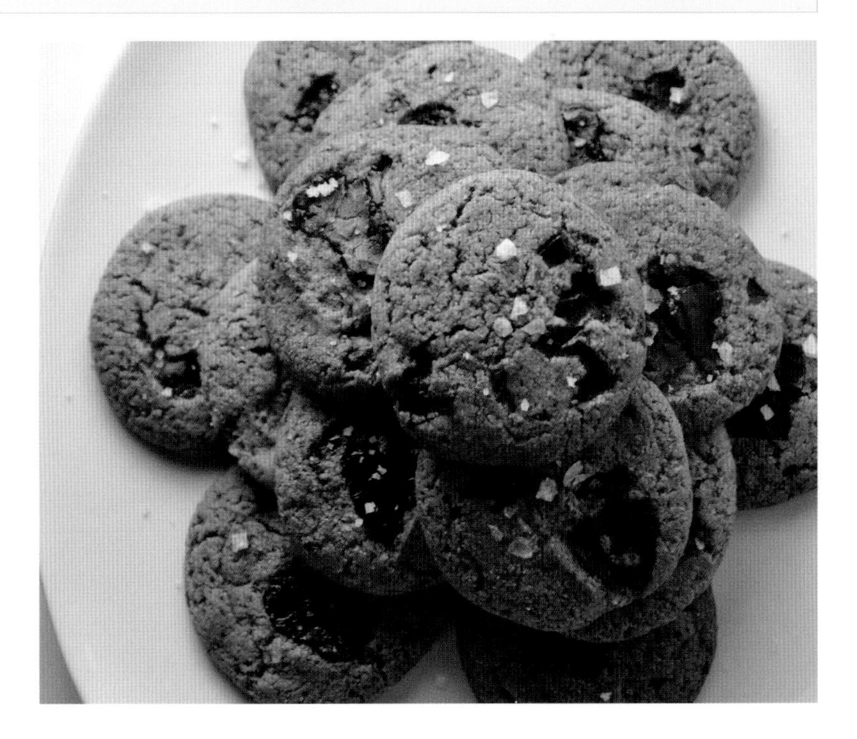

SALTED DARK CHOCOLATE–DIPPED PB COOKIES

PREP: 35 MINUTES | COOK: 10 MINUTES | MAKES: 36 SERVINGS (1 COOKIE EQUALS 1 SERVING)

For the Peanut Butter Cookies

½ cup palm shortening
½ cup creamy, no-sugar-added natural peanut butter (substitute almond butter if you have a peanut allergy)
1 cup coconut sugar
1 teaspoon baking powder
¼ teaspoon sea salt
⅛ teaspoon baking soda
1 egg
2 tablespoons coconut cream
1 teaspoon vanilla extract
2 cups blanched almond flour

For the Salted Dark Chocolate Dip

1 (9-ounce) bag stevia-sweetened dark chocolate chips (such as Lily's brand)
2 tablespoons coconut oil
1 tablespoon coarse sea salt

1. Preheat the oven to 350 degrees F. Line 2 or 3 baking sheets with parchment paper.
2. For the peanut butter cookies: In the bowl of an electric mixer, beat the palm shortening and peanut butter on high for 30 seconds. Add the coconut sugar, baking powder, sea salt, and baking soda. Beat on medium for 2 minutes, scraping down the sides of the bowl as needed. Beat in the egg, coconut cream, and vanilla. Beat in the almond flour until everything is well incorporated.
3. Drop the dough by rounded tablespoons 2 inches apart on the prepared baking sheets. Use a fork dipped in coconut oil to make a crisscross on the top of each cookie. Bake for 8 to 10 minutes, until the edges are lightly browned. Transfer the parchment paper with the cookies onto a wire rack to cool. Once the cookies are cool, transfer the parchment paper with the cookies to the freezer for 10 minutes.
4. For the salted dark chocolate dip: While the cookies cool, melt the chocolate chips and coconut oil in a double boiler over medium heat, stirring often until smooth, about 5 minutes. Dip the cold cookies halfway into the chocolate, and then place on a parchment paper–lined baking sheet (make sure that it fits in your freezer!). Sprinkle the coarse sea salt on the chocolate. Place the dipped cookies in the freezer for about 15 minutes, until set.

Quick Tip: Store leftovers in the freezer or the fridge to keep the chocolate set.

NUTRITION

Calories: 118 | Fat: 9 g | Carbohydrates: 8 g | Sodium: 193 mg | Fiber: 1 g | Protein: 2 g | Sugar: 5 g

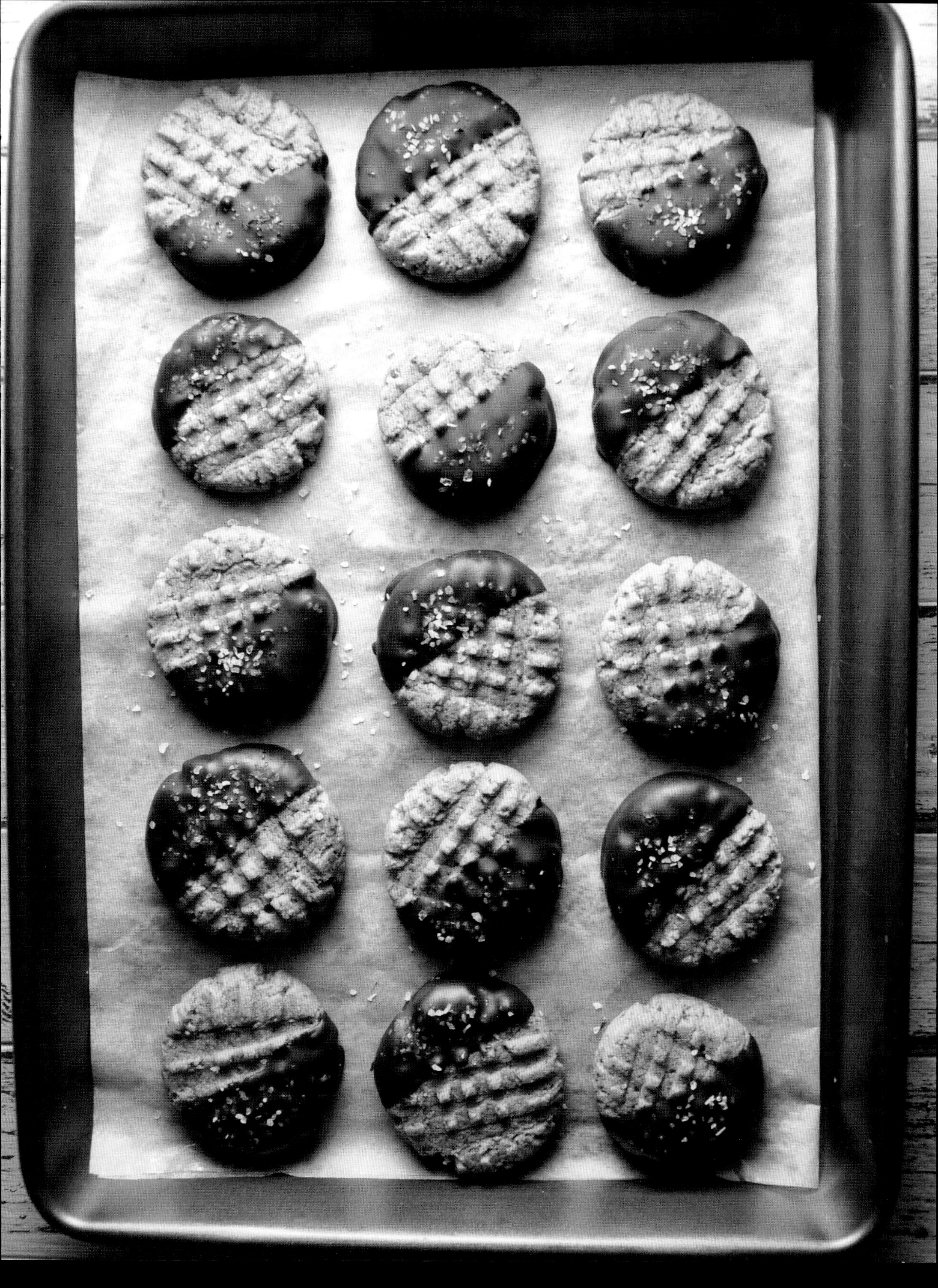

MEXICAN BROWNIES

PREP: 20 MINUTES | COOK: 25 MINUTES | MAKES: 20 SERVINGS

Coconut oil for greasing
1 cup blanched almond flour
¼ cup unsweetened cocoa powder
½ teaspoon sea salt
½ teaspoon baking powder
¼ teaspoon ground cayenne pepper
1 cup stevia-sweetened dark chocolate chips (such as Lily's brand)
1 cup coconut oil
1¼ cups coconut sugar
1 teaspoon instant espresso powder
3 eggs, beaten
1 teaspoon vanilla extract
Powdered erythritol sweetener, such as confectioners' Swerve, for garnish (optional)

1. Preheat the oven to 350 degrees F. Line the bottom of a 9 × 9-inch baking pan with parchment paper and lightly grease the paper with coconut oil.
2. In a large mixing bowl, whisk together the almond flour, cocoa powder, salt, baking powder, and cayenne. Mix well.
3. Melt the chocolate chips, coconut oil, coconut sugar, and espresso powder in a saucepan over low heat, about 5 minutes. Remove the pan from the heat and stir in the eggs and vanilla. Mix in the flour mixture.
4. Pour the batter into the prepared pan and bake for 25 minutes, until the middle doesn't jiggle when you shake the pan. Set the pan on a wire rack to cool completely. Cut the brownies into 20 squares. If desired, sift some powdered erythritol sweetener over the top as a garnish.

Quick Tip: Mexican brownies have a little kick from cayenne pepper. I highly recommend giving this exciting flavor combination a try. However, if you are simply not a fan of spiciness, leave out the cayenne pepper and enjoy the chocolate.

NUTRITION

Calories: 193 | Fat: 15 g | Carbohydrates: 16 g | Sodium: 77 mg | Fiber: 2 g | Protein: 2 g | Sugar: 6 g

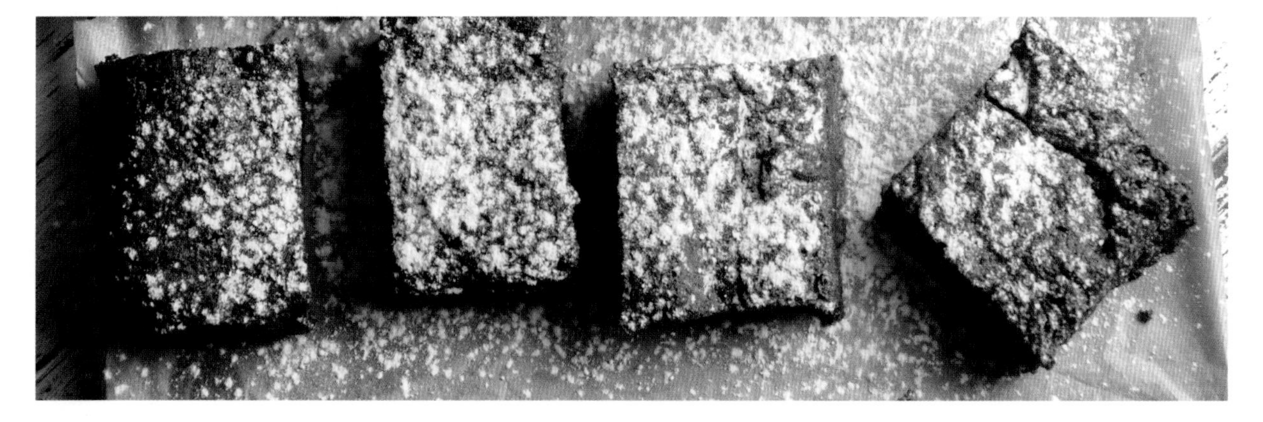

CHICKPEA PECAN BLONDIES

PREP: 15 MINUTES | COOK: 25 MINUTES | MAKES: 16 SERVINGS

- Coconut oil for greasing
- 3 tablespoons unsalted butter
- ¾ cup coconut sugar
- 2 eggs
- 1 teaspoon vanilla extract
- 1 (15-ounce) can unsalted chickpeas, drained and rinsed
- 3 tablespoons nut butter (tahini, natural peanut butter, or almond butter)
- 2 tablespoons full-fat unsweetened coconut milk
- ⅓ cup blanched almond flour
- ½ teaspoon baking powder
- ½ teaspoon sea salt
- ⅓ cup toasted pecans, chopped, plus more for garnish

1. Preheat the oven to 350 degrees F. Line the bottom of an 8 × 8-inch baking pan with parchment paper and lightly grease the paper with coconut oil.
2. Melt the butter in a small saucepan over medium heat. Cook, stirring often, until lightly browned, about 5 minutes. Transfer to a bowl and cool for 10 minutes. Whisk in the coconut sugar, eggs, and vanilla.
3. Combine the chickpeas, nut butter, and coconut milk in a food processor and pulse until smooth, scraping down the sides of the bowl as needed. Stir into the butter mixture.
4. In a small mixing bowl, whisk together the almond flour, baking powder, and salt. Add to the butter mixture. Mix well, then fold in the pecans.
5. Pour the batter into the prepared pan and bake for 25 minutes, until the middle doesn't jiggle when you shake the pan. Set the pan on a wire rack to cool completely. Cut the blondies into 16 squares. Add more pecans for garnish.

Quick Tip: These are made with ¾ cup of coconut sugar; however, if you would like to reduce the sugar impact and calories, use granular erythritol, such as Swerve, instead. You could also make these with half coconut sugar and half Swerve.

NUTRITION

Calories: 137

Fat: 8 g

Carbohydrates: 14 g

Sodium: 130 mg

Fiber: 2 g

Protein: 3 g

Sugar: 9 g

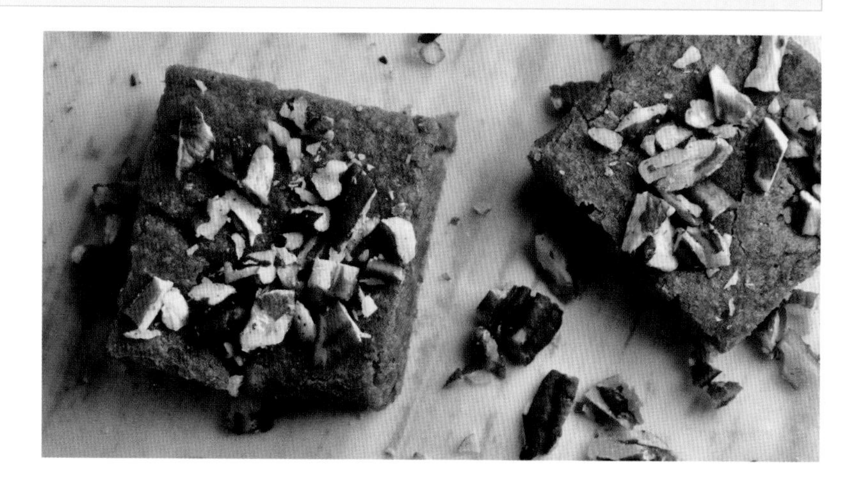

NO-BAKE SALTED CARAMEL BARS

PREP: 30 MINUTES | COOK/FREEZE: 40 MINUTES | MAKES: 30 SERVINGS

For the Cookie Layer

2½ cups raw pecans
8 pitted dates, soaked in hot water for 10 minutes, then drained
2 tablespoons blanched almond flour
1 teaspoon coconut flour
¼ teaspoon sea salt
¼ cup granular erythritol (such as Swerve)
3 tablespoons coconut oil, melted

For the Caramel Layer

½ cup coconut sugar
½ cup granular erythritol
2 tablespoons full-fat unsweetened coconut milk
2 tablespoons coconut oil
1 tablespoon vanilla extract
Pinch of sea salt
½ teaspoon baking soda

For the Chocolate Layer

2 cups stevia-sweetened chocolate chips (such as Lily's brand)
2 tablespoons coconut oil

For the Topping

⅓ cup dry-roasted macadamia nuts, chopped
Coarse sea salt

1. For the cookie layer: Place a large skillet over medium heat. Spread the pecans over the skillet and toast, stirring often, for 8 to 10 minutes, until golden. Remove from the heat.
2. Transfer the toasted pecans to a food processor and pulse until fine. Add the remaining cookie layer ingredients. Pulse until a dough forms.
3. For the caramel layer: In a skillet over medium heat, combine the coconut sugar, granular erythritol, coconut milk, coconut oil, vanilla, and sea salt. Once the mixture begins to boil, decrease the heat to low and continue to cook, stirring often, for 5 minutes.
4. Remove the skillet from the heat and whisk in the baking soda. The mixture will turn a lighter color and become creamy. Return the pan to low heat and cook, stirring often, for 2 minutes.
5. Remove the caramel from the heat and allow it to cool and thicken for 5 minutes.
6. For the chocolate layer: In a double boiler, melt the chocolate chips and coconut oil, about 5 minutes. Stir until the mixture is smooth, then remove from the heat.
7. To assemble the bars, line the bottom and sides of a 9 × 9-inch baking pan with parchment paper, so that the parchment paper hangs over the sides. (These will be your "handles" to easily pull the caramel bars from the pan once they're done.) Lightly rub the parchment paper with coconut oil.
8. Press the cookie dough into the prepared pan, flattening to create an even layer of dough. Place in the freezer for 5 minutes to harden.
9. Pour the caramel layer over the cookie layer and spread to evenly coat. Place in the freezer for 5 minutes. Pour the chocolate over the top of the caramel and carefully spread to evenly cover.
10. For the topping: Sprinkle the bars with the macadamia nuts and coarse sea salt.
11. Place the pan in the freezer for 10 minutes, until the top chocolate layer sets.

12. Use the parchment paper handles to ease the set mixture out of the pan. Transfer it to a cutting board and slice it into 30 bite-size bars.

Quick Tip: I like to keep extras in the freezer to maintain freshness.

NUTRITION

Calories: 180 | Fat: 15 g | Carbohydrates: 15 g | Sodium: 56 mg | Fiber: 4 g | Protein: 2 g | Sugar: 4 g

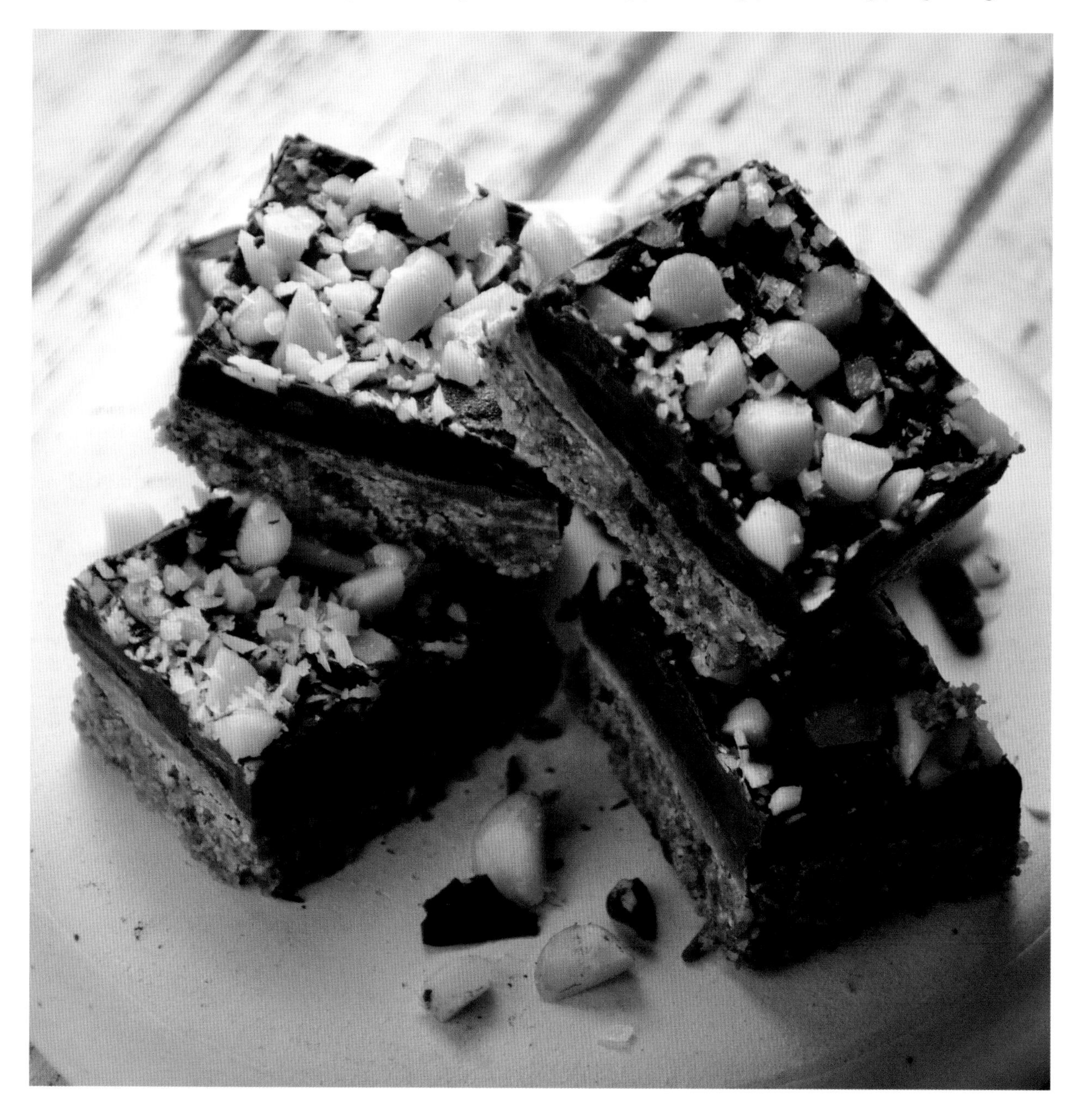

FRUIT MINI TARTS

PREP: 40 MINUTES | COOK/CHILL: 80 MINUTES | MAKES: 20 SERVINGS

For the Custard

8 egg yolks
1 cup honey
1 tablespoon coconut flour
3 (13.66-ounce) cans full-fat unsweetened coconut milk
1 teaspoon vanilla extract
¼ teaspoon grated lemon zest

For the Sugar Cookie Crust

Vegetable oil spray
½ cup coconut oil
½ cup palm shortening
1 cup coconut sugar
1 teaspoon baking soda
1 teaspoon cream of tartar
¼ teaspoon sea salt
3 egg yolks
½ teaspoon vanilla extract
1 cup blanched almond flour
¼ cup coconut flour
2 tablespoons arrowroot starch

For the Fruit Toppings

2 kiwifruits, peeled and sliced
½ cup pomegranate arils
½ cup raspberries
½ cup blackberries
½ cup blueberries
½ cup red grapes
1 cup strawberries, thinly sliced
Fresh mint leaves, for garnish

1. For the custard: Make the custard the night before you plan to assemble and serve the tarts. Combine the egg yolks and honey in a medium saucepan. Whisk together until smooth. Mix in the coconut flour.
2. Combine the coconut milk, vanilla, and lemon zest in a separate medium saucepan. Place the coconut milk mixture over medium heat. Bring to a boil and then remove from the heat.
3. Gradually whisk the hot coconut milk mixture into the egg yolk mixture, stirring while you pour. Place the mixture on low heat, stirring constantly, for 5 minutes. Don't boil; just simmer.
4. Remove the saucepan from the heat and cool for a few minutes. Continue to stir the custard occasionally as it cools. Once the custard has cooled to room temperature, chill it in the fridge overnight, until you are ready to assemble the tarts. (If you are not making the tarts, you can serve the custard on its own, garnished with fresh fruit and mint leaves.)
5. For the sugar cookie crust: Preheat the oven to 350 degrees F. Spray 20 muffin tin cups with vegetable oil spray, and place paper muffin liners in the cups.
6. In the bowl of an electric mixer, beat the coconut oil and palm shortening on high speed for 30 seconds. Add the coconut sugar, baking soda, cream of tartar, and salt. Beat until combined, scraping the sides of the bowl occasionally. Beat in the egg yolks and vanilla until combined. Beat in the almond flour, coconut flour, and arrowroot starch. Chill the dough in the fridge for 15 minutes.
7. Divide the chilled cookie dough into 20 pieces. Press each piece of cookie dough into the bottom of a paper muffin liner and 1 inch up the sides. Bake for about 12 minutes, until the crusts are golden and browned on the top and the edges. Remove from the oven and cool for 10 minutes. Place the cooled crusts in the fridge for 30 minutes, or up to overnight. It's important that your crusts are fully chilled before assembling the tarts.
8. Spoon the custard into each chilled crust.

9. For the fruit toppings: Decorate the tops of the tarts with the fresh fruit. Chill in the refrigerator for 30 minutes before serving. It's also possible to freeze these tarts for 1 hour before serving. This will help to keep all the toppings in place. Remove from the freezer and set out at room temperature. Garnish each tart with a mint leaf.

Quick Tip: It's really important that both the custard and the cookie crust are nice and cold when you assemble your fruit tarts. Plan to make the custard the night before so it has a chance to chill overnight. Bake the cookie crust at least a few hours before you plan to decorate the tarts so it can cool completely and chill in the fridge. Spread a generous tablespoon of custard on each crust, and then decorate with the fresh fruit. Have fun!

It's possible to keep leftovers in the freezer for up to two weeks. Store in an airtight container, or wrap well with plastic wrap. Take the tarts out of the freezer 10 minutes before serving so that they reach that perfect cold-but-not-too-frozen state for optimal enjoyment.

Quick Tip: This recipe calls for egg yolks only. Once you've separated the eggs, keep the whites to use in other dishes, such as *Instant Pot Egg White Bites* (page 112) or egg white omelets with bacon.

NUTRITION

Calories: 192 | Fat: 14 g | Carbohydrates: 16 g | Sodium: 61 mg | Fiber: 2 g | Protein: 1 g | Sugar: 9 g

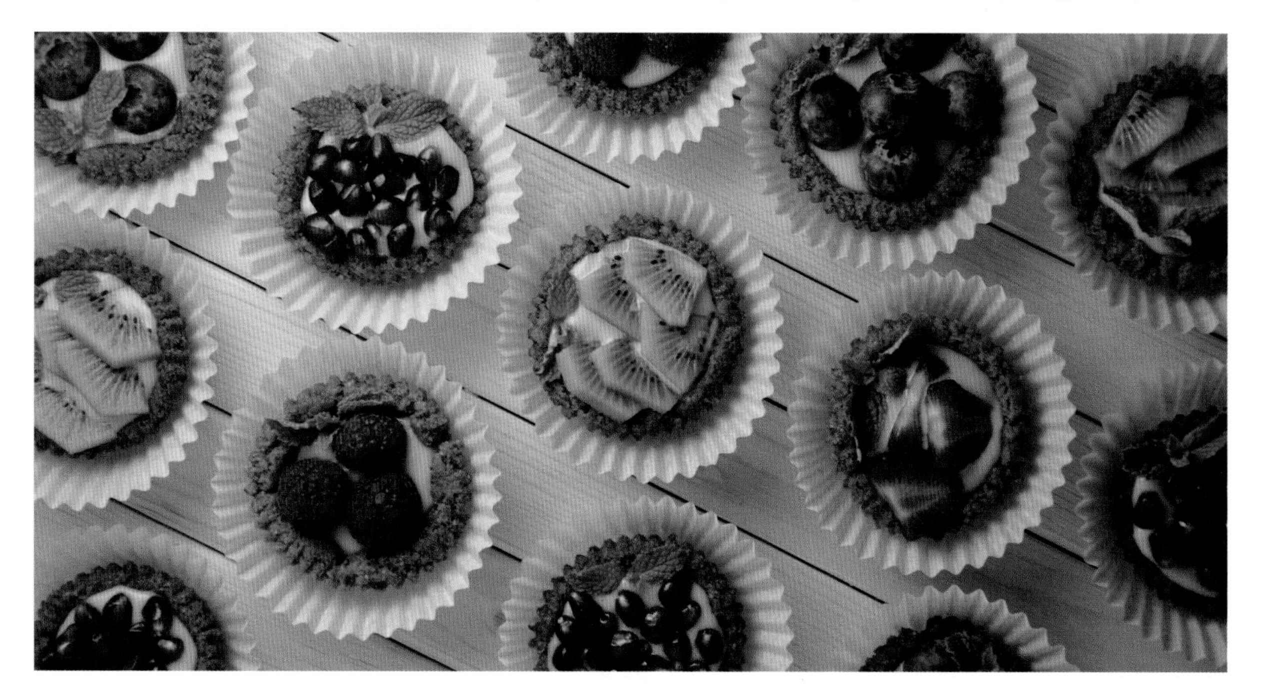

LEMON POPPY SEED CREPES

PREP: 10 MINUTES | COOK: 8 MINUTES | MAKES: 12 SERVINGS

6 eggs
1 (13.66-ounce) can full-fat unsweetened coconut milk
¼ cup coconut flour
¼ cup flaxseed meal
½ teaspoon baking soda
½ teaspoon sea salt
5 drops liquid stevia or 1 tablespoon granular erythritol (such as Swerve)
1 tablespoon grated lemon zest, plus more for garnish (optional)
1 tablespoon poppy seeds
Coconut oil for greasing
Powdered erythritol, such as confectioners' Swerve, for garnish (optional)

1. Preheat a medium nonstick skillet over medium-low heat.
2. Combine the eggs, coconut milk, coconut flour, flaxseed, baking soda, salt, stevia, and lemon zest in a high-speed blender and mix until smooth. Stir in the poppy seeds. Let the batter sit for 10 minutes.
3. Coat the skillet with coconut oil. Pour ⅓ cup of batter into the skillet and swirl the pan to spread it into a circle. Allow to cook until set, approximately 2 minutes, then flip to brown the other side. Repeat with all the batter to make 12 crepes. Top with additional grated lemon zest and powdered erythritol, if you like.

Quick Tip: These are tasty served with a filling of yogurt and fresh berries, such as blueberries or sliced strawberries.

NUTRITION

Calories: 100 | Fat: 9 g | Carbohydrates: 2 g | Sodium: 112 mg
Fiber: 1 g | Protein: 5 g | Sugar: 0 g

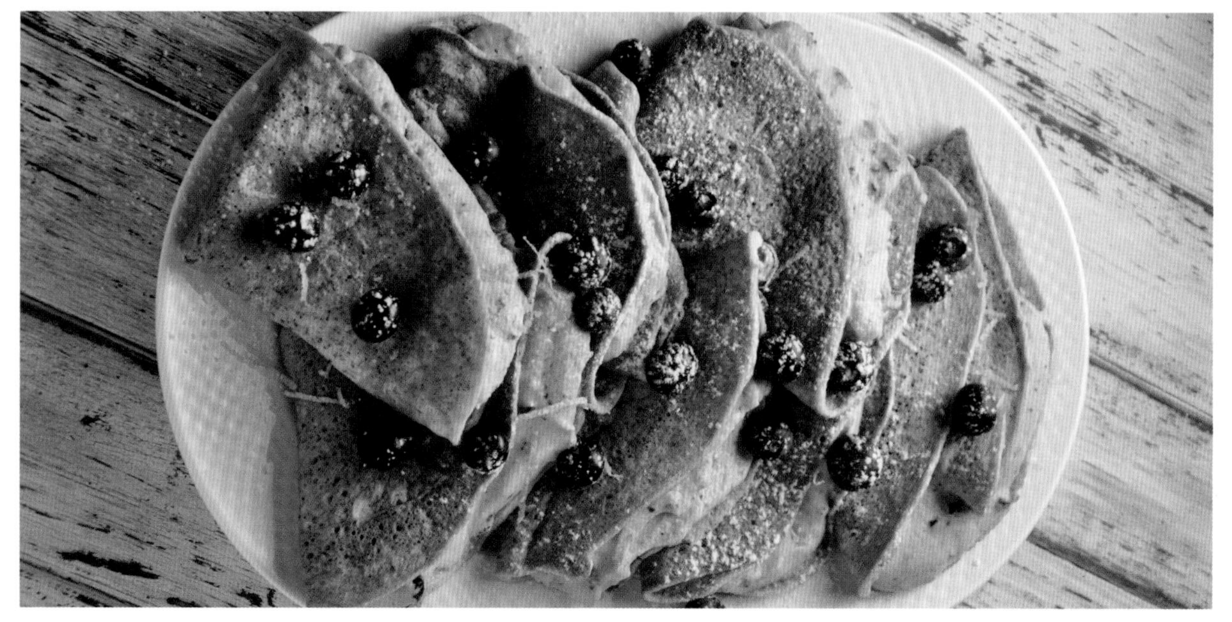

COCONUT PANNA COTTA

PREP: 6 HOURS | COOK: 3 MINUTES/CHILL 6 HOURS | MAKES: 4 SERVINGS

½ cup chopped fresh mango
1 teaspoon white balsamic vinegar
2 tablespoons cold water
1½ teaspoons unflavored gelatin
1 cup full-fat unsweetened coconut milk
2 tablespoons granular erythritol
3 tablespoons unsweetened flaked coconut
½ teaspoon vanilla extract
1 cup plain full-fat Greek yogurt
¼ cup coconut cream
4 sprigs fresh mint

1. In a medium bowl, combine the mango and vinegar. Place in the fridge.
2. Combine the water and gelatin in a small bowl and set aside.
3. Heat a saucepan over medium heat and add the coconut milk, granular erythritol, flaked coconut, and vanilla. Bring to a simmer, about 3 minutes. Remove from the heat, strain over a medium bowl, and discard the solids. Whisk in the gelatin mixture, yogurt, and coconut cream. Divide into four bowls and chill in the fridge for 6 hours. Top with the mango and fresh mint.

Quick Tip: Make this dessert ahead of time to chill until you are ready to enjoy.

NUTRITION

Calories: 196 | Fat: 13 g | Carbohydrates: 2.6 g | Sodium: 118 mg | Fiber: 2 g | Protein: 29 g | Sugar: 21 g

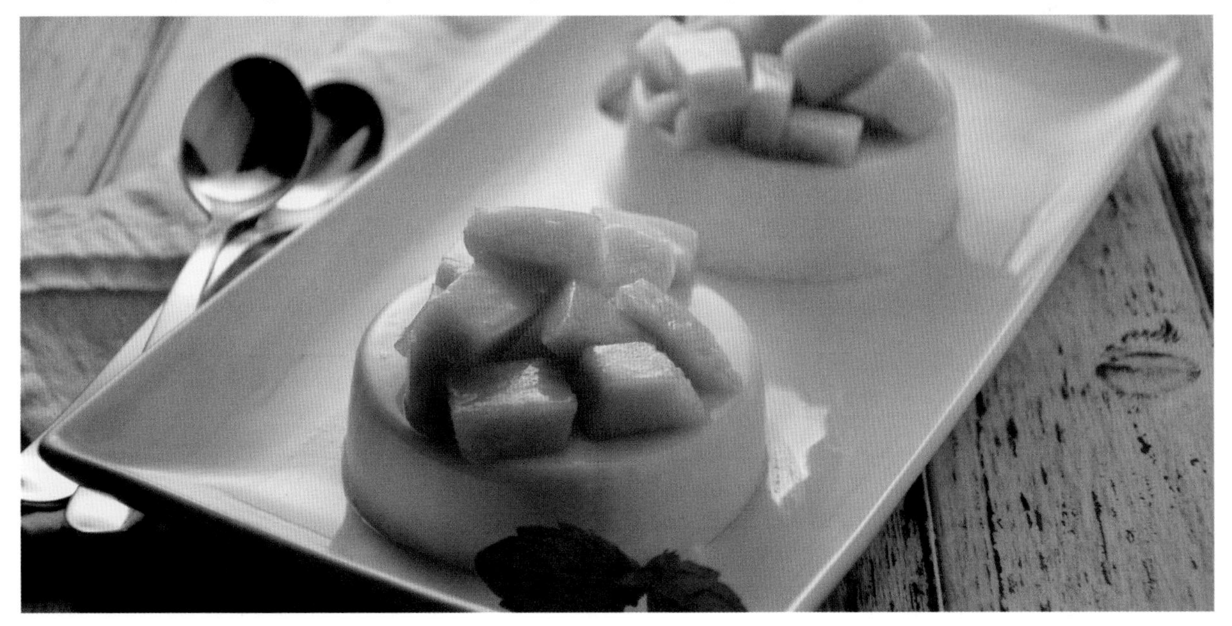

CHOCOLATE VERY CHERRY ICE CREAM

PREP: 10 MINUTES | MAKES: 4 SERVINGS

- 3 overripe bananas, peeled, cut into 1-inch pieces, and frozen
- ¼ cup full-fat unsweetened coconut milk
- Pinch of sea salt
- ¼ cup fresh Bing cherries, pitted and halved, chilled
- ¼ cup chopped stevia-sweetened dark chocolate bar (such as Lily's brand), chilled

1. Combine the frozen bananas, coconut milk, and salt in a food processor and process until the smooth, creamy consistency of soft serve ice cream is achieved. Stir in the cherries and chocolate and serve immediately, or place in a freezer-safe container and freeze until serving.

Quick Tip: Blend 3 frozen bananas with ¼ cup of coconut milk and use as the base for any combination of ice cream flavors. You can also blend in a few fresh berries or chopped tropical fruit in place of the cherries.

NUTRITION

Calories: 165 | Fat: 7 g | Carbohydrates: 27 g | Sodium: 134 mg | Fiber: 6 g | Protein: 2 g | Sugar: 12 g

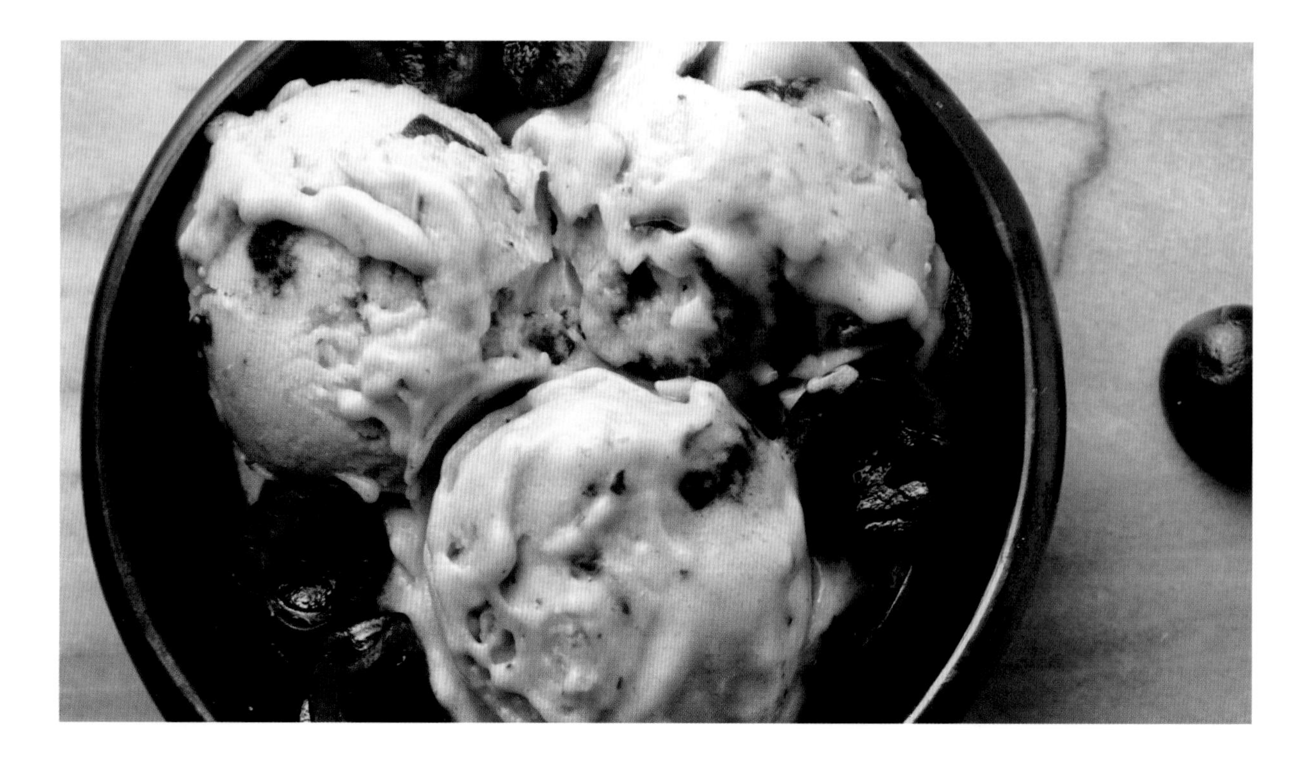

PRE-BEDTIME FAT-BURNING SNACKS

CHILI-SPICED NUTS

PREP: 10 MINUTES | COOK: 20 MINUTES | MAKES: 16 (¼-CUP) SERVINGS

- 4 cups mixed nuts (pecans, almonds, pistachios, walnuts, cashews, and/or Brazil nuts)
- 1 teaspoon sea salt
- 1 teaspoon ground cumin
- 1 teaspoon sweet paprika
- 1 teaspoon chili powder
- ½ teaspoon garlic powder
- ¼ teaspoon ground ginger
- ¼ teaspoon black pepper
- ¼ cup coconut sugar
- ¼ cup water
- 1 tablespoon coconut oil

1. Preheat the oven to 350 degrees F. Line a rimmed baking sheet with foil.
2. In a large bowl, combine the nuts, salt, cumin, paprika, chili powder, garlic powder, ginger, and pepper.
3. In a small skillet over medium heat, combine the coconut sugar, water, and coconut oil. Mix until the sugar has dissolved, about 1 minute. Pour the mixture over the nuts and spices. Mix until fully coated.
4. Spread the coated nuts over the prepared baking sheet in a single layer. Bake for 10 minutes and then stir. Bake for an additional 10 minutes, until golden.

Quick Tip: Place ¼-cup portions of these dynamite spiced nuts in individual ziplock bags for convenience and portion control.

NUTRITION

Calories: 135 | Fat: 12 g | Carbohydrates: 6 g | Sodium: 139 mg | Fiber: 2 g | Protein: 4 g | Sugar: 3 g

ALL-SPICED-UP ROASTED CHICKPEAS

PREP: 5 MINUTES | COOK: 50 MINUTES | MAKES: 6 SERVINGS

2 (15-ounce) cans chickpeas, drained, rinsed, and patted dry
1 tablespoon olive oil
½ teaspoon sea salt
½ teaspoon garlic powder
½ teaspoon sweet paprika
½ teaspoon black pepper
Pinch of ground cayenne pepper

1. Preheat the oven to 400 degrees F and position a rack in the center of the oven.
2. Spread the chickpeas over a rimmed baking sheet. Roast for 5 minutes, until any excess water dries.
3. Remove the pan from the oven and drizzle the chickpeas with the olive oil and salt. Return to the oven for 20 to 30 minutes, or until crunchy, shaking the pan every 10 minutes. Turn the oven off and leave in the oven for 15 minutes.
4. Remove the pan from the oven and sprinkle the chickpeas with the garlic, paprika, black pepper, and cayenne. Toss to coat.

Quick Tip: If you have fresh herbs on hand, chop some up and throw them into your pan of roasting chickpeas for an added burst of flavor.

NUTRITION

Calories: 188 | Fat: 4 g | Sodium: 575 mg | Carbohydrates: 32 g | Fiber 6.3 g | Protein: 7 g | Sugar: 0 g

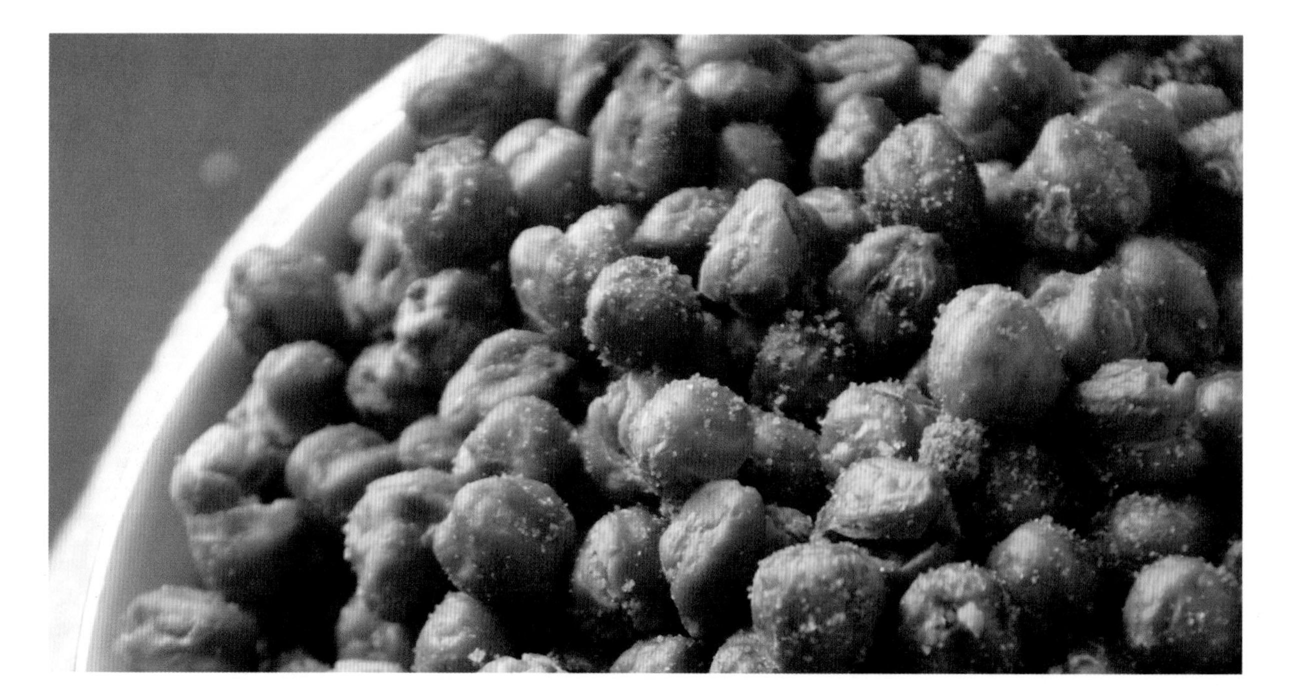

TERIYAKI MEATBALLS

PREP: 15 MINUTES | COOK: 17 MINUTES | MAKES: 6 SERVINGS

1 tablespoon chopped fresh garlic
2 tablespoons chopped fresh ginger
¼ cup chopped scallions, plus more for garnish
1 pound extra-lean ground beef
1 teaspoon sea salt
1 tablespoon toasted sesame oil
3 tablespoons coconut aminos
1 tablespoon honey
1 tablespoon white wine vinegar
½ teaspoon arrowroot starch
3 tablespoons water
Sesame seeds, for garnish

1. Combine the garlic, ginger, and scallions in a food processor. Pulse until well combined and finely minced.
2. Transfer the garlic mixture to a large bowl and add the ground beef and salt. Use your hands to mix until well combined. Form the mixture into 20 meatballs, about 1 inch in diameter.
3. In a large skillet over medium-high heat, heat the sesame oil. Add the meatballs and cook, shaking often, until browned on all sides and cooked through, about 15 minutes. Remove the meatballs and set aside on a plate.
4. Add the coconut aminos, honey, and vinegar to the skillet (still on medium-high heat). In a small bowl, whisk the arrowroot starch and water together until the starch is fully dissolved. Add to the skillet, mix, and simmer until the mixture has thickened, about 2 minutes. Return the meatballs to the skillet and cover them with the sauce. Serve immediately, garnished with scallions and sesame seeds.

Quick Tip: I like to make two batches at a time of these tasty meatballs and save the leftovers!

NUTRITION

Calories: 189 | Fat: 7 g | Carbohydrates: 6 g | Sodium: 372 mg | Fiber: 3 g | Protein: 23 g | Sugar: 3 g

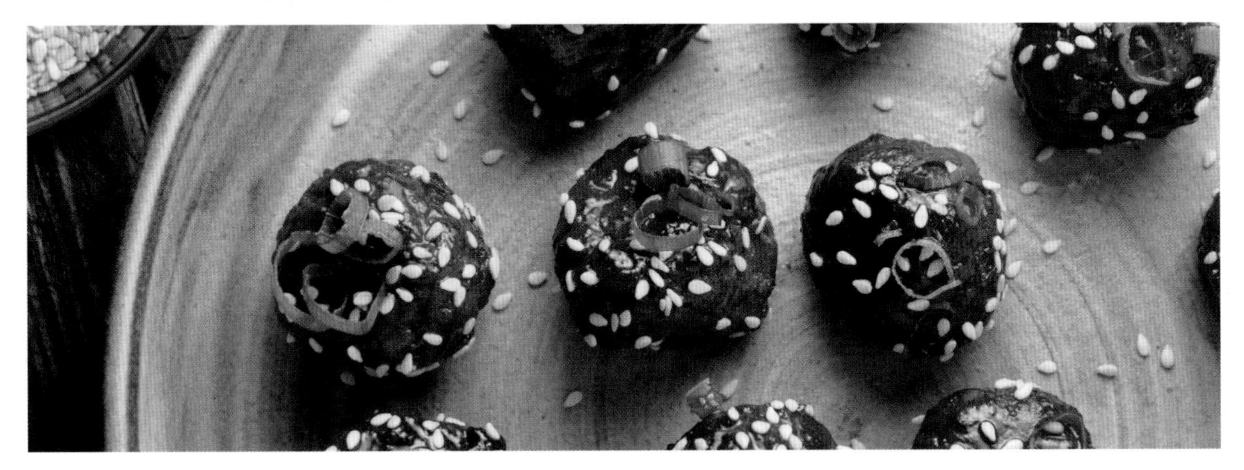

HOMEMADE BEEF JERKY

PREP: 24 HOURS, 10 MINUTES | COOK: 6 HOURS | MAKES: 30 SERVINGS

2 pounds lean flank steak, frozen
2 cups coconut aminos
2 cups unsweetened apple juice
½ cup pure maple syrup
1 tablespoon liquid smoke
2 tablespoons black pepper
1 tablespoon onion powder
2 teaspoons smoked paprika
2 teaspoons garlic powder
3 tablespoons sesame seeds

1. Using a mandoline slicer, slice the frozen flank steak into strips about ¼ inch thick, slicing with the grain.
2. Combine all the remaining ingredients in a large food storage container. Add the steak slices. Cover tightly and refrigerate for 24 hours.
3. Set your oven to 160 degrees F. Cover the bottom of the oven with foil—this gets messy! Pat any excess marinade off each steak strip, then lay the strips directly across your oven racks. Wipe any excess marinade from the foil-lined oven bottom. Place a wooden spoon in the crack of the oven door to keep it slightly propped open.
4. Allow the steak to dehydrate for 3 hours. Flip each piece over and dehydrate for another 3 hours. Your jerky is done when you're able to easily rip a piece off.
5. This jerky will keep in a ziplock bag, without refrigeration, for 3 months.

Quick Tip: It's important to use a mandoline slicer to ensure that your jerky is thin and evenly sliced. Exercise caution and care when using this sharp kitchen tool.

NUTRITION
Calories: 62
Fat: 2 g
Carbohydrates: 2 g
Sodium: 83 mg
Fiber: 0 g
Protein: 7 g
Sugar: 3 g

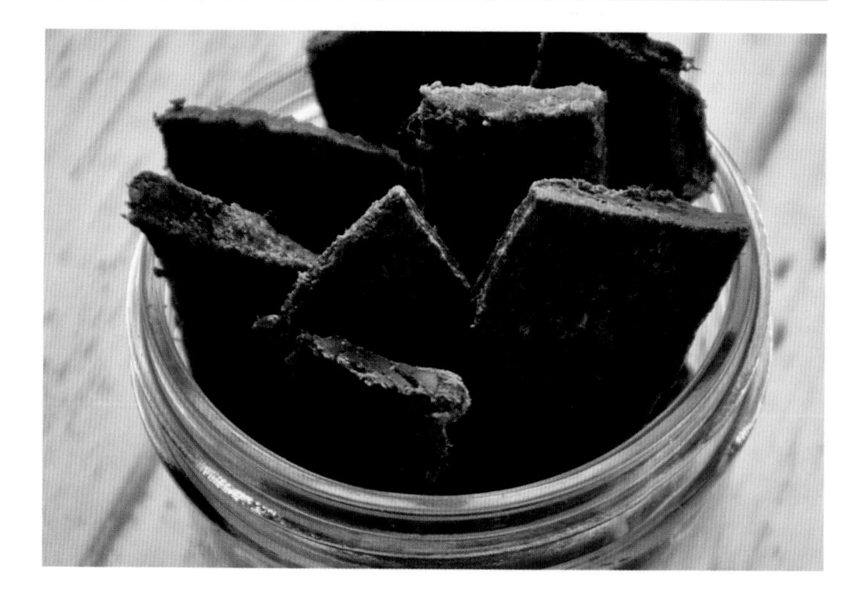

CREAMY APPLE CELERY SALAD

PREP: 12 MINUTES | CHILL: 10 MINUTES | MAKES: 4 SERVINGS

- 2 cups cored and chopped apples
- ¼ cup thinly sliced celery
- 1 tablespoon golden raisins
- 2 teaspoons lemon juice
- 1 cup nonfat plain Greek yogurt
- ¼ cup Vanilla Cream BioTrust Low Carb Protein Powder Blend
- ¼ teaspoon ground cinnamon

1. Combine the apples, celery, and raisins in a medium bowl. Toss with the lemon juice.
2. In another medium bowl, combine the yogurt, protein powder, and cinnamon. Mix until fully combined. Add the apple mixture and mix well. Chill for 10 minutes and then serve.

Quick Tip: While any type of apple will work in this salad, I find that Pink Lady, Honeycrisp, or SweeTango tastes the best.

NUTRITION

Calories: 224 | Fat: 1 g | Carbohydrates: 44 g | Sodium: 66 mg | Fiber: 7 g | Protein: 14 g | Sugar: 33 g

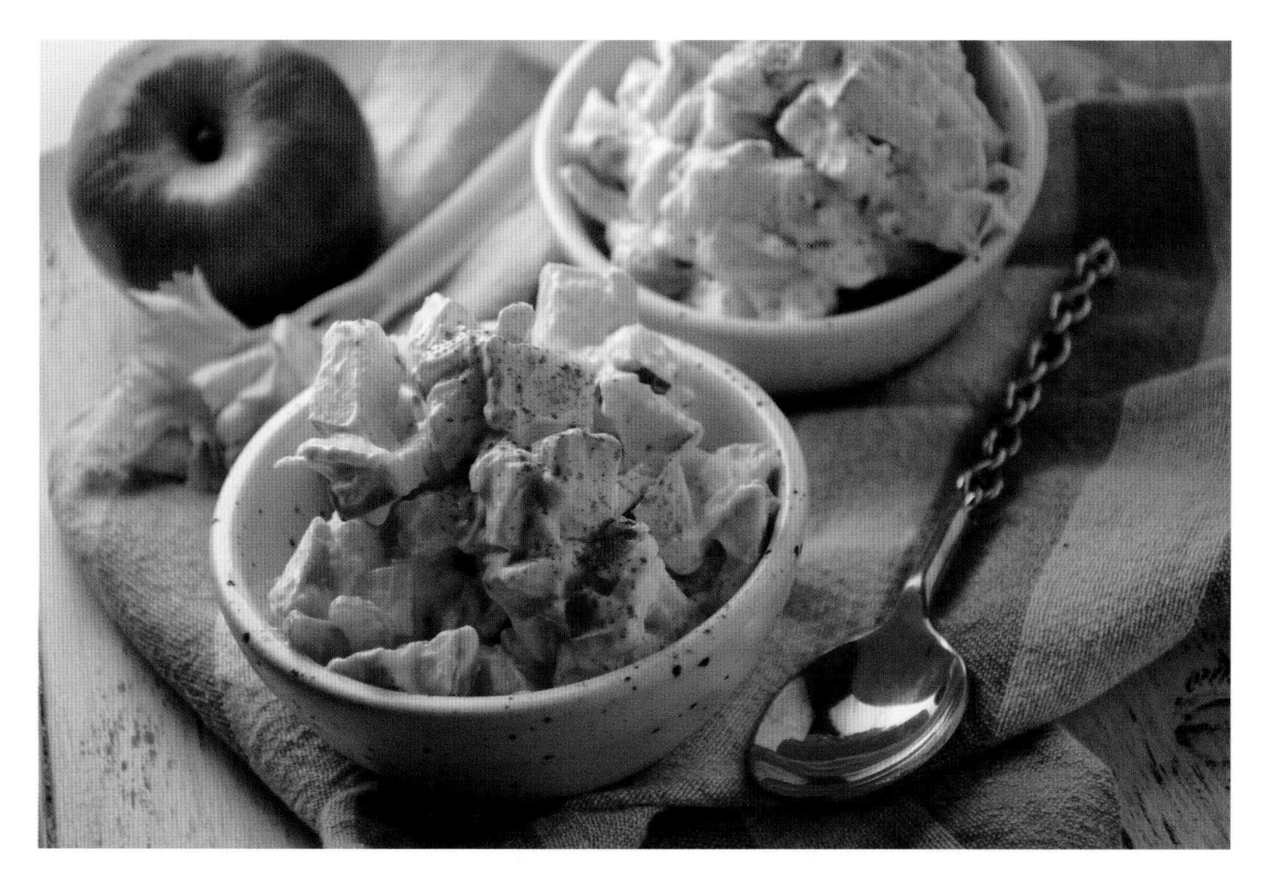

BLACKBERRY CHIA SEED PUDDING

PREP: 5 MINUTES | CHILL: OVERNIGHT | MAKES: 4 SERVINGS

1 (13.66-ounce) can full-fat unsweetened coconut milk
2 tablespoons granular erythritol
1 teaspoon vanilla extract
½ cup frozen or fresh blackberries
¼ cup chia seeds
Dollop of full-fat Greek yogurt and strawberries, for garnish (optional)

1. In a food processor, combine the coconut milk, granular erythritol, and vanilla. Blend until smooth.
2. Add the blackberries and process until bright purple and fully incorporated. Fold in the chia seeds.
3. Divide the mixture between four cups and chill overnight, or for up to 3 days, before serving. If desired, garnish with strawberries and yogurt.

NUTRITION

Calories: 287 | Fat: 26 g | Carbohydrates: 16 g | Sodium: 119 mg | Fiber: 7 g | Protein: 4 g | Sugar: 8 g

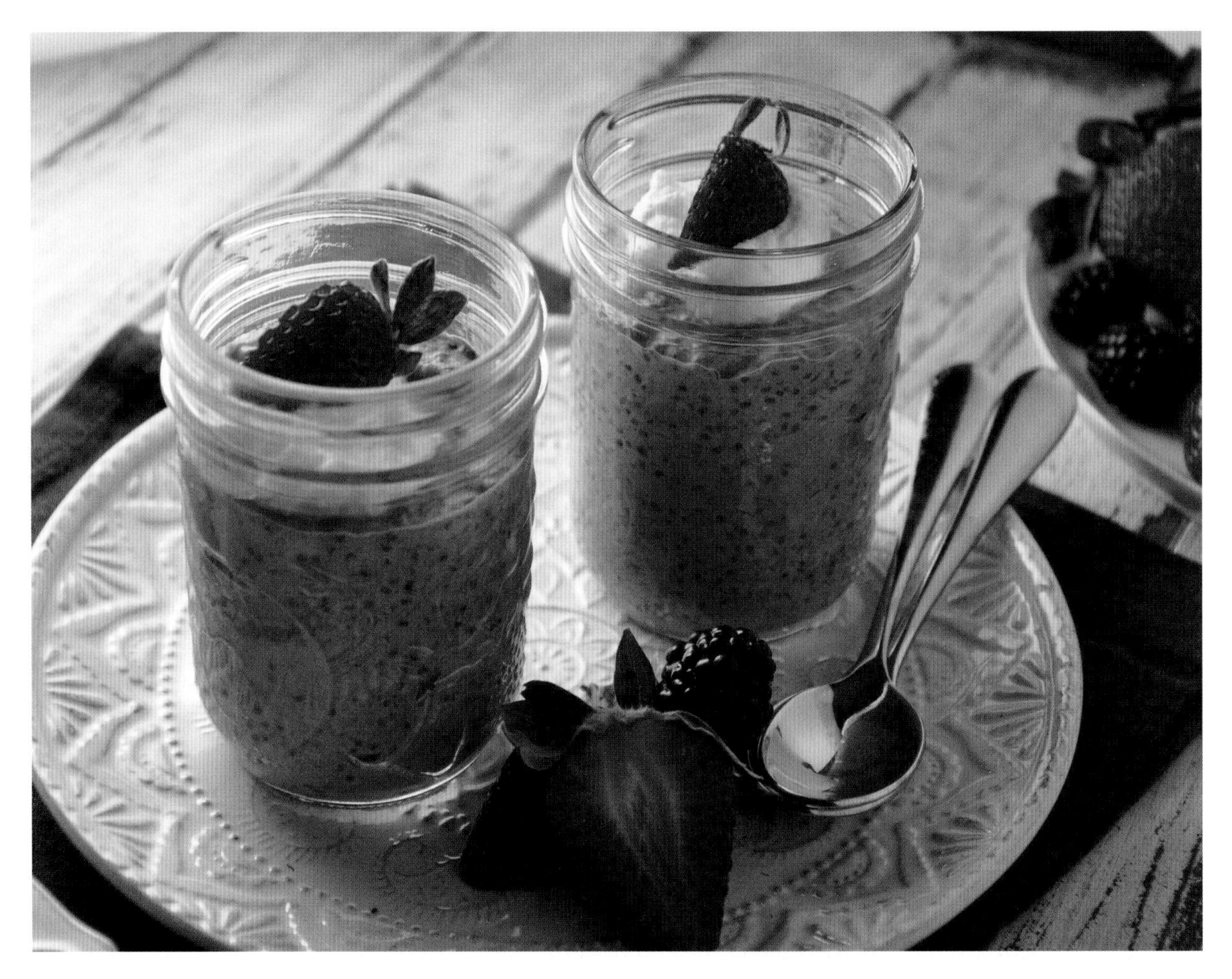

FROZEN DESSERT BARK

PREP: 15 MINUTES | FREEZE: 3 HOURS | MAKES: 3 SERVINGS

- 2 cups full-fat plain Greek yogurt
- 1 teaspoon honey
- 10 drops liquid stevia
- ⅛ teaspoon almond extract
- 3 tablespoons stevia-sweetened mini dark chocolate chips (such as Lily's brand), divided
- 5 fresh strawberries, halved and sliced
- 2 tablespoons unsweetened flaked coconut

1. Find a baking sheet that fits in your freezer and line it with parchment paper.
2. In a medium bowl, mix the yogurt, honey, stevia, almond extract, and 1 tablespoon of the chocolate chips.
3. Spread the mixture ½ inch thick over the prepared sheet. Sprinkle with the strawberries, coconut, and remaining 2 tablespoons chocolate chips. Place in the freezer for 3 hours, until completely frozen.
4. Remove from the freezer and cut or break the dessert bark into pieces. Store in a ziplock bag in the freezer.

NUTRITION

Calories: 174 | Fat: 6 g | Carbohydrates: 14 g | Sodium: 50 mg | Fiber: 2 g | Protein: 16 g | Sugar: 4 g

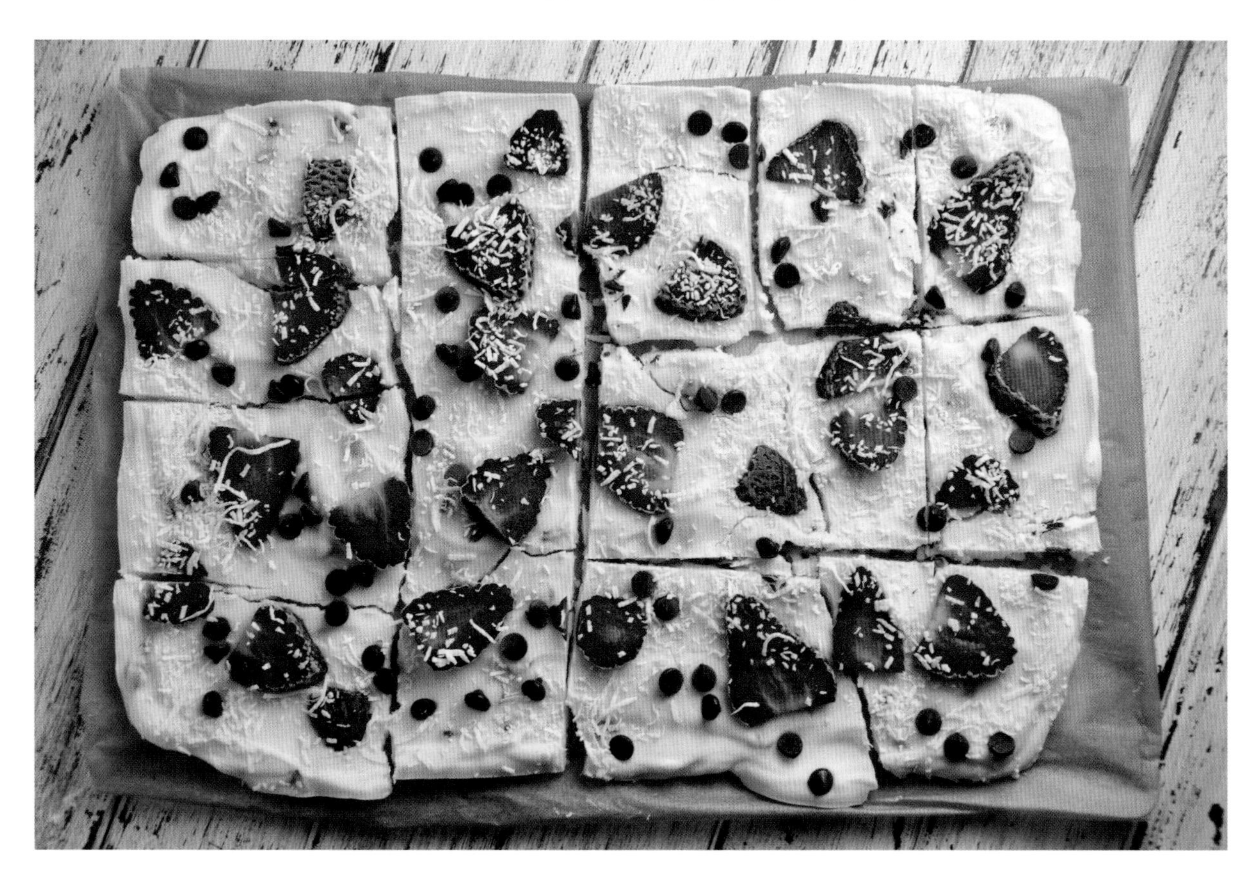

CHOCOLATE BUTTONS

PREP: 15 MINUTES | COOK: 10 MINUTES | MAKES: 24 SERVINGS (2 BUTTONS IS 1 SERVING)

1 (9-ounce) bag stevia-sweetened dark chocolate chips (such as Lily's brand)
1 tablespoon coconut oil
½ cup pistachios, finely chopped
48 pecan halves
1 teaspoon coarse sea salt

1. In a double boiler, melt the chocolate chips and coconut oil until smooth, about 5 minutes.
2. In two mini whoopie pie pans or mini muffin tins, divide the chopped pistachios among 48 cups, using ½ teaspoon in each cup. Top each cup with a spoonful of the melted chocolate mixture.
3. Press a pecan half into the top of each button and sprinkle with a pinch of coarse sea salt. Place the buttons in the fridge or freezer to harden (about 1 hour). Store in a ziplock bag in the freezer.

Quick Tip: Keep your buttons in a ziplock bag in the freezer.

NUTRITION

Calories: 124 | Fat: 12 g | Carbohydrates: 5 g | Sodium: 43 mg | Fiber: 3 g | Protein: 2 g | Sugar: 0 g

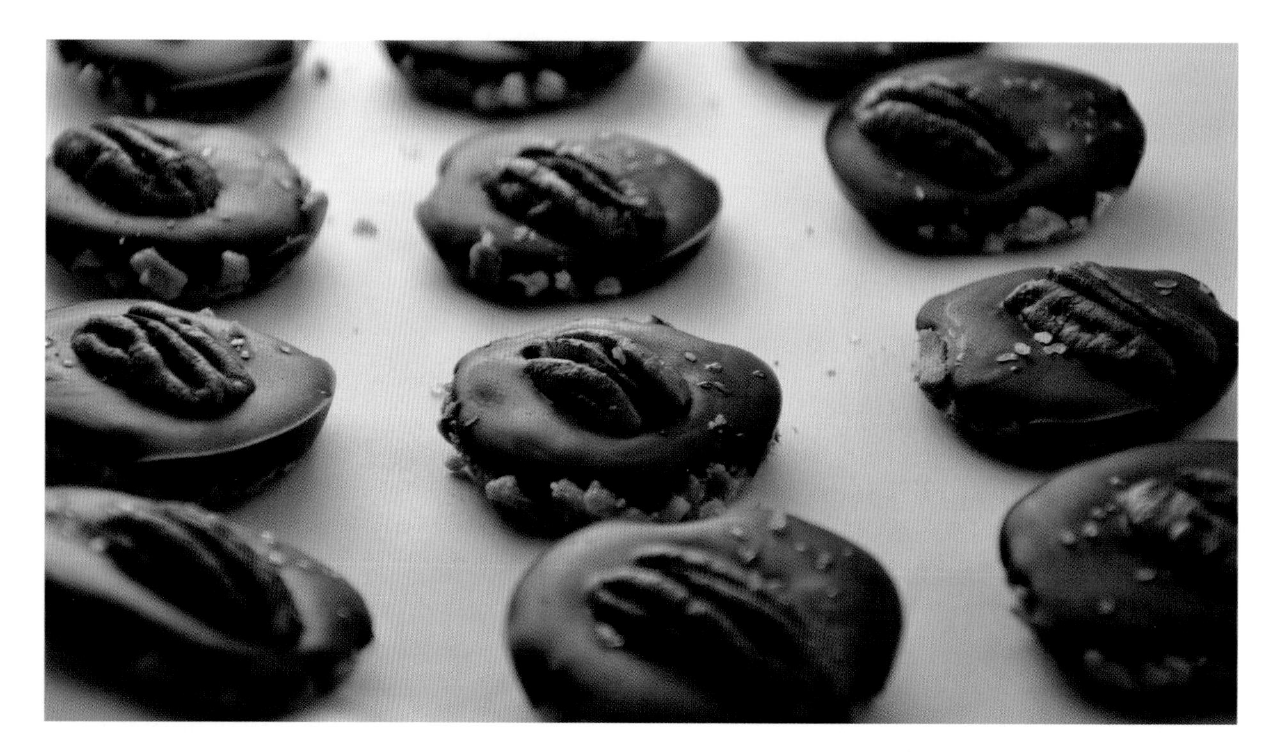

CHOCOLATE NUT BUTTER PROTEIN BARS

PREP: 15 MINUTES | CHILL: 15 MINUTES | MAKES: 20 SERVINGS

- 1 tablespoon coconut oil, plus more for greasing
- 1 cup full-fat unsweetened coconut milk
- 1 cup nut butter (tahini, natural peanut butter, or almond butter)
- ½ cup dates, pitted
- 2 cups uncooked rolled oats
- 2 cups Vanilla Cream or Milk Chocolate BioTrust Low Carb Protein Powder Blend
- ½ cup stevia-sweetened dark chocolate chips (such as Lily's brand)

1. Line the bottom and sides of a 9 × 9-inch baking pan with parchment paper, so that the parchment paper hangs over the sides. (These will be your "handles" to easily pull the protein bars from the pan once they're done.) Lightly rub the parchment paper with coconut oil.
2. Combine the coconut milk and nut butter in a small saucepan over low heat. Cook, stirring often, until fully combined and smooth, about 5 minutes. Remove from the heat and allow to cool.
3. Blend the dates in a food processor until smooth. Add the nut butter mixture, oats, and protein powder and pulse until fully incorporated. Press the dough into the prepared pan and place in the freezer for 10 minutes. Cut into 20 bars.
4. Combine the chocolate chips and coconut oil in a small saucepan over low heat, stirring constantly until melted, about 2 minutes. Drizzle the melted chocolate over the protein bars. Chill until the chocolate sets, about 5 minutes. Store in the fridge.

NUTRITION

Calories: 171 | Fat: 10 g | Carbohydrates: 13 g | Sodium: 83 mg | Fiber: 3 g | Protein: 15 g | Sugar: 4 g

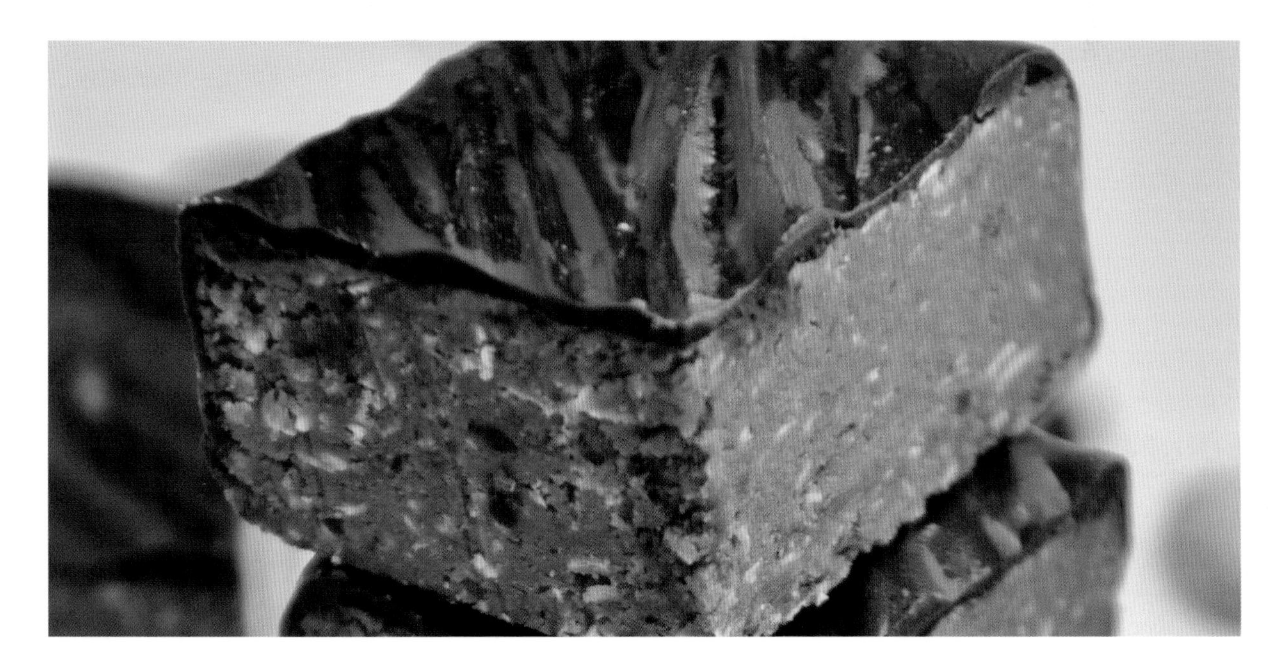

LEMON BLUEBERRY PROTEIN BARS

PREP: 15 MINUTES | COOK/CHILL: 15 MINUTES | MAKES: 20 SERVINGS

3 tablespoons coconut oil, melted, plus more for greasing
1 cup full-fat unsweetened coconut milk
1 cup almond butter
½ cup dried blueberries
2 cups uncooked rolled oats
1 tablespoon grated lemon zest
2 cups Vanilla Cream BioTrust Low Carb Protein Powder Blend
1 tablespoon powdered erythritol (such as confectioners' Swerve)

1. Line the bottom and sides of a 9 × 9-inch baking pan with parchment paper, so that the parchment paper hangs over the sides. (These will be your "handles" to easily pull the protein bars from the pan once they're done.) Lightly rub the parchment paper with coconut oil.
2. Combine the coconut milk and almond butter in a small saucepan over low heat. Cook, stirring often, until fully combined and smooth, about 5 minutes. Remove from the heat and allow to cool.
3. Blend the dried blueberries in a food processor until smooth. Add the almond butter mixture, oats, lemon zest, and protein powder and pulse until fully incorporated. Press the dough into the prepared pan and place in the freezer for 10 minutes. Cut into 20 bars.
4. Whisk the coconut oil and powdered erythritol together in a small bowl. Drizzle over the protein bars. Chill until the glaze sets, about 5 minutes. Store in the fridge.

NUTRITION
Calories: 80
Fat: 5 g
Carbohydrates: 5 g
Sodium: 23 mg
Fiber: 1 g
Protein: 12 g
Sugar: 1 g

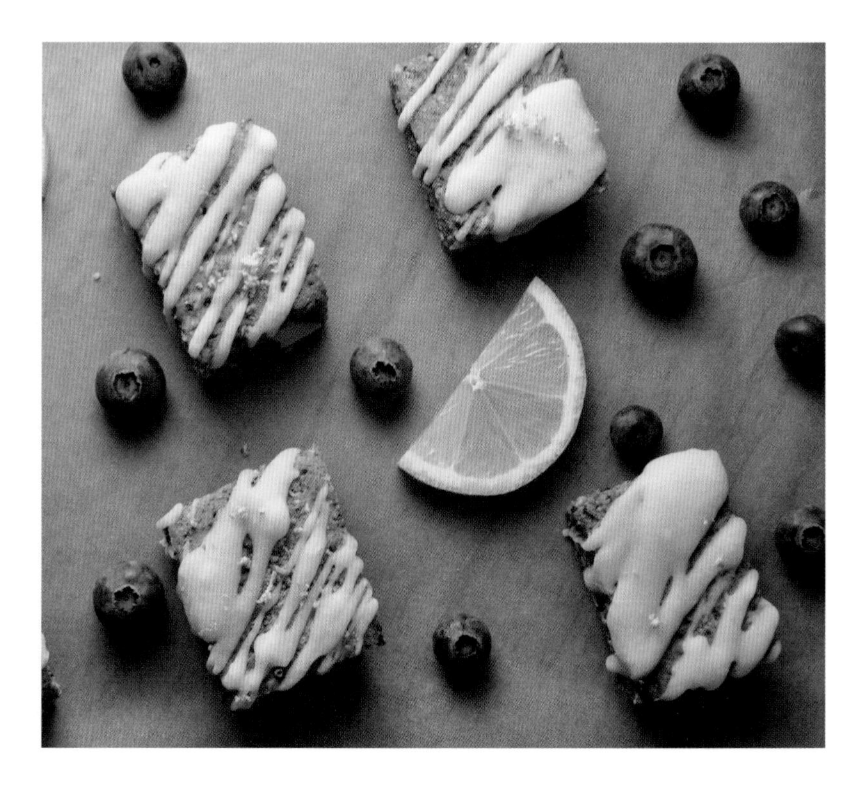

DARK CHOCOLATE GRANOLA

PREP: 10 MINUTES | COOK: 20 MINUTES | MAKES: 16 (¼-CUP) SERVINGS

3 tablespoons coconut oil, plus more for greasing
1 tablespoon honey
1 tablespoon vanilla extract
½ teaspoon almond extract
1 cup unsweetened flaked coconut
1 cup walnuts, chopped
1 cup pecans, chopped
½ cup sprouted pumpkin seeds
½ cup macadamia nuts, chopped
¼ cup unsweetened cocoa powder
2 tablespoons flaxseed meal
2 tablespoons ground chia seeds (optional)
2 teaspoons ground cinnamon
1 teaspoon ground nutmeg
Sea salt, to taste

1. Preheat the oven to 300 degrees F. Lightly grease a baking sheet with coconut oil.
2. In a small saucepan over low heat, melt the coconut oil and honey together, about 1 minute. Remove from the heat. Mix in the vanilla and almond extracts.
3. In a large bowl, combine all the remaining ingredients. Mix in the coconut oil mixture until the ingredients are evenly coated.
4. Spread the granola over the prepared pan. Bake for 10 minutes, stir, and then bake for about 10 minutes more, until golden brown.

Quick Tip: This granola is so tasty that it's easy to end up eating more of it than you intend. To stick with your perfect portion, use a ¼-cup scoop to divide the granola into individual ziplock bags right after it cools. Grab a single portion for your bedtime snack! It tastes great with sliced bananas too.

NUTRITION

Calories: 235
Fat: 22 g
Carbohydrates: 6 g
Sodium: 57 mg
Fiber: 4 g
Protein: 5 g
Sugar: 2 g

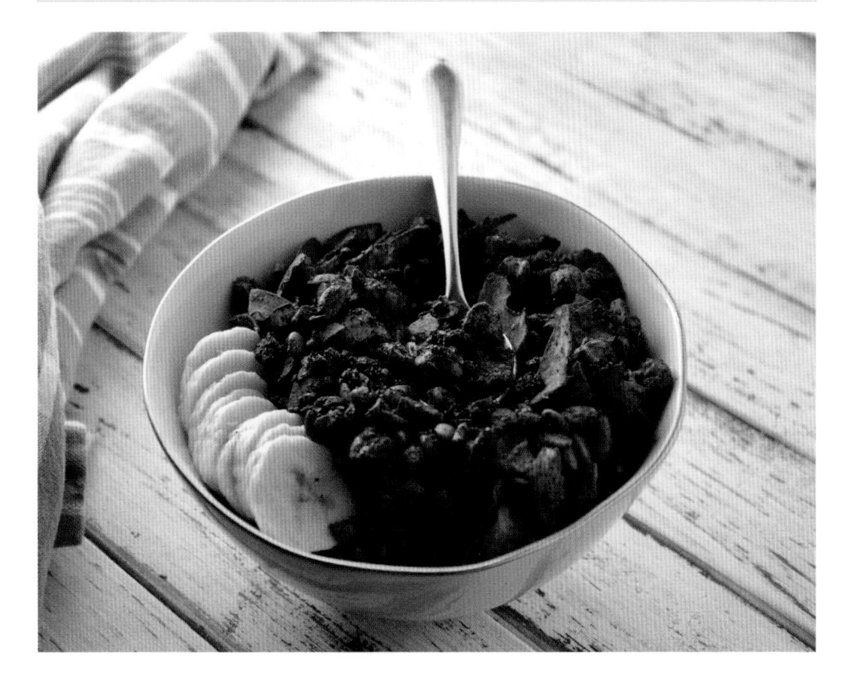

ORANGE SPICED GRANOLA

PREP: 8 MINUTES | COOK: 40 MINUTES | MAKES: 24 (¼-CUP) SERVINGS

- 3 tablespoons coconut oil, plus more for greasing
- 1 teaspoon raw honey
- ¼ cup fruit-only orange marmalade
- 2 tablespoons freshly squeezed orange juice
- 1 tablespoon vanilla extract
- ¼ teaspoon almond extract
- 2 cups unsweetened flaked coconut
- 2 cups sliced almonds
- 1 cup pecans, roughly chopped
- 2 tablespoons flaxseed meal
- 1 teaspoon ground cinnamon
- ½ teaspoon ground ginger
- 1 orange, zested
- Pinch of sea salt
- ½ cup dried cranberries (no added sugar) or crimson raisins

1. Preheat the oven to 300 degrees F. Lightly grease baking sheet with coconut oil.
2. In a small saucepan over low heat, melt the coconut oil, honey, and marmalade together, about 1 minute. Remove from the heat. Mix in the orange juice and vanilla and almond extracts.
3. In a large bowl, combine all the remaining ingredients. Mix in the coconut oil mixture until the ingredients are evenly coated.
4. Spread the granola over the prepared pan. Bake for 20 minutes, stir, and bake for about 20 minutes more, until golden brown.

NUTRITION

Calories: 168 | Fat: 15 g | Carbohydrates: 7 g | Sodium: 15 mg | Fiber: 3 g | Protein: 3 g | Sugar: 3 g

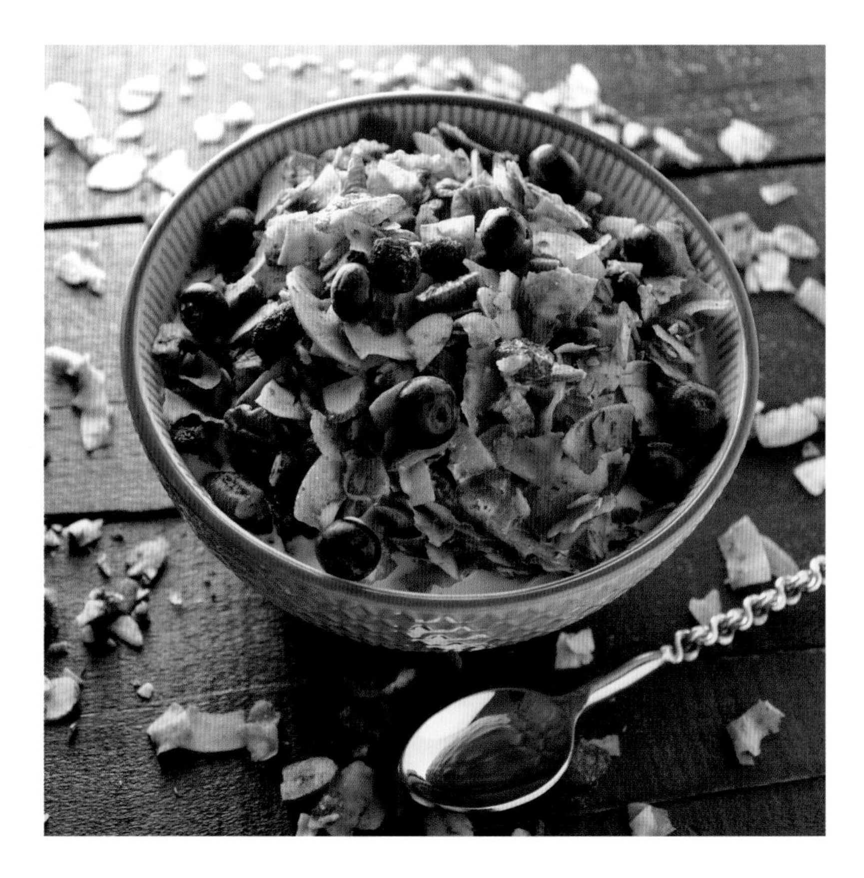

COOKIE BUTTER PROTEIN SMOOTHIE

PREP: 5 MINUTES | MAKES: 1 SERVING

1 cup unsweetened almond milk
1 *Chocolate Chunk Cookie* (page 175)
¼ teaspoon vanilla extract
2 scoops Vanilla Cream BioTrust Low Carb Protein Powder Blend
Handful of ice cubes
Liquid stevia, to taste

1. Blend all the ingredients in a high-speed blender until smooth. Serve immediately.

NUTRITION

Calories: 271 | Fat: 12 g | Carbohydrates: 14 g | Sodium: 241 mg | Fiber: 4 g | Protein: 27 g | Sugar: 5 g

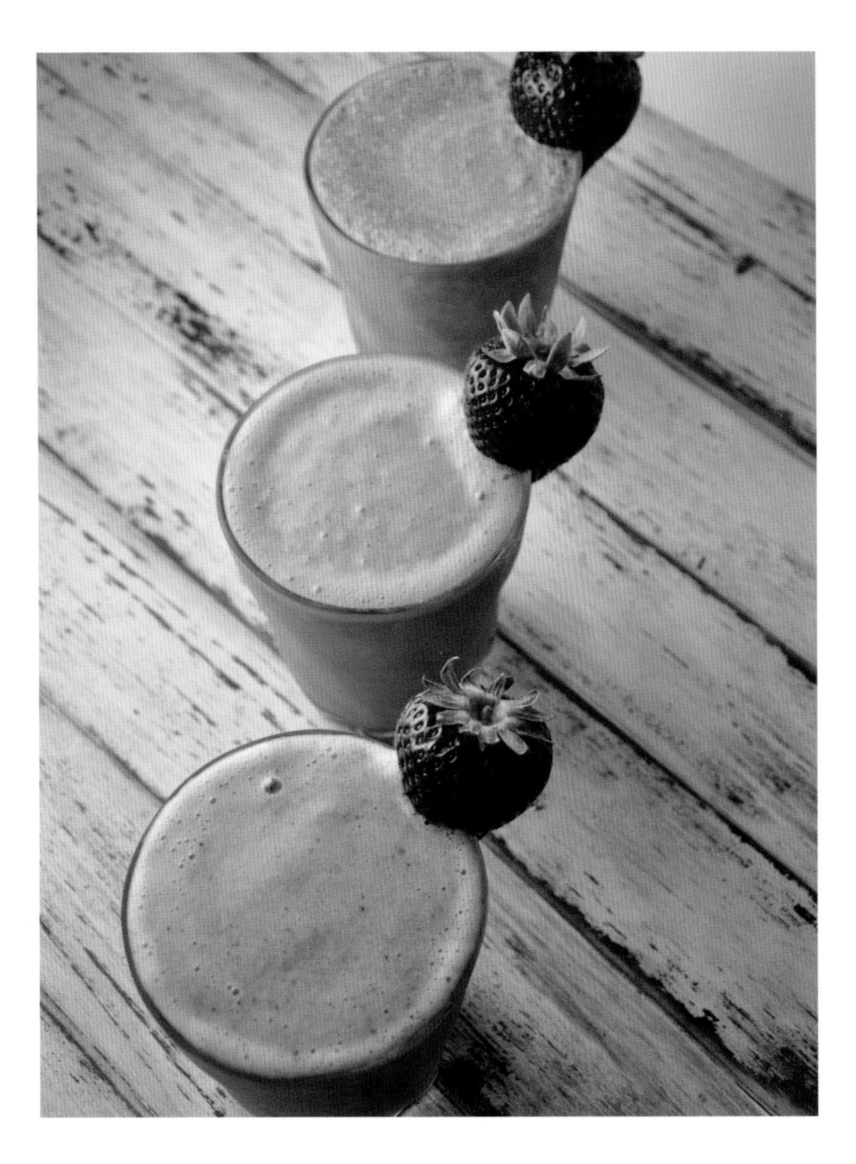

NUT BUTTER BANANA PROTEIN SMOOTHIE

PREP: 5 MINUTES | MAKES: 1 SERVING

1 cup unsweetened almond milk
1 tablespoon nut butter (tahini, natural peanut butter, or almond butter)
½ frozen banana
2 scoops Vanilla Cream BioTrust Low Carb Protein Powder Blend
Handful of ice cubes
Liquid stevia, to taste

1. Blend all the ingredients in a high-speed blender until smooth. Serve immediately.

NUTRITION

Calories: 336 | Fat: 13 g | Carbohydrates: 25 g | Sodium: 153 mg | Fiber: 7 g | Protein: 31 g | Sugar: 9 g

CHOCOLATE NUT BUTTER SMOOTHIE

PREP: 5 MINUTES | MAKES: 1 SERVING

1 cup unsweetened almond milk
1 tablespoon nut butter (tahini, natural peanut butter, or almond butter)
1 teaspoon unsweetened cocoa powder
2 scoops Milk Chocolate BioTrust Low Carb Protein Powder Blend
Handful of ice cubes
Liquid stevia, to taste

1. Blend all the ingredients in a high-speed blender until smooth. Serve immediately.

NUTRITION

Calories: 283 | Fat: 13 g | Carbohydrates: 12 g | Sodium: 153 mg | Fiber: 5 g | Protein: 30 g | Sugar: 2 g

CREAMY CAFÉ MOCHA PROTEIN SMOOTHIE

PREP: 5 MINUTES | MAKES: 1 SERVING

½ cup chilled black coffee
½ cup unsweetened almond milk
2 scoops Café Mocha BioTrust Low Carb Protein Powder Blend
1 teaspoon unsweetened cocoa powder
1 teaspoon instant coffee
Handful of ice cubes
Liquid stevia, to taste

1. Blend all the ingredients in a high-speed blender until smooth. Serve immediately.

NUTRITION

Calories: 175 | Fat: 5 g | Carbohydrates: 9 g | Sodium: 183 mg | Fiber: 5 g | Protein: 26 g | Sugar: 1 g

CINNAMON ALMOND PROTEIN SMOOTHIE

PREP: 5 MINUTES | MAKES: 1 SERVING

1 cup unsweetened almond milk
1 tablespoon almond butter
¼ teaspoon ground cinnamon
⅛ teaspoon almond extract (optional)
2 scoops Vanilla Cream BioTrust Low Carb Protein Powder Blend
Handful of ice cubes
Liquid stevia, to taste

1. Blend all the ingredients in a high-speed blender until smooth. Serve immediately.

NUTRITION

Calories: 287 | Fat: 14 g | Carbohydrates: 12 g | Sodium: 151 mg | Fiber: 6 g | Protein: 29 g | Sugar: 2 g

SPICED OATMEAL PROTEIN SMOOTHIE

PREP: 5 MINUTES | MAKES: 1 SERVING

1 cup unsweetened almond milk
1 tablespoon uncooked rolled oats
¼ teaspoon ground cinnamon
Pinch of ground nutmeg
Pinch of ground ginger
Pinch of sea salt
2 scoops Vanilla Cream BioTrust Low Carb Protein Powder Blend
Handful of ice cubes
Liquid stevia, to taste

1. Blend all the ingredients in a high-speed blender until smooth. Serve immediately.

NUTRITION

Calories: 205 | Fat: 5 g | Carbohydrates: 13 g | Sodium: 151 mg | Fiber: 5 g | Protein: 27 g | Sugar: 1 g

STRAWBERRY BANANA PROTEIN SMOOTHIE

PREP: 5 MINUTES | MAKES: 1 SERVING

1 cup unsweetened almond milk
½ frozen banana
½ cup frozen strawberries
½ cup plain full-fat Greek yogurt
2 scoops Vanilla Cream BioTrust Low Carb Protein Powder Blend

1. Blend all the ingredients in a high-speed blender until smooth. Serve immediately.

NUTRITION

Calories: 328 | Fat: 5 g | Carbohydrates: 36 g | Sodium: 151 mg | Fiber: 8 g | Protein: 36 g | Sugar: 16 g

MATCHA PROTEIN SMOOTHIE

PREP: 5 MINUTES | MAKES: 1 SERVING

1 cup unsweetened almond milk
½ cup frozen strawberries
1 cup fresh spinach
¼ cup plain full-fat Greek yogurt
1 tablespoon matcha green tea powder
2 scoops Vanilla Cream BioTrust Low Carb Protein Powder Blend
Handful of ice cubes
Liquid stevia, to taste

1. Blend all the ingredients in a high-speed blender until smooth. Serve immediately.

NUTRITION

Calories: 232 | Fat: 5 g | Carbohydrates: 12 g | Sodium: 175 mg | Fiber: 8 g | Protein: 30 g | Sugar: 8 g

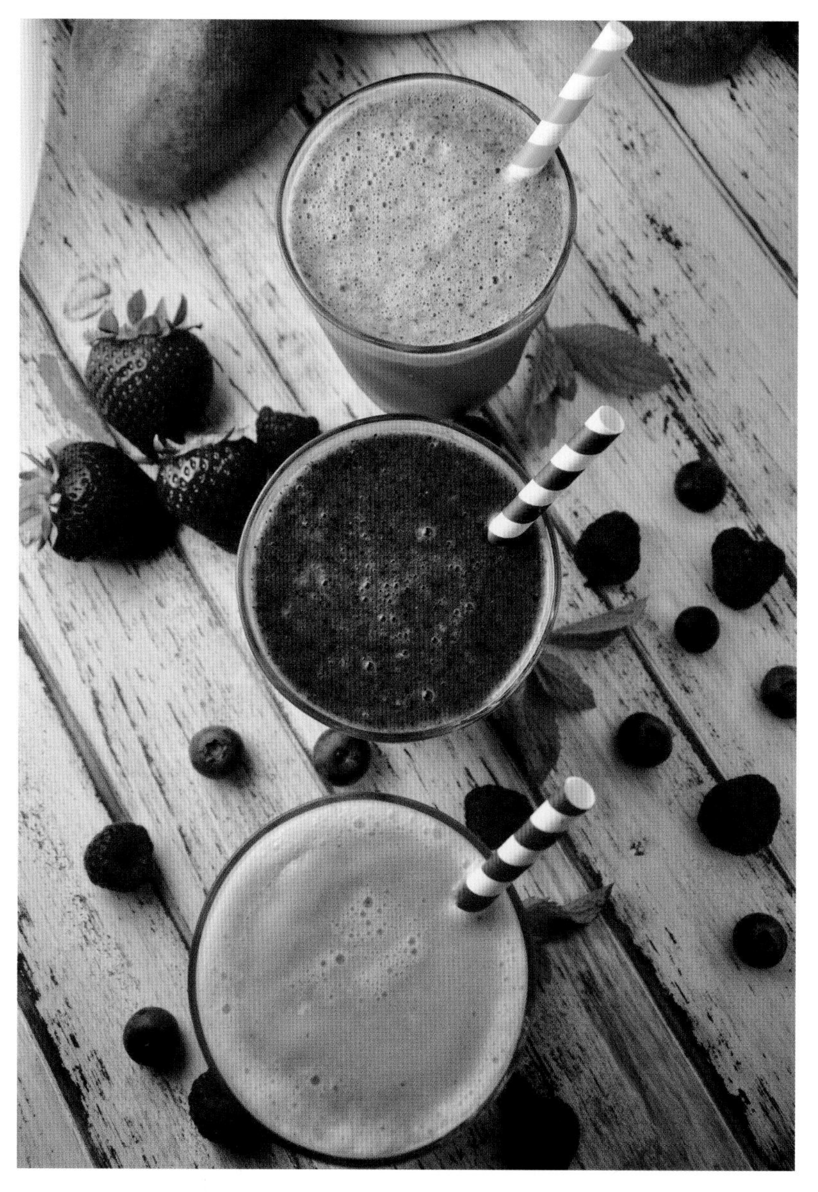

PEACH MANGO PROTEIN SMOOTHIE

PREP: 5 MINUTES | MAKES: 1 SERVING

- 1 cup unsweetened almond milk
- ½ cup frozen peach slices
- ½ cup frozen mango chunks
- ½ cup plain full-fat Greek yogurt
- 2 scoops Vanilla Cream BioTrust Low Carb Protein Powder Blend

1. Blend all the ingredients in a high-speed blender until smooth. Serve immediately.

NUTRITION

Calories: 337 | Fat: 5 g | Carbohydrates: 36 g | Sodium: 151 mg | Fiber: 8 g | Protein: 36 g | Sugar: 16 g

PIÑA COLADA PROTEIN SMOOTHIE

PREP: 5 MINUTES | MAKES: 1 SERVING

- ½ cup full-fat unsweetened coconut milk
- ½ cup water
- ½ cup fresh pineapple chunks
- 2 scoops Vanilla Cream BioTrust Low Carb Protein Powder Blend
- Handful of ice cubes
- Liquid stevia, to taste

1. Blend all the ingredients in a high-speed blender until smooth. Serve immediately.

NUTRITION

Calories: 266 | Fat: 10 g | Carbohydrates: 19 g | Sodium: 150 mg | Fiber: 6 g | Protein: 26 g | Sugar: 9 g

CHEAT DAY TREATS

GINGERBREAD-SPICED WAFFLES

PREP: 15 MINUTES | COOK: 15 MINUTES | MAKES: 16 SERVINGS

1 cup blanched almond flour
1 tablespoon coconut flour
1 teaspoon baking soda
½ teaspoon ground ginger
½ teaspoon ground cinnamon
¼ teaspoon ground cloves
Pinch of sea salt
4 eggs
½ cup full-fat unsweetened coconut milk
2 tablespoons molasses
1 teaspoon vanilla extract
¼ teaspoon liquid stevia
Coconut oil for greasing

1. Preheat a waffle maker.
2. In a medium bowl, combine the almond flour, coconut flour, baking soda, ginger, cinnamon, cloves, and salt.
3. In another medium bowl, beat the eggs. Mix in the coconut milk, molasses, vanilla, and stevia. Add the egg mixture all at once to the flour mixture. Stir just until moistened.
4. Use a paper towel to carefully rub coconut oil on your preheated waffle maker. Cook the batter according to the manufacturer's directions.

Quick Tip: Feel free to whip this batter into pancakes instead of waffles if that's more your style. They taste phenomenal either way. I like to top these with raspberries and a little maple syrup.

NUTRITION
Calories: 90
Fat: 4 g
Carbohydrates: 4 g
Sodium: 69 mg
Fiber: 1 g
Protein: 2 g
Sugar: 2 g

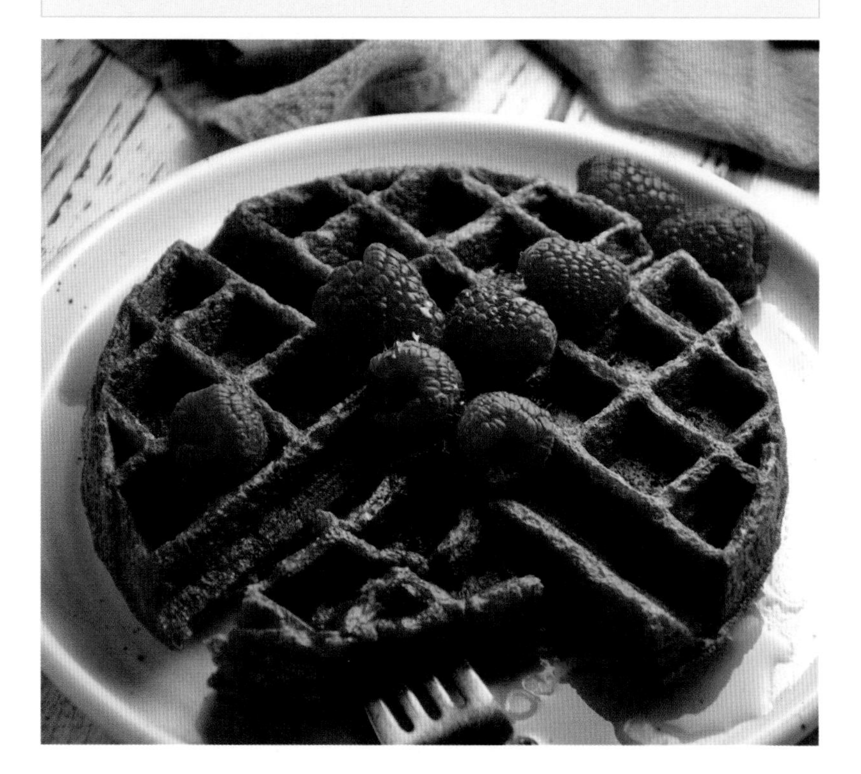

COCONUT CASHEW PROTEIN PANCAKES

PREP: 15 MINUTES | COOK: 8 MINUTES | MAKES: 12 SERVINGS

½ cup Vanilla Cream BioTrust Low Carb Protein Powder Blend
½ cup uncooked rolled oats
½ teaspoon baking soda
¼ teaspoon sea salt
½ teaspoon liquid stevia (or ½ banana)
1 teaspoon vanilla extract
3 tablespoons chopped cashews
¼ cup unsweetened shredded coconut, toasted and divided
4 eggs
1 cup low-fat cottage cheese
½ cup full-fat unsweetened coconut milk
Coconut oil for greasing

1. Preheat a pancake griddle or a large skillet over medium-high heat.
2. Combine the protein powder, oats, baking soda, salt, stevia, vanilla, cashews, 2 tablespoons of the coconut, eggs, cottage cheese, and coconut milk in a food processor. Pulse to combine until smooth.
3. Let the batter sit for 10 to 15 minutes to help your pancakes bind together.
4. Use a paper towel to carefully rub coconut oil on your preheated griddle or skillet. Reduce the heat to medium. Use a ¼-cup measuring cup to scoop the batter onto the griddle in nice big circles. When bubbles form (about a minute), flip the pancakes to cook on the other side. Sprinkle with the remaining 2 tablespoons coconut.

NUTRITION

Calories: 139 | Fat: 9 g | Carbohydrates: 5 g | Sodium: 231 mg | Fiber: 1 g | Protein: 9 g | Sugar: 1 g

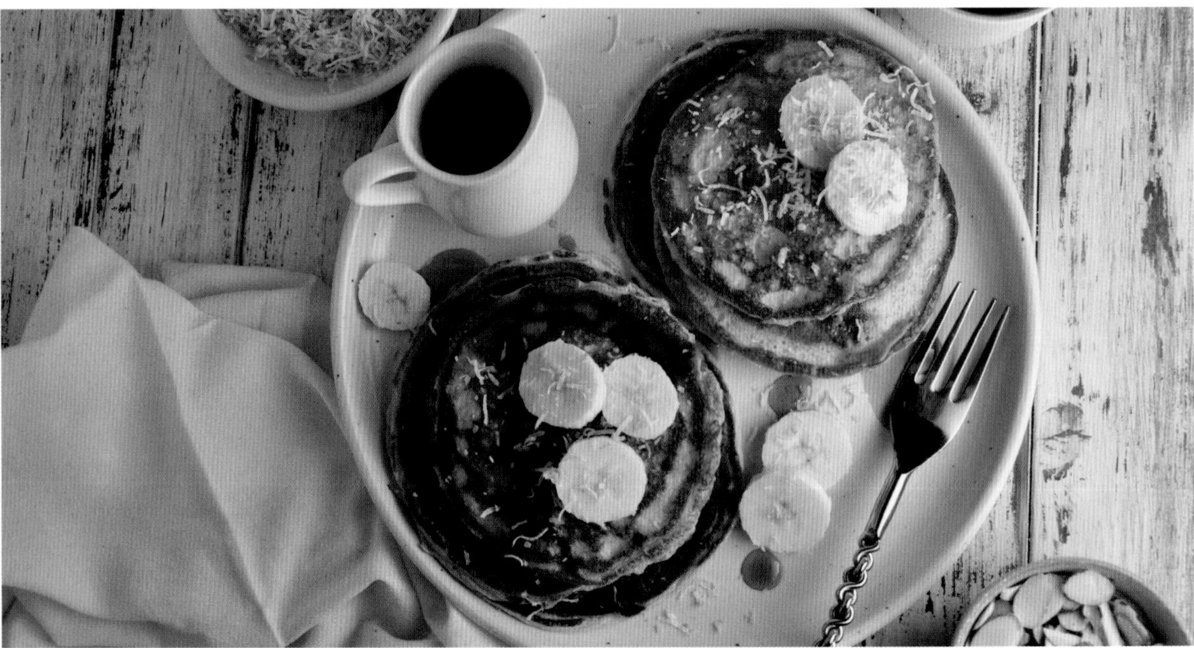

SWEET POTATO PANCAKES

PREP: 15 MINUTES | COOK: 8 MINUTES | MAKES: 20 SERVINGS

- 1 cup blanched almond flour
- 1 cup arrowroot starch
- 1½ teaspoons ground cinnamon
- ½ teaspoon ground nutmeg
- ½ teaspoon sea salt
- 1 cup baked and mashed sweet potato
- 1 (13.66-ounce) can full-fat unsweetened coconut milk
- 3 eggs, slightly beaten
- 2 tablespoons coconut oil, melted, plus more for greasing

1. Preheat a pancake griddle or a large skillet over medium-high heat.
2. In a medium bowl, combine the almond flour, arrowroot starch, cinnamon, nutmeg, and salt.
3. In another medium bowl, combine the mashed sweet potato, coconut milk, eggs, and coconut oil. Mix until fully combined. Add the dry ingredients to the wet ones and mix until fully incorporated. Let the batter sit for 10 to 15 minutes to help your pancakes bind together.
4. Use a paper towel to carefully rub coconut oil on your preheated griddle or skillet. Reduce the heat to medium. Use a ¼-cup measuring cup to scoop the batter onto the griddle in nice big circles. When bubbles form (about 1 minutes), flip the pancakes to cook on the other side.

NUTRITION

Calories: 124 | Fat: 9 g | Carbohydrates: 8 g | Sodium: 64 mg | Fiber: 2 g | Protein: 3 g | Sugar: 1 g

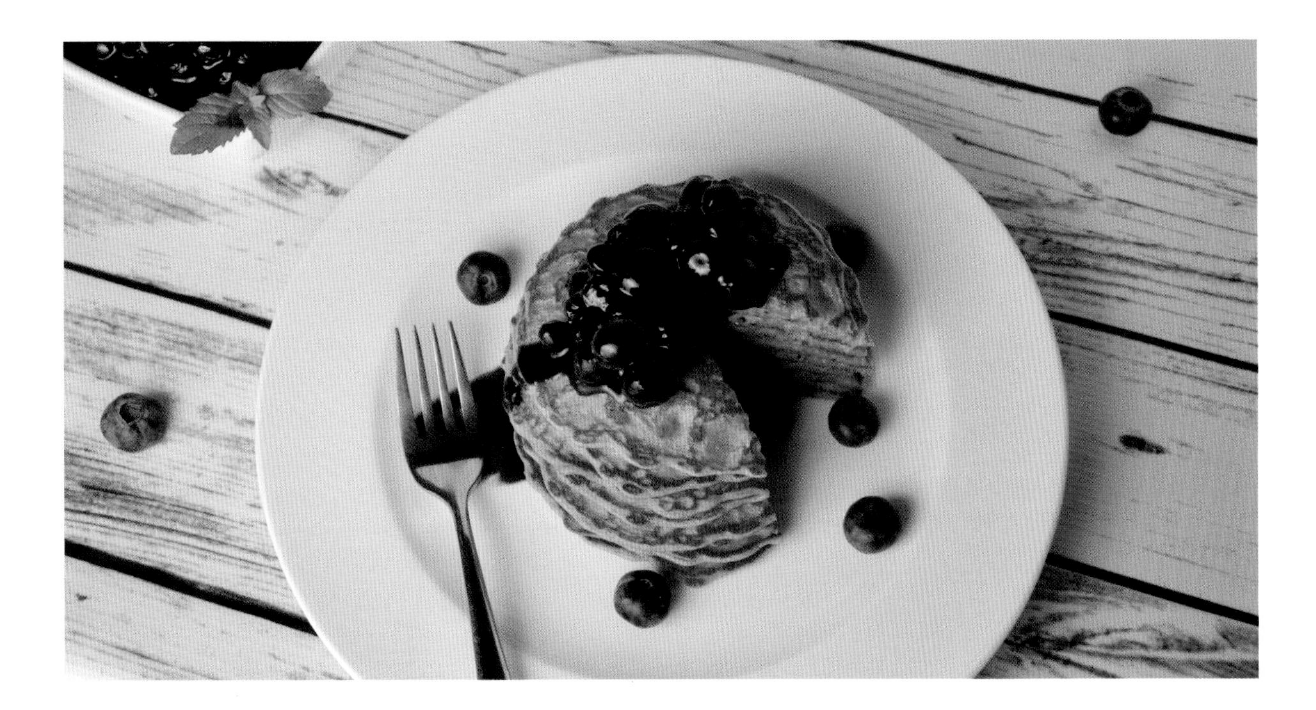

QUINOA PANCAKES

PREP: 15 MINUTES | COOK: 8 MINUTES | MAKES: 20 SERVINGS

1 cup cooked quinoa
1 cup blanched almond flour
¼ cup arrowroot starch
1½ teaspoons baking powder
½ teaspoon sea salt
2 eggs, slightly beaten
1 (13.66-ounce) can full-fat unsweetened coconut milk
1 tablespoon coconut sugar
1 tablespoon vanilla extract
Coconut oil for greasing

1. Preheat a pancake griddle or a large skillet over medium-high heat.
2. In a medium bowl, combine the quinoa, almond flour, arrowroot starch, baking powder, and salt.
3. In another medium bowl, combine the eggs, coconut milk, coconut sugar, and vanilla. Mix until fully combined. Add the dry ingredients to the wet ones and mix until fully incorporated. Let the batter sit for 10 to 15 minutes to help your pancakes bind together.
4. Use a paper towel to carefully rub coconut oil on your preheated griddle or skillet. Reduce the heat to medium. Use a ¼-cup measuring cup to scoop the batter onto the griddle in nice big circles. When bubbles form (about 1 minute), flip the pancakes to cook on the other side.

Quick Tip: While serving pancakes hot off the griddle is always best, having frozen pancakes to toss into the toaster during the morning rush is a great option for a quick on-the-go breakfast. Serve with fresh fruit, toasted pecans, and a drizzle of pure maple syrup.

NUTRITION

Calories: 119 | Fat: 7 g | Carbohydrates: 10 g | Sodium: 58 mg | Fiber: 2 g | Protein: 4 g | Sugar: 1 g

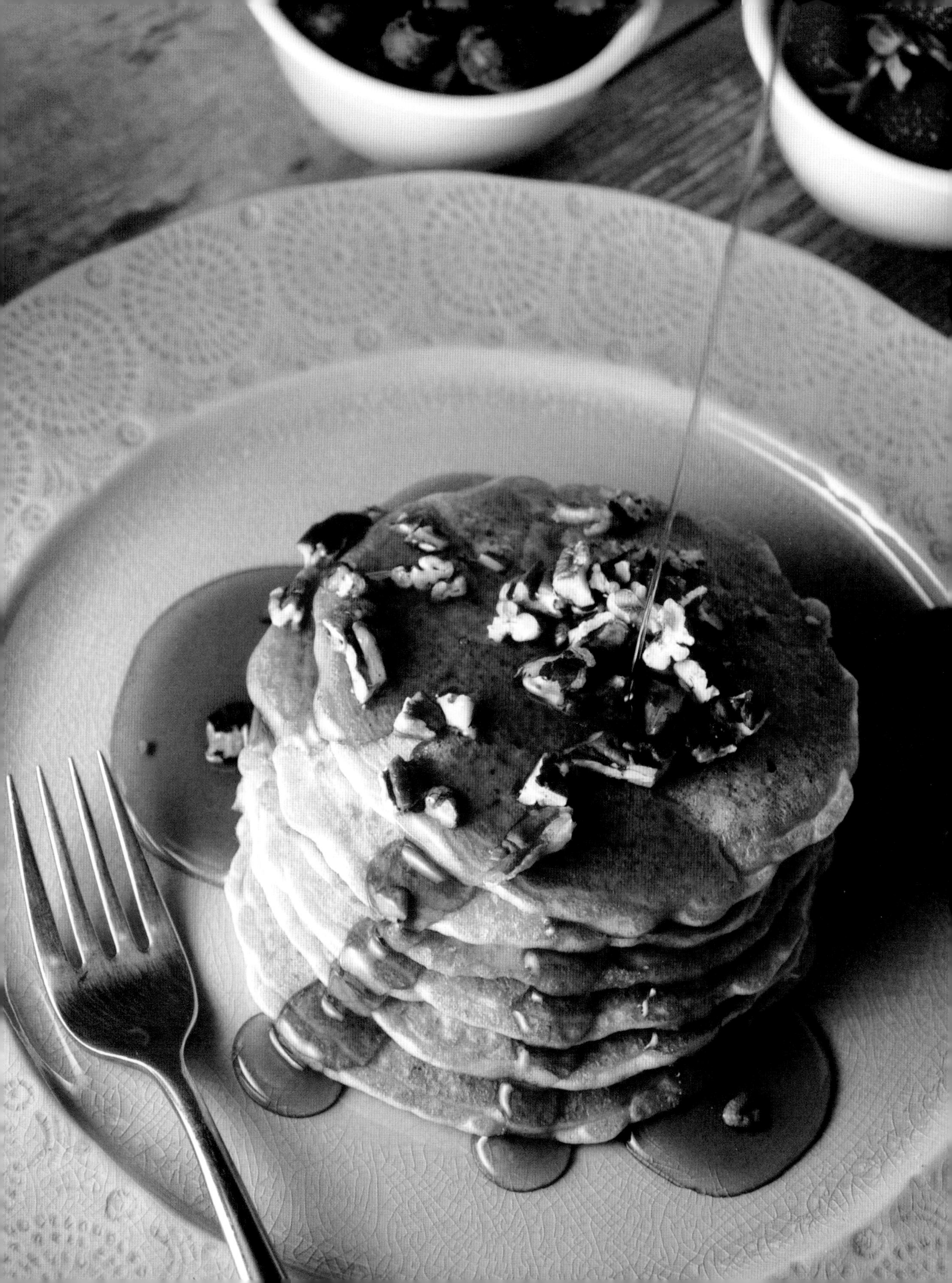

APPLE SPICE PROTEIN DOUGHNUTS

PREP: 20 MINUTES | COOK: 10 MINUTES | MAKES: 12 DOUGHNUTS

For the Apple Spice Topping

1 teaspoon coconut oil
¼ cup finely chopped apple
1 teaspoon pure maple syrup
¼ teaspoon ground cinnamon
Pinch of sea salt

For the Doughnuts

½ cup Vanilla Cream BioTrust Low Carb Protein Powder Blend
2 tablespoons coconut flour
½ teaspoon baking powder
¼ teaspoon ground cinnamon
2 egg whites, at room temperature
1 tablespoon coconut oil, melted

For the Glaze

3 tablespoons coconut oil, melted
1 tablespoon powdered erythritol (such as confectioners' Swerve)
Sea salt and ground cinnamon for sprinkling

1. For the apple spice topping: In a small skillet over medium heat, heat the coconut oil. Add the apple and cook, stirring often, until very soft, about 5 minutes. Add the syrup, cinnamon, and salt. Continue to cook for another 2 minutes. Remove from the heat and allow to cool.
2. For the doughnuts: Preheat the oven to 325 degrees F. Combine the protein powder, coconut flour, baking powder, and cinnamon together in a medium bowl. Add the egg whites and coconut oil and mix well until a dough forms.
3. Use a piping bag, or a ziplock bag with the corner cut off, to pipe the dough into a silicone 12-mold mini doughnut pan. Evenly sprinkle the apple spice topping over the tops of the doughnuts, and lightly press into the dough. Bake for 8 minutes.
4. Cool slightly, remove from the mold, and place on a plate lined with parchment paper. Place the doughnuts in the freezer while you prepare the glaze.
5. For the glaze: Combine the glaze ingredients in a medium bowl with a fork. Dip each cooled doughnut into the glaze and place back on the parchment paper–lined plate until set. Sprinkle with sea salt and ground cinnamon.

NUTRITION

Calories: 81 | Fat: 6 g | Carbohydrates: 5 g | Sodium: 25 mg | Fiber: 1 g | Protein: 5 g | Sugar: 2 g

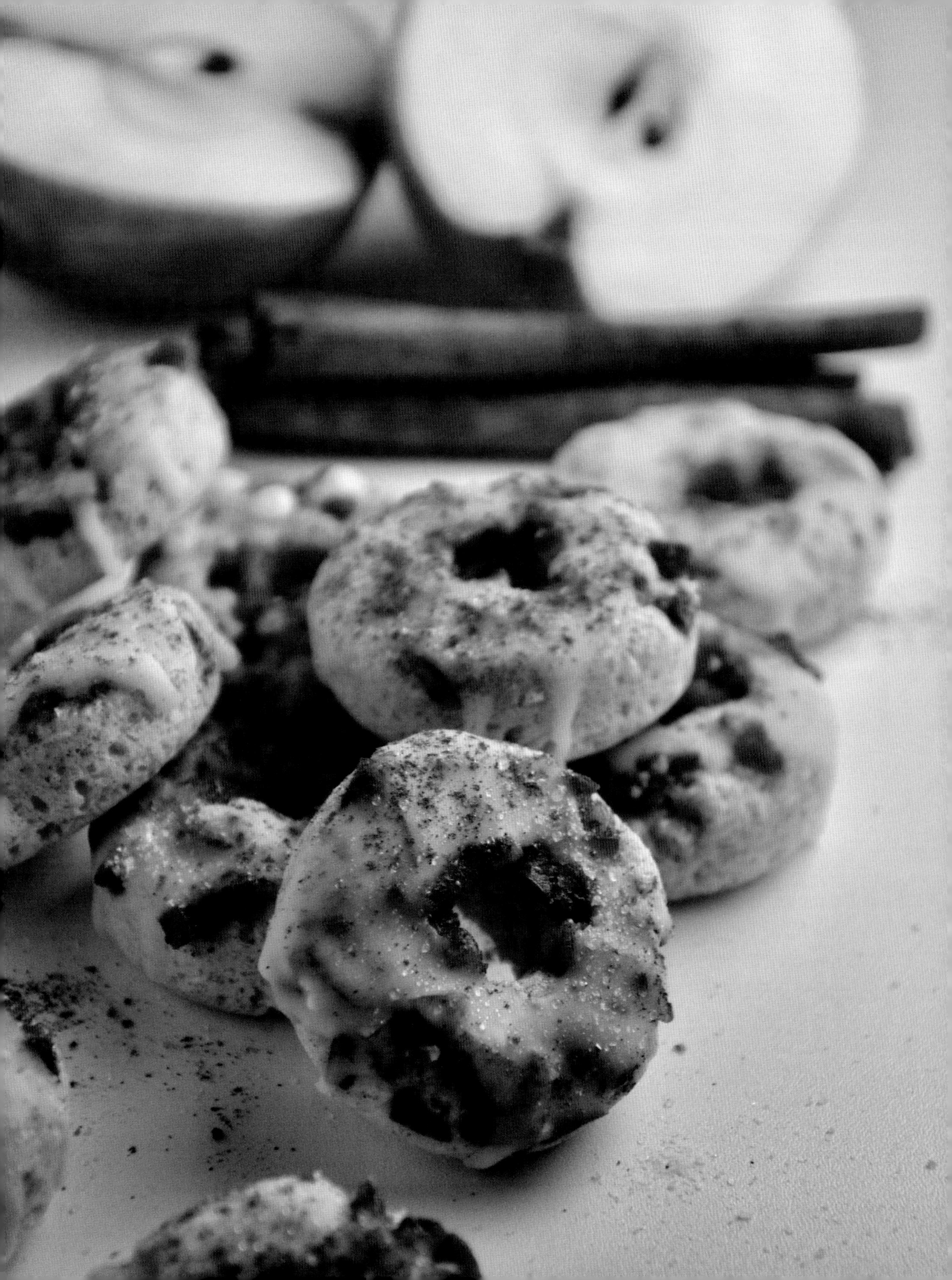

Acknowledgments

Simply put, this book wouldn't exist without the help and collaboration of so many, and within the paragraphs that follow I want to recognize those individuals formally for their tremendous assistance in making this book an incredible reality.

To start, I'd like to thank my great friend and literary agent, Heather Jackson. Heather, your faith in me going back 13 years is the reason we got to do this book together. I'm grateful to you for your friendship and for being the best possible advocate and coach in my corner that one could ever ask for. That, and you're brilliant at what you do. Thank you so much for playing such a huge role in the story of my life! Here's to many more wonderful years together!

To the amazing publishing team at BenBella, you have been a joy to work with. Glenn Yeffeth, thank you for believing in this project from the very beginning; we've created something special because of that. Claire Schulz, our amazing editor, you took the manuscript from good to *great* and really made the pages sing. Thank you so much for taking the intentional time; your passion shines through your work. To the design team, inside and out, thank you for creating something beautiful that we can all be proud to hold in our hands.

I'd also like to thank Maggie Greenwood-Robinson, our collaborator, who worked tirelessly behind the scenes putting my thoughts and vision and programming into a manuscript that I couldn't be more thrilled with. Without you, this book would have been nearly impossible for me to pull off while running and operating so many other companies full-time, plus doing the most important job of all—being a present father and husband. Thank you.

Speaking of other companies, I want to thank my brother from another mother and BioTrust cofounder, Josh Bezoni, for bringing the life-changing opportunity that was and is BioTrust to the table. That will certainly have a huge impact on the success of this book, and in turn on the continued success of our mission. I'm grateful for all we have been through, and all that is to come. Decades more of helping people all over the world—that's where the true fulfillment is.

To my friend and creator of all the wonderful recipes and beautiful photos in this book, Diana Keuilian, thank you for being who you are. Thank you for putting your heart and soul into every single recipe, and for being dedicated to producing only the best. Thank you for your cheerful spirit and great attitude, no matter what is asked of you. This book wouldn't be half of what it is without you, literally!

To the Transformation Insider team, thank you for being available to pull research and to help with and direct everything that was asked of you and more. I am grateful to be surrounded by the best of the best people in business and in life. Your help was invaluable.

To my beautiful, kind, patient, and loving wife, Lisa, who has supported me through every up and down that my career has brought, thank you for being the rock by my side, for being the most amazing mother to our two girls, and for always being my biggest cheerleader; you are loved more than you know. Thank you for trusting me, through all my wild projects and ideas, including this one. Thank you for being you. My life would be close to empty without you and our family.

And lastly, but in all actuality number one by leaps and bounds, thank you, Lord, for blessing me with the air in my lungs, for the ability to write, for the passion to help others, for the opportunity to learn through failures and to celebrate wins, and, most important, for salvation through your son, Jesus Christ. I am nothing without you. I don't take this life for granted. I don't take this opportunity for granted. Use it for your glory.

And to everyone reading, you're the real rock stars! Without you, there is no reason to even write this book. May it help and inspire you, and ultimately help direct you down the path of the life that you were born to live—a life with purpose, a life where you're making a difference in your family, in your relationships, in your career, and in the world around you. It all starts with you!

References

INTRODUCTION

Kant, A. K., et al. 1997. "Evening Eating and Subsequent Long-Term Weight Change in a National Cohort." *International Journal of Obesity and Related Metabolism Disorders* 21: 407.

Kinsey, A. W., and M. J. Ormsbee. 2015. "The Health Impact of Nighttime Eating: Old and New Perspectives." *Nutrients* 7: 2648–62.

Sofer, S., et al. 2011. "Greater Weight Loss and Hormonal Changes After 6 Months with Carbohydrates Eaten Mostly at Dinner." *Obesity* 19: 2006–14.

CHAPTER 1: WHY YOU SHOULD ALWAYS EAT AFTER 7 PM

Aragones, G., et al. 2016. "Modulation of Leptin Resistance by Food Compounds." *Molecular Nutrition & Food Research* 60: 1789–803.

Calcagno, M., et al. 2019. "The Thermic Effect of Food: A Review." *Journal of the American College of Nutrition* 25: 1–5.

Groen, B. B., et al. 2012. "Intragastric Protein Administration Stimulates Overnight Muscle Protein Synthesis in Elderly Men." *American Journal of Physiology—Endocrinology and Metabolism* 302: E52–60.

Haghighatdoost, F., et al. 2018. "Effect of Green Tea on Plasma Leptin and Ghrelin Levels: A Systematic Review and Meta-analysis of Randomized Controlled Clinical Trials." *Nutrition* 45: 17–23.

Halson, S. L. 2014. "Sleep in Elite Athletes and Nutritional Interventions to Enhance Sleep." *Sports Medicine* 44 (Supplement 1): 13–23.

Kouw, I. W., et al. 2017. "Protein Ingestion Before Sleep Increases Overnight Muscle Protein Synthesis Rates in Healthy Older Men: A Randomized Controlled Trial." *Journal of Nutrition* 147: 2252–61.

Mayo Clinic Staff. 2017. "Caffeine: How Much Is Too Much?" March 8, mayoclinic.org.

Nonino-Borges, C. B, et al. 2007. "Influence of Meal Time on Salivary Circadian Cortisol Rhythms and Weight Loss in Obese Women." *Nutrition* 23: 385–91.

Palou, M., et al. 2015. "Pectin Supplementation in Rats Mitigates Age-Related Impairment in Insulin and Leptin Sensitivity Independently of Reducing Food Intake." *Molecular Nutrition & Food Research* 59: 2022–33.

Peuhkuri, K. 2012. "Diet Promotes Sleep Duration and Quality." *Nutrition Research* 32: 309–19.

Res, P. T., et al. 2012. "Protein Ingestion Before Sleep Improves Postexercise Overnight Recovery." *Medicine and Science in Sports and Exercise* 44: 1560–69.

Sofer, S., et al. 2013. "Changes in Daily Leptin, Ghrelin and Adiponectin Profiles Following a Diet with Carbohydrates Eaten at Dinner in Obese Subjects." *Nutrition, Metabolism, and Cardiovascular Diseases* 23: 744–50.

Stote, K. S., et al. 2007. "A Controlled Trial of Reduced Meal Frequency Without Caloric Restriction in Healthy, Normal-Weight, Middle-Aged Adults." *American Journal of Clinical Nutrition* 85: 981–88.

Waller, S. M. 2004. "Evening Ready-to-Eat Cereal Consumption Contributes to Weight Management." *Journal of the American College of Nutrition* 23: 316–21.

CHAPTER 2: THE *REAL* TRUTH ABOUT BREAKFAST

Barberio, A. M., et al. 2017. "Fluoride Exposure and Indicators of Thyroid Functioning in the Canadian Population: Implications for Community Water Fluoridation." *Journal of Epidemiology and Community Health* 71: 1019–25.

Betts, J. A., et al. 2016. "Is Breakfast the Most Important Meal of the Day?" *Proceedings of the Nutrition Society* 75: 464–74.

Boschmann, M., et al. 2003. "Water-Induced Thermogenesis." *Journal of Clinical Endocrinology & Metabolism* 88: 6015–19.

Brandhorst, S., et al. 2015. "A Periodic Diet That Mimics Fasting Promotes Multi-system Regeneration, Enhanced Cognitive Performance, and Healthspan." *Cell Metabolism* 22: 86–99.

Brown, J. E., et al. 2013. "Intermittent Fasting: A Dietary Intervention for Prevention of Diabetes and Cardiovascular Disease?" *British Journal of Diabetes and Vascular Disease* 13: 68–72.

Camacho, S., et al. 2015. "Anti-obesity and Anti-hyperglycemic Effects of Cinnamaldehyde via Altered Ghrelin Secretion and Functional Impact on Food Intake and Gastric Emptying." *Scientific Reports* 21: 7919.

Cho, S., et al. 2003. "The Effect of Breakfast Type on Total Daily Energy Intake and Body Mass Index: Results from the Third National Health and Nutrition Examination Survey (NHANES III)." *Journal of the American College of Nutrition* 22: 296–302.

Dhurandhar, E. J., et al. 2014. "The Effectiveness of Breakfast Recommendations on Weight Loss: A Randomized Controlled Trial." *American Journal of Clinical Nutrition* 100: 507–13.

Gabel, K., Varady, K., et al. 2018. "Effects of 8-Hour Time Restricted Feeding on Body Weight and Metabolic Disease Risk Factors in Obese Adults: A Pilot Study." *Nutrition and Healthy Aging* 4: 345–53.

Halberg, N. 2005. "Effect of Intermittent Fasting and Refeeding on Insulin Action in Healthy Men." *Journal of Applied Physiology* 99: 2128–36.

Horne, B. D., et al. 2015. "Health Effects of Intermittent Fasting: Hormesis or Harm? A Systematic Review." *American Journal of Clinical Nutrition* 102: 464–70.

Huang, J., et al. 2014. "The Anti-obesity Effects of Green Tea in Human Intervention and Basic Molecular Studies." *European Journal of Clinical Nutrition* 68: 1075–87.

Kempel, M. C., et al. 2012. "Intermittent Fasting Combined with Calorie Restriction Is Effective for Weight Loss and Cardioprotection in Obese Women." *Nutrition Journal* 11: 98.

Khan, N., and H. Mukhtar. 2019. "Tea Polyphenols in Promotion of Human Health." *Nutrients* 11: 39.

Kleiner, S. M. 1999. "Water: An Essential but Overlooked Nutrient." *Journal of the American Dietetic Association* 99: 200–206.

Malone, M., and G. Tsai. 2018. "The Evidence for Herbal and Botanical Remedies, Part 1." *Journal of Family Practice* 67: 10–16.

Nieber, K. 2017. "The Impact of Coffee on Health." *Planta Medica* 83: 1256–63.

O'Keefe, J. H., et al. 2018. "Coffee for Cardioprotection and Longevity." *Progress in Cardiovascular Disease* 61: 38–42.

Reed, J. A., et al. 2008. "Effects of Peppermint Scent on Appetite Control and Caloric Intake." *Appetite* 51: 393.

Rupasinghe, H. P., et al. 2016. "Phytochemicals in Regulating Fatty Acid β-Oxidation: Potential Underlying Mechanisms and Their Involvement in Obesity and Weight Loss." *Pharmacology & Therapeutics* 165: 153–63.

Schusdziarra, V., et al. 2011. "Impact of Breakfast on Daily Energy Intake: An Analysis of Absolute Versus Relative Breakfast Calories." *Nutrition Journal* 10: 5.

Sievert, K., et al. 2019. "Effect of Breakfast on Weight and Energy Intake: Systematic Review and Meta-analysis of Randomised Controlled Trials." *British Medical Journal* 364: 142.

CHAPTER 3: ENERGIZING LUNCHES AND FAT-BURNING DINNERS WITH PORTION VOLUMIZATION

Ebbeling, C. B., et al. 2012. "Effects of Dietary Composition on Energy Expenditure During Weight-Loss Maintenance." *Journal of the American Medical Association* 307: 2627–34.

Farnsworth, E., et al. 2003. "Effect of a High-Protein, Energy-Restricted Diet on Body Composition, Glycemic Control, and 41 Lipid Concentrations in Overweight and Obese Hyperinsulinemic Men and Women." *American Journal of Clinical Nutrition* 78: 31–39.

Gannon, M. C., et al. 2003. "An Increase in Dietary Protein Improves the Blood Glucose Response in Persons with Type 2 Diabetes." *American Journal of Clinical Nutrition* 78: 734–41.

Gannon, M. C., and F. Q. Nuttall. 2004. "Effect of a High-Protein, Low-Carbohydrate Diet on Blood Glucose Control in People with Type 2 Diabetes." *Diabetes* 53: 2375–82.

Halton, T. L., and F. B. Hu. 2004. "The Effects of High Protein Diets on Thermogenesis, Satiety and Weight Loss: A Critical Review." *Journal of the American College of Nutrition* 23: 373–85.

Layman, D. K. 2003. "The Role of Leucine in Weight Loss Diets and Glucose Homeostasis." *Journal of Nutrition* 133: 261S–67S.

Layman, D. K., and J. I. Baum. 2004. "Dietary Protein Impact on Glycemic Control During Weight Loss." *Journal of Nutrition* 134: 968S–73S.

Leidy, H. J. 2014. "Increased Dietary Protein as a Dietary Strategy to Prevent and/or Treat Obesity." *Missouri Medicine* 111: 54–58.

Mangano, K. M., et al. 2014. "Dietary Protein Is Beneficial to Bone Health Under Conditions of Adequate Calcium Intake: An Update on Clinical Research." *Current Opinion in Clinical Nutrition and Metabolic Care* 17: 69–74.

Noreen, E. E., et al. 2010. "Effects of Supplemental Fish Oil on Resting Metabolic Rate, Body Composition, and Salivary Cortisol in Healthy Adults." *Journal of the International Society of Sports Nutrition* 7: 31.

Ortinau, L. C., et al. 2014 "Effects of High-Protein vs. High-Fat Snacks on Appetite Control, Satiety, and Eating Initiation in Healthy Women." *Nutrition Journal* 13: 97.

Siri-Tarino, P. W., et al. 2010. "Meta-analysis of Prospective Cohort Studies Evaluating the Association of Saturated Fat with Cardiovascular Disease." *American Journal of Clinical Nutrition* 91: 535–46.

Soenen, S., et al. 2013. "Normal Protein Intake Is Required for Body Weight Loss and Weight Maintenance, and Elevated Protein Intake for Additional Preservation of Resting Energy Expenditure and Fat Free Mass." *Journal of Nutrition* 143: 591–96.

Tang, M., et al. 2014. "Diet-Induced Weight Loss: The Effect of Dietary Protein on Bone." *Journal of the Academy of Nutrition and Dietetics* 114: 72–85.

Westerterp, K. R. 2004. "Diet Induced Thermogenesis." *Nutrition & Metabolism* 1: 5.

Westerterp-Plantenga, M. S., et al. 1999. "Satiety Related to 24 h Diet-Induced Thermogenesis During High Protein/ Carbohydrate vs High Fat Diets Measured in a Respiration Chamber." *European Journal of Clinical Nutrition* 53: 495–502.

CHAPTER 4: THE POWER OF LATE-NIGHT SNACKS

Auborn, K. J., et al. 2003. "Indole-3-Carbinol Is a Negative Regulator of Estrogen." *Journal of Nutrition* 133 (7 Supplement): 2470S–75S.

Bradlow, H. L., et al. 1994. "Long-Term Responses of Women to Indole-3-Carbinol or a High Fiber Diet." *Cancer Epidemiology Biomarkers & Prevention* 3: 591–95.

Cassady, B. A., et al. 2009. "Mastication of Almonds: Effects of Lipid Bioaccessibility, Appetite, and Hormone Response." *American Journal of Clinical Nutrition* 89: 794–800.

Choi, K.-M., et al. 2014. "Sulforaphane Attenuates Obesity by Inhibiting Adipogenesis and Activating the AMPK Pathway in Obese Mice." *Journal of Nutritional Biochemistry* 25: 201–7.

DeFuria, J., et al. 2009. "Dietary Blueberry Attenuates Whole-Body Insulin Resistance in High Fat-Fed Mice by Reducing Adipocyte Death and Its Inflammatory Sequelae." *Journal of Nutrition* 139: 1510–16.

D'Eon, T. M., et al. 2005. "Estrogen Regulation of Adiposity and Fuel Partitioning. Evidence of Genomic and Non-genomic Regulation of Lipogenic and Oxidative Pathways." *Journal of Biological Chemistry* 280: 35983–91.

Fowke, J. H., et al. 2000. "Brassica Vegetable Consumption Shifts Estrogen Metabolism in Healthy Postmenopausal Women." *Cancer Epidemiology Biomarkers & Prevention* 9: 773–79.

Fujioka, K., et al. 2006. "The Effects of Grapefruit on Weight and Insulin Resistance: Relationship to the Metabolic Syndrome." *Journal of Medicinal Food* 9: 49–54.

Fulgoni, V. L., et al. 2013. "Avocado Consumption Is Associated with Better Diet Quality and Nutrient Intake, and Lower Metabolic Syndrome Risk in US Adults: Results from the National Health and Nutrition Examination Survey (NHANES) 2001–2008." *Nutrition Journal* 12: 1.

Garrido, M., et al. 2010. "Jerte Valley Cherry-Enriched Diets Improve Nocturnal Rest and Increase 6-Sulfatoxymelatonin and Total Antioxidant Capacity in the Urine of Middle-Aged and Elderly Humans." *Journals of Gerontology. Series A, Biological Sciences and Medical Sciences* 65: 909–14.

Jung, U. J., et al. 2003. "Naringin Supplementation Lowers Plasma Lipids and Enhances Erythrocyte Antioxidant Enzyme Activities in Hypercholesterolemic Subjects." *Clinical Nutrition* 22: 561–68.

Kahn, B. B., and J. S. Flier. 2000. "Obesity and Insulin Resistance." *Journal of Clinical Investigation* 106: 473–481.

Kall, M. A., et al. 1996. "Effects of Dietary Broccoli on Human *In Vivo* Drug Metabolizing Enzymes: Evaluation of Caffeine, Oestrone and Chlorzoxazone Metabolism." *Carcinogenesis* 17: 793–99.

Kelley, D. S., et al. 2018. "A Review of the Health Benefits of Cherries." *Nutrients* 10: E368.

Kouw, I. W., et al. 2017. "Protein Ingestion Before Sleep Increases Overnight Muscle Protein Synthesis Rates in Healthy Older Men: A Randomized Controlled Trial." *Journal of Nutrition* 147: 2252–61.

Lo Verme, J., et al. 2005. "Regulation of Food Intake by Oleoylethanolamide." *Cellular and Molecular Life Sciences* 62: 708–16.

Lee, J.-H., et al. 2012. "Sulforaphane Induced Adipolysis via Hormone Sensitive Lipase Activation, Regulated by AMPK Signaling Pathway." *Biochemical and Biophysical Research Communications* 426: 492–97.

Lin, H.-H., et al. 2011. "Effect of Kiwifruit Consumption on Sleep Quality in Adults with Sleep Problems." *Asia Pacific Journal of Clinical Nutrition* 20: 169–74.

Mattes, R. D., et al. 2008. "Impact of Peanuts and Tree Nuts on Body Weight and Healthy Weight Loss in Adults." *Journal of Nutrition* 138: 1741S–45S.

Mattes, R. D., and M. L. Dreher. 2010. "Nuts and Healthy Body Weight Maintenance Mechanisms." *Asia Pacific Journal of Clinical Nutrition* 19: 137–41.

McLeay, Y., et al. 2012. "Effect of New Zealand Blueberry Consumption on Recovery from Eccentric Exercise-Induced Muscle Damage." *Journal of the International Society of Sports Nutrition* 9: 19.

Michnovicz, J. J., and H. L. Bradlow. 1991. "Altered Estrogen Metabolism and Excretion in Humans Following Consumption of Indole-3-Carbinol." *Nutrition and Cancer* 16: 59–66.

Moghe, S. S., et al. 2012. "Effect of Blueberry Polyphenols on 3T3-F442A Preadipocyte Differentiation." *Journal of Medicinal Food* 15: 448–52.

Pigeon, W. R., et al. 2010. "Effects of a Tart Cherry Juice Beverage on the Sleep of Older Adults with Insomnia: A Pilot Study." *Journal of Medicinal Food* 13: 579–83.

Richard, A. J., et al. 2013. "Naringenin Inhibits Adipogenesis and Reduces Insulin Sensitivity and Adiponectin Expression in Adipocytes." *Evidence-Based Complementary Alternative Medicine* 2013: 1–10.

Sanchez, M., et al. 2014. "Effect of *Lactobacillus rhamnosus* CGMCC1.3724 Supplementation on Weight Loss and Maintenance in Obese Men and Women." *British Journal of Nutrition* 111: 1507–19.

Schwartz, G. J., et al. 2008. "The Lipid Messenger OEA Links Dietary Fat Intake to Satiety." *Cell Metabolism* 8: 281–88.

Silver, H. J., et al. 2011. "Effects of Grapefruit, Grapefruit Juice and Water Preloads on Energy Balance, Weight Loss, Body Composition, and Cardiometabolic Risk in Free-Living Obese Adults." *Nutrition & Metabolism* 8: 8.

Tapsell, L., et al. 2009. "The Effect of a Calorie Controlled Diet Containing Walnuts on Substrate Oxidation During 8-Hours in a Room Calorimeter." *Journal of the American College of Nutrition* 28: 611–17.

Tsuda, T. 2008. "Regulation of Adipocyte Function by Anthocyanins; Possibility of Preventing the Metabolic Syndrome." *Journal of Agricultural and Food Chemistry* 56: 642-46.

Wien, M., et al. 2013. "A Randomized 3 × 3 Crossover Study to Evaluate the Effect of Hass Avocado Intake on Post-ingestive Satiety, Glucose and Insulin Levels, and Subsequent Energy Intake in Overweight Adults." *Nutrition Journal* 12: 155.

Yoshida, H., et al. 2013. "Citrus Flavonoid Naringenin Inhibits TLR2 Expression in Adipocytes." *Journal of Nutritional Biochemistry* 24: 1276–84.

Zygmunt, K., et al. 2010. "Naringenin, a Citrus Flavonoid, Increases Muscle Cell Glucose Uptake via AMPK." *Biochemical and Biophysical Research Communications* 398: 178–83.

CHAPTER 5: CHEAT YOUR WAY THIN

Aragones, G., et al. 2016. "Modulation of Leptin Resistance by Food Compounds." *Molecular Nutrition & Food Research* 60: 1789-803.

Palou, M., et al. 2015. "Pectin Supplementation in Rats Mitigates Age-Related Impairment in Insulin and Leptin Sensitivity Independently of Reducing Food Intake." *Molecular Nutrition & Food Research* 59: 2022-33.

CHAPTER 7: THE ACCELERATION PHASE

Laaksonen, D. E., et al. 2003. "Changes in Abdominal Subcutaneous Fat Water Content with Rapid Weight Loss and Long-Term Weight Maintenance in Abdominally Obese Men and Women." *International Journal of Obesity and Related Metabolic Disorders* 27: 677–83.

Nackers, L. M., et al. 2010. "The Association Between Rate of Initial Weight Loss and Long-Term Success in Obesity Treatment: Does Slow and Steady Win the Race?" *International Journal of Behavioral Medicine* 17: 161–67.

CHAPTER 9: THE LIFESTYLE PHASE

Larsen, T. M., et al. 2010. "Diets with High or Low Protein Content and Glycemic Index for Weight-Loss Maintenance." *New England Journal of Medicine* 363: 2102–13.

CHAPTER 10: SUPPLEMENT FOR SUCCESS

Babault, N., et al. 2015. "Pea Proteins Oral Supplementation Promotes Muscle Thickness Gains During Resistance Training: A Double-Blind, Randomized, Placebo-Controlled Clinical Trial vs. Whey Protein." *Journal of the International Society of Sports Nutrition* 12: 3.

Choi, F. D., et al. 2019. "Oral Collagen Supplementation: A Systematic Review of Dermatological Applications." *Journal of Drugs in Dermatology* 18: 9–16.

Devries, M. C., and S. M. Phillips. 2015. "Supplemental Protein in Support of Muscle Mass and Health: Advantage Whey." *Journal of Food Science* 80 (Supplement 1): A8–A15.

Gómez Candela, C., et al. 2011. "Importance of a Balanced Omega 6/Omega 3 Ratio for the Maintenance of Health: Nutritional Recommendations." *Nutrición Hospitalaria* 26: 323–29.

Linares, D. M., et al. 2016. "Beneficial Microbes: The Pharmacy in the Gut." *Bioengineered* 7: 11–20.

Munro, I. A., and M. L. Garg. 2013. "Prior Supplementation with Long Chain Omega-3 Polyunsaturated Fatty Acids Promotes Weight Loss in Obese Adults: A Double-Blinded Randomised Controlled Trial." *Food & Function* 4: 650–58.

Nan-Nong, S., et al. 2016. "Natural Dietary and Herbal Products in Anti-obesity Treatment." *Molecules* 21: 1351.

Okla, M., et al. 2017. "Dietary Factors Promoting Brown and Beige Fat Development and Thermogenesis." *Advances in Nutrition* 8: 473–83.

Rao, V., et al. 2011. "*In Vitro* and *In Vivo* Antioxidant Properties of the Plant-Based Supplement Greens+™." *International Journal of Molecular Sciences* 12: 4896–908.

Stubbs, B. J., et al. 2017. "On the Metabolism of Exogenous Ketones in Humans." *Frontiers in Physiology* 8: 848.

Willoughby, D., et al. 2018. "Body Composition Changes in Weight Loss: Strategies and Supplementation for Maintaining Lean Body Mass, a Brief Review." *Nutrients* 10: 12.

Index

Recipe Index

T

W

About the Author

Joel Marion, CISSN, NSCA-CPT, is a five-time best-selling e-book author who has been featured all over the media throughout his 18-year career, including in the pages of more than 20 popular national newsstand magazines such as *Men's Fitness*, *Woman's Day*, *Oxygen*, *Clean Eating*, *MuscleMag International*, and *Muscle & Fitness Hers*.

Joel is also the cofounder of BioTrust Nutrition, one of the fastest-growing and largest e-commerce supplement companies in the United States, and the host of the top-ranked podcast, *Born to Impact*. Today Joel lives in Florida with his wife, Lisa, and two beautiful daughters, Lily and Gabby, and is dedicated to the mission of helping more than 100 million people all over the world find their purpose and live the life they were born to live.

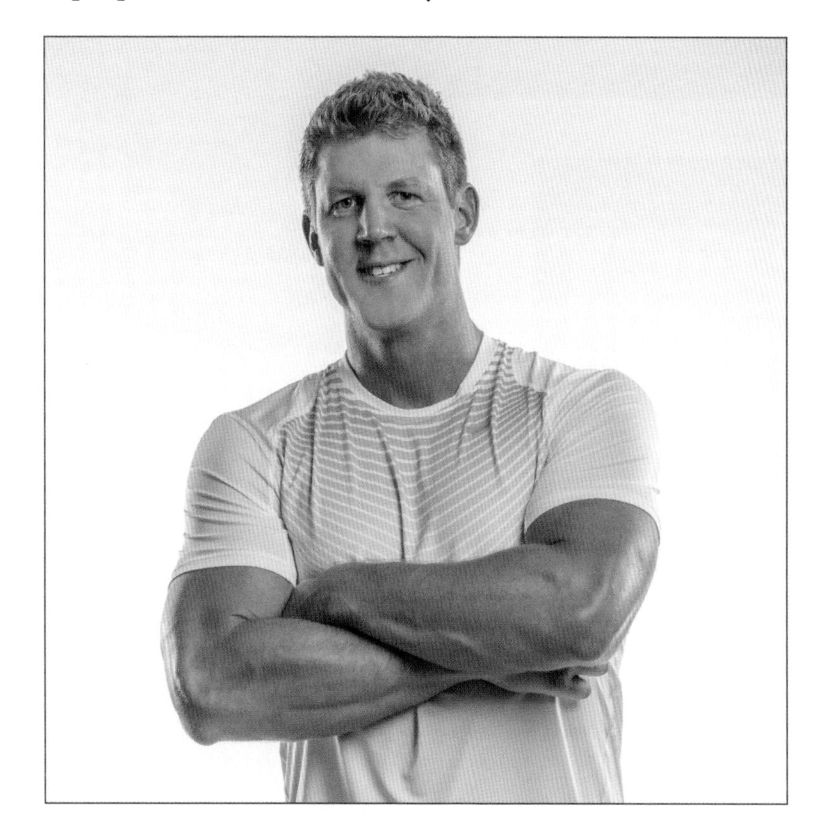